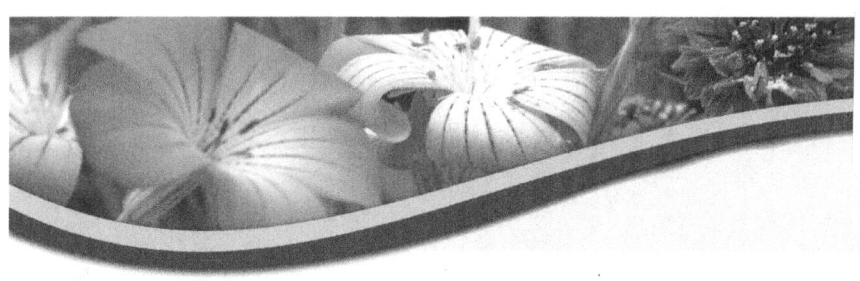

My Gift: Myself

A Guide to Excellence

in

End of Life Care

by

JoAnne Chitwood, R.N.

Volunteer Manual

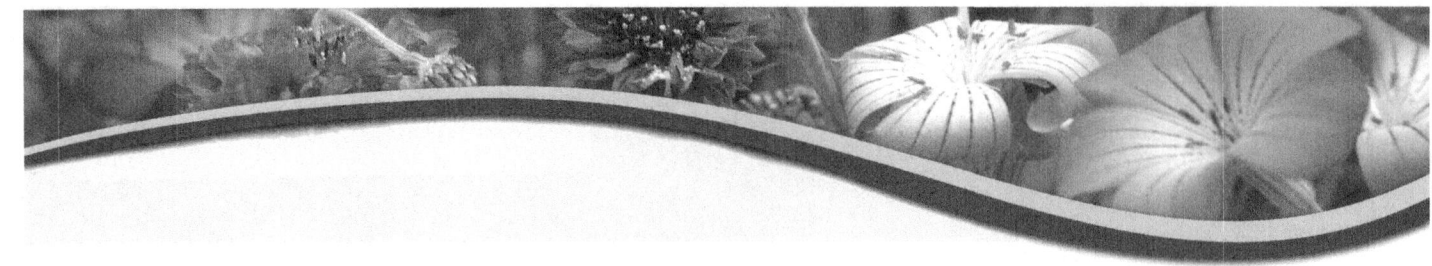

Border Mountain Books

An imprint of Promise Productions

Wasilla, Alaska 99687

© 2018 JoAnne Chitwood

bordermountain@msn.com

www.bordermountain.com

Edited by Leandra Collier and Greg Thrall

Cover Design by Greg Thrall

All images used in this book ©jupiterimagescorporation

All rights reserved. No portion of this book may be copied or saved by any electronic means without express permission of the publishers.

Printed in the United States of America

Notice:

No part of this book is intended to take the place of professional health care, nor does it negate the caregiver's resonsibility to provide care within the constraints of their professional scope of practice. Information within this book is offered with no guarantee on the part of the author or Promise Publications. The author and publisher disclaim all liability in connection with use of this book.

Dedication

To Mary

May your legacy bring healing to the hurting

and hope to the forgotten

"And now abides faith, hope, and love;

but the greatest of these is love."

-The Bible

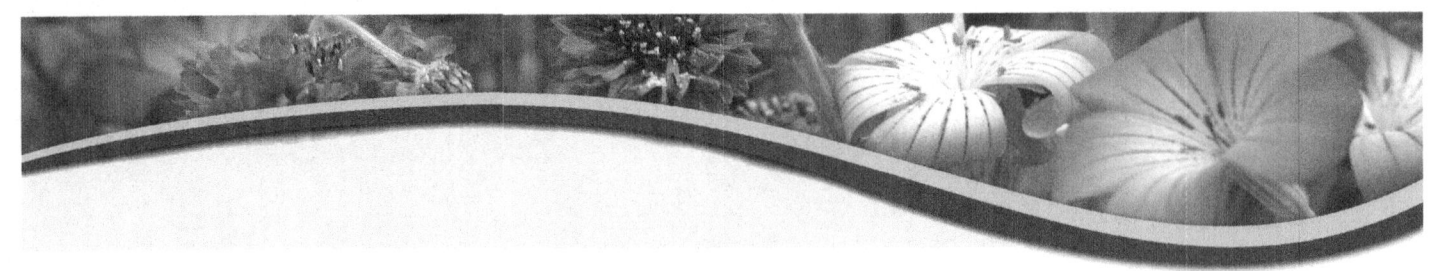

Contents

1. What's It All About? *Concepts in End of Life Care* 1

2. What Can I Do? *Activities and Interventions* 24

3. The Greatest Gift *Learning to Listen with Love* 68

4. Physical Care *When a Patient is Dying* 100

5. Things of the Spirit *Providing Spiritual Care* 146

6. A Time for Grief *Understanding Bereavement* 178

7. Caring for You *Focusing on Healthy Self Care* 220

Other Goodies 250

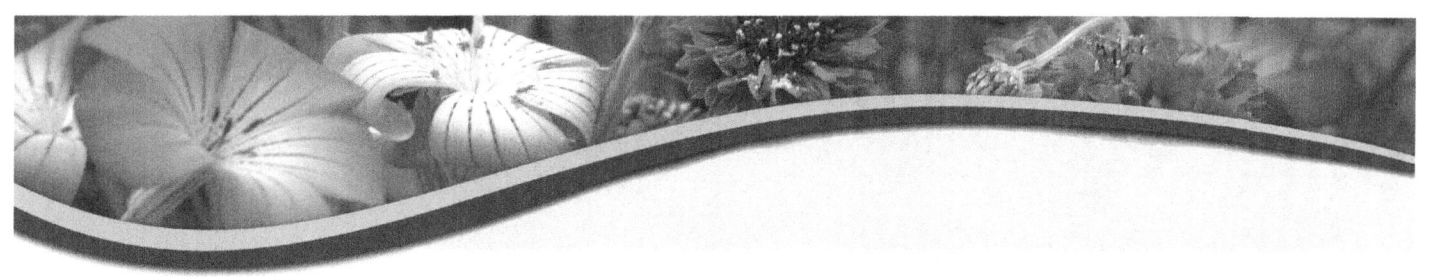

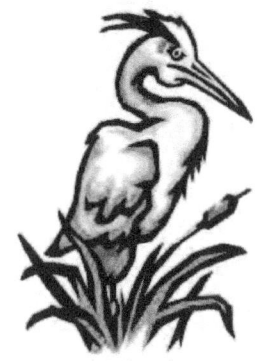

H olds the dignity of the patient sacred

O ffers hope and affirms life

S urrounds the patient with a familiar environment

P articipates with the family in providing care

I nitiates and maintains pain and symptom control

C ares for the emotional needs of the family unit

E xtends bereavement care for a year after death

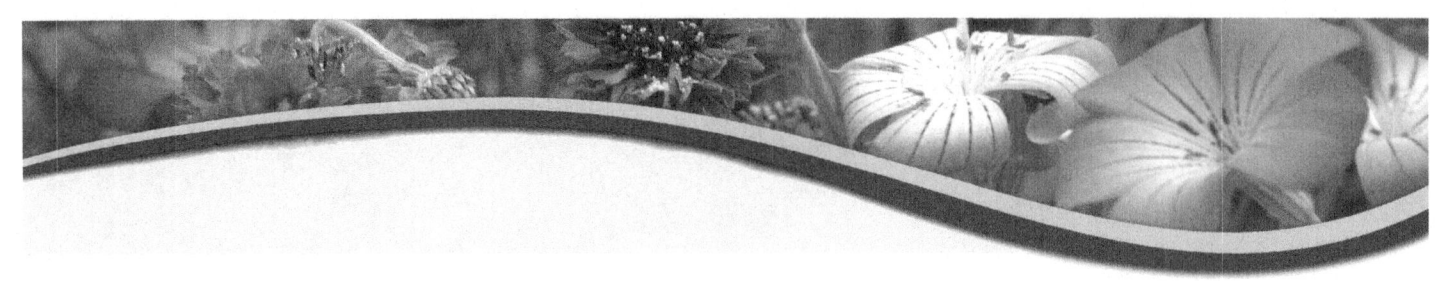

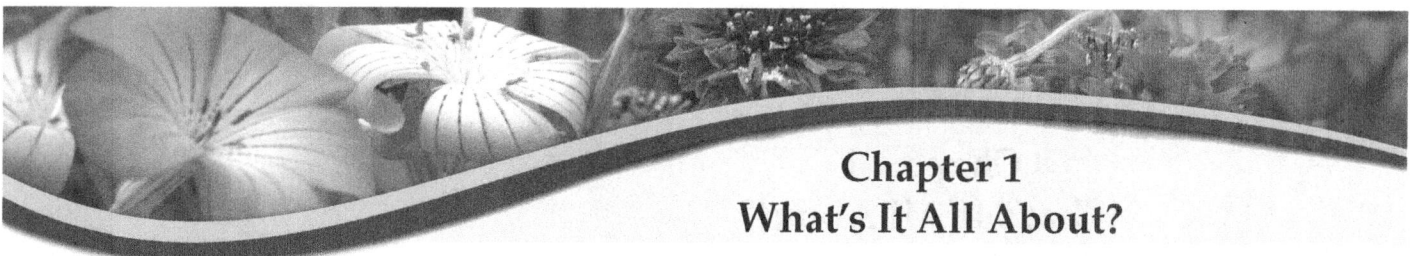

**Chapter 1
What's It All About?**

1. What's It All About?

Concepts in End of Life Care

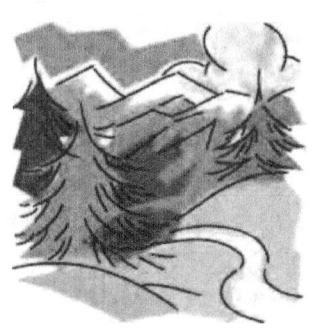

"Just the facts, please..."

A woman stands at the bedside of a dying man. Her eyes fill with tears as he, her husband of 65 years, takes his last breath. She begins to speak softly to him, gently touching his hands, running her fingers over each of his, telling him how much she has loved his strong hands and how he used them to provide for her and for their family. She is saying good-bye.

She feels deep sadness, but also a strong sense of satisfaction. Everything that could have been done for her husband's comfort and for her support has been offered to her. She realizes that this transition in her life could have been much different if she hadn't had the loving support of her local hospice team. Especially her beloved volunteer, who stayed with her in the long hours before her husband's death.

Without the presence of knowledgeable, skilled, and dedicated end of life care givers, she would have been alone in a frightening and unfamiliar landscape. She would be facing profound loss and difficult medical decisions without support or guidance.

Death comes to each one of us, someday, somehow. None of us knows when that time will come. Some of us plan for it and some of us don't. Some of us think about the implications that a terminal illness might have on our plans, hopes, dreams and relationships. Some of us prefer to live in the moment and leave those possibilities in the realm of the unknown until they actually occur.

And occur they will. More than 5 million people die each year. One in ten of those deaths is from cancer, many of the others from AIDS, chronic diseases, and other life-threatening conditions. Many are in long term care facilities. Many more are choosing to die at home surrounded by their children and grandchildren, pets, and familiar personal items.

All would benefit greatly from caregivers who understand the special needs of a dying person.

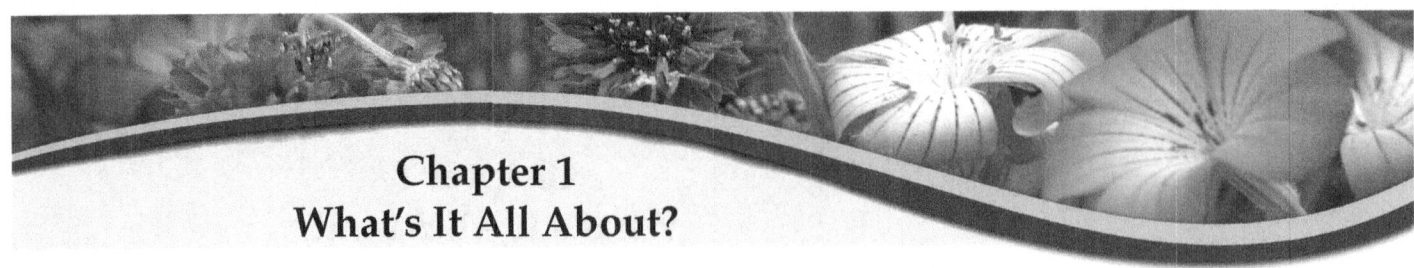

Chapter 1
What's It All About?

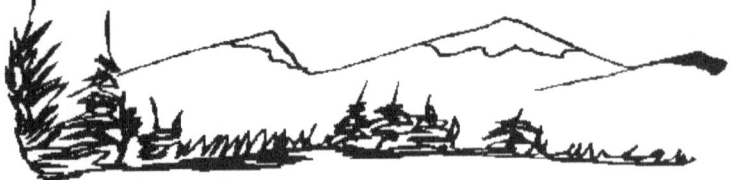

About Hospice

Hospice was a term used centuries ago to describe places of refuge along the rough, rugged paths of the Swiss Alps. In these shelters, weary and wounded travelers found rest and loving care. Although hospice today is a system of care rather than a particular place, it still provides support, respite, and relief to weary travelers; those walking the path of a terminal illness and the loved ones who suffer with them.

The focus of hospice is on the individual and the involved family rather than on the disease. It is the goal of the hospice staff to provide for the whole person, emotionally, physically, and spiritually. Care focuses on restoring dignity and a sense of personal fulfillment to the dying by allowing choices, listening, and caring.

To provide the very best care possible, a multi-disciplinary team shares the responsibilities involved in attending to the needs of hospice patients and their families. The hospice team, made up of a medical director, the patient's primary physician, nurses, social workers, pharmacists, chaplains, home care aides, volunteers, therapists, and others, meets at least every two weeks to discuss ways to best support every hospice family's needs.

Although hospice care is not for everyone (some situations and problems are more medically complicated and the patient or family may not opt for palliative care) it offers many advantages. Some of these basic components of hospice are:

- 24-hour consultation with nursing staff, as needed
- State-of-the-art pain and symptom management
- Emotional support and counseling
- Spiritual Support
- Bereavement support
- Medications needed for pain and symptom management
- Equipment needed for comfort
- Assistance with physical care
- Therapies as needed
- Volunteers as support

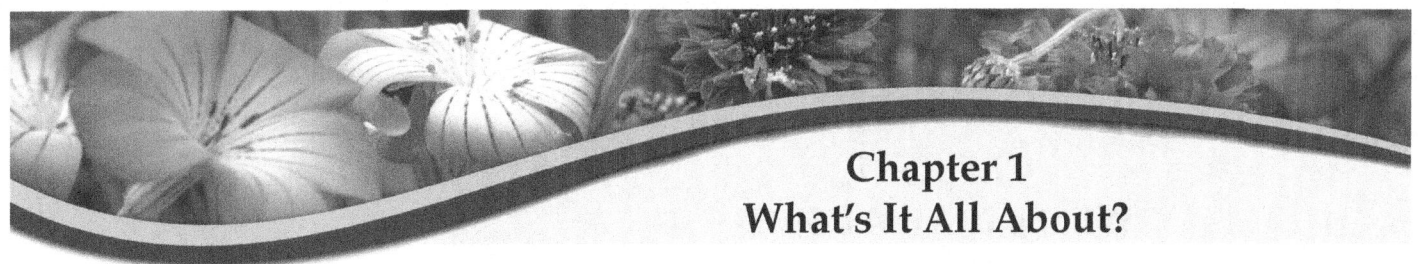

Chapter 1
What's It All About?

Some questions you may be asking...

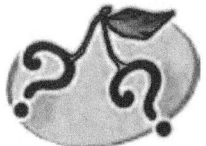 **Who started the hospice movement and where did it begin?**

The very first hospice, St. Christopher's in London, England, was started in 1967 by Dame Cicely Saunders. She was the first to recognize that terminally ill patients weren't getting the specialized care they needed. All too often, the medical community emphasized cure at all costs and viewed death as defeat and failure. Because of this attitude of denial of death as part of the cycle of life, terminal patients were frequently isolated. A "conspiracy of silence" was practiced where the diagnosis, prognosis, and any discussion of these tended to be withheld.

The worst fallout from this tendency to "treat the doctor instead of the patient" (pay more attention to the physician's comfort level than the patient's) usually occurred in the area of pain management. Pain tended to be treated with limited amounts of medication only when the pain became severe. Physicians feared psychological dependence and physical addiction to the drugs used to control pain. A cancer diagnosis was a dreaded death sentence because it almost certainly meant uncontrolled pain and stigma.

St. Christopher's hospice began the daunting task of changing society's attitudes toward the dying process, and in 1974 the first hospice was established in the United States in New Haven, Connecticut by Florence Wald, R.N., a former dean at Yale University school of nursing. The first medical director was Dr. Sylvia Lack. In the decades since that first hospice opened its doors, thousands of others have sprung up in every corner of the nation.

In recent years, the hospice concept has spread internationally with the needs of patients in every part of the globe for improved end of life care gaining international attention. Access to trained hospice and palliative care professionals in many of the world's nations is a serious problem. Studies show that over 100 million people in the world, dying of a terminal illnessand often in severe pain, are not getting palliative care. Help the Hospicesin the UK and the International Association for Hospice and Palliative Care based in Houston, Texas are organizations dedicated to improving the accessibility of hospice care, including adequate pain management in all parts of the world.

"Just the facts, please..."

Chapter 1
What's It All About?

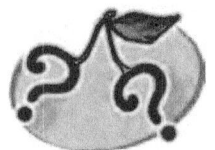 **Does a person have to be at home to have hospice support?**

Hospice patients usually prefer to remain at home, surrounded by family and pets, amid familiar sights, sounds, and smells. Hospice is primarily geared to helping people stay home. Needed equipment and supplies are offered, as well as the assistance of the hospice team. Sometimes, however, it is impossible for the patient to stay at home and in these cases family may opt for an adult foster care or nursing home placement. In most cases, hospice can still provide care and support to the patient and family with adjustments made according to the care situation.

Should the care provider in the home setting become exhausted and need a break from caring for the patient, hospice offers respite care in a nursing home or hospital for a few days (usually five) to allow the care provider to rest. Many cities in the U.S. have inpatient hospice centers where hospice patient's can go when symptoms are out of control or family is unable to provide care at home. These centers focus on providing a home-like atmosphere and amenities for the family's comfort as they stay close in the final days of their loved one's life.

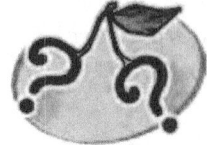 **What are the criteria for admitting a patient to hospice services?**

To be accepted onto the hospice program, a patient must have:

- *A diagnosed terminal illness*
- *An acceptance of the concept of palliative care*
- *Life expectancy of six months or less*
- *Definite and definable needs*
- *The availability of a committed primary care provider*
- *An attending physician who is supportive of the hospice concept*
- *A place of residence that is within the hospice' service area*
- *Acceptance onto services by the interdisciplinary team (The decision may be made by the core team, consisting of the medical director, a spiritual counselor, a social worker, and a nurse. This group also meets once a month or so to review policies and make program decisions)*

"Just the facts, please..."

Chapter 1
What's It All About?

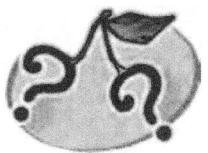 ## Who pays for hospice services?

The majority of people who use hospice services are on Medicare. The Medicare Hospice Benefit is available to any Medicare beneficiary that meets hospice criteria and lives close to a Medicare certified hospice. Under this benefit, the hospice is paid a per diem rate for every day the patient is on services and the hospice team provides staff support, medications that are controlling the patient's pain and other symptoms related to the terminal diagnosis, any equipment the patient may need for comfort and safety, and respite care as needed.

Many private insurance companies now provide hospice coverage for their beneficiaries. Some follow the Medicare model and pay a per diem rate, asking the hospice to provide services to the patient identical to those available under Medicare. Others prefer to pay for individual visits by hospice team members. Many hospices provide services free of charge to those in their community who have no insurance coverage and need the support and symptom management expertise that hospice offers. Donations from the community often help to offset the cost of providing these services.

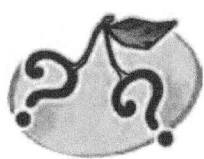 ## Who initiates the referral to hospice?

Anyone can make a request for hospice services by contacting the hospice office or the patient's physician and asking for a hospice evaluation.

If the request comes to the hospice office first, the patient care coordinator makes the appropriate follow-up telephone calls to be sure the physician wishes the patient to be evaluated. The hospice team will make the final determination as to whether or not hospice is appropriate for this particular person. This decision is based on the admission criteria.

The hospice movement in the United States is based on the belief promoted by Dr. Josephina Magno, a hospice pioneer:

"If we cannot comprehend why we must die... and cannot control when we die, we can at least to some extent control how we will die."

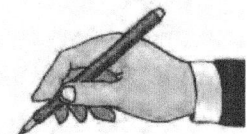

"Just the facts, please..."

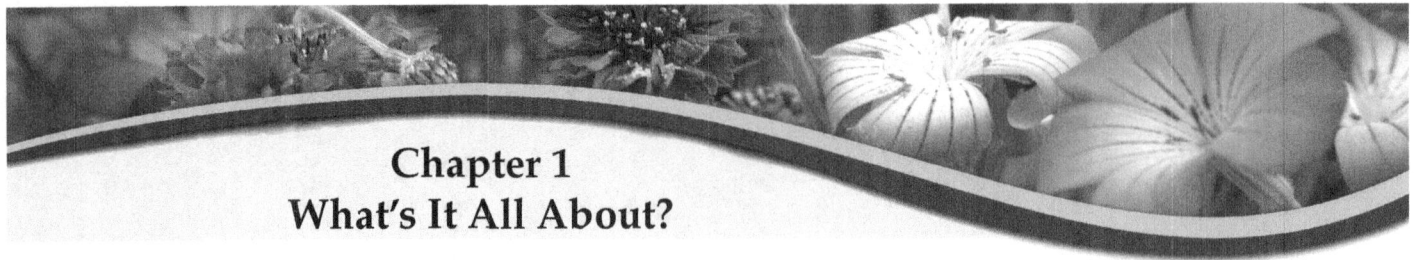

Chapter 1
What's It All About?

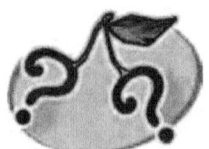 **How does the hospice team interact to provide care to terminally ill patients and their families?**

Continuity of care is a major focus in hospice. Team members meet at least once every two weeks for an interdisciplinary team meeting to discuss each hospice family and share ideas about how to provide the best care possible. Each problem that comes up is examined by the team from as many different perspectives as there are team members present.

A Case History:

> Betsy Miller, a 79 year old woman with end stage heart disease, has been restless at night and is experiencing pain in her back. Her daughter is worried about her kidneys, since she has a history of kidney failure as well. The hospice team brings up her case in team meeting.
>
> The nurse, June Felding, shares that Mrs. Miller's blood sugars have been elevated and she is running a low grade fever. Dr. Roberts, the medical director, suggests giving her a low dose of morphine for the pain and adding a mild sedative. He orders a urinalysis to check for infection. Ms. Felding makes a notation to increase her nursing visits from once a week to three times a week until the symptoms are resolved.
>
> The volunteer coordinator, Bob Wild, reports that Mrs. Miller's volunteer, Rose, has noticed an increase in the patient's anxiety and restlessness since the daughter's arrival from out of town.
>
> Chaplain John Ross speaks up and suggests that the tension the patient is experiencing could be attributed to something she is worried about talking to her daughter about, and asks the social worker, Wanda Townsend, if she has had a chance to talk to the patient this week. Ms. Townsend adds a visit to Mrs. Miller to her list of patients to visit that afternoon.

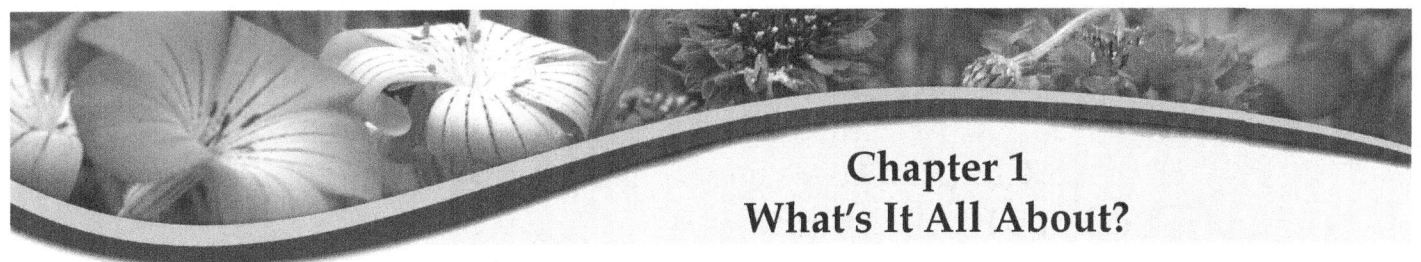

Chapter 1
What's It All About?

 *At the Heart of the Matter*

Exercise:

Referring to the story of the "Alps Traveler" on the DVD, answer the following questions. Be prepared to discuss your answers with the group if you are comfortable doing so.

1. Have you known someone who has had a terminal illness? Did they have the support they needed to deal with their diagnosis? Why or why not?

2. Who could the traveler represent?

At the Heart of the Matter

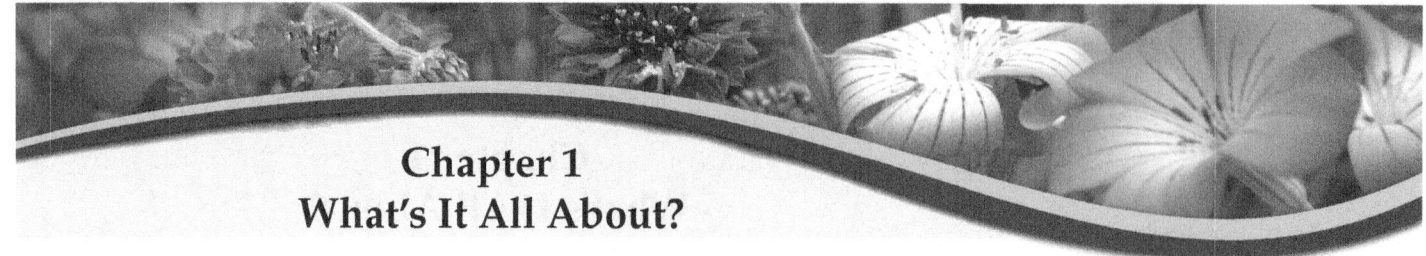

Chapter 1
What's It All About?

3. What do you think the heavy door that is so hard to open could symbolize?

4. Who do you think the monk in the story could represent? The dog? Why?

5. Imagine again the traveler's tired, bruised feet. What do you think the condition of his feet and the healing balm and bandages applied to them by the monk could symbolize?

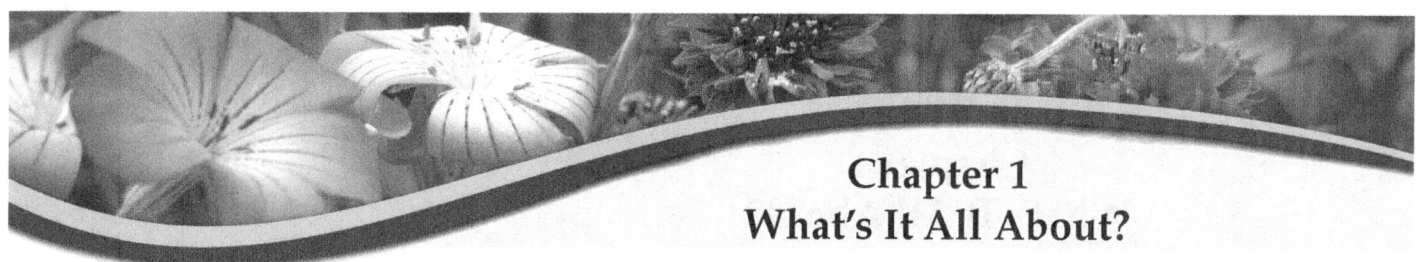

Chapter 1
What's It All About?

6. What could the warm blanket and the comfortable chair by the fire imply?

7. In light of the hospice concept, what could the map of the path ahead and the information about weather conditions and other places of shelter that the monk shared with the traveler represent?

8. In what ways does the Alps Traveler story remind you of an experience someone you know has had with hospice?

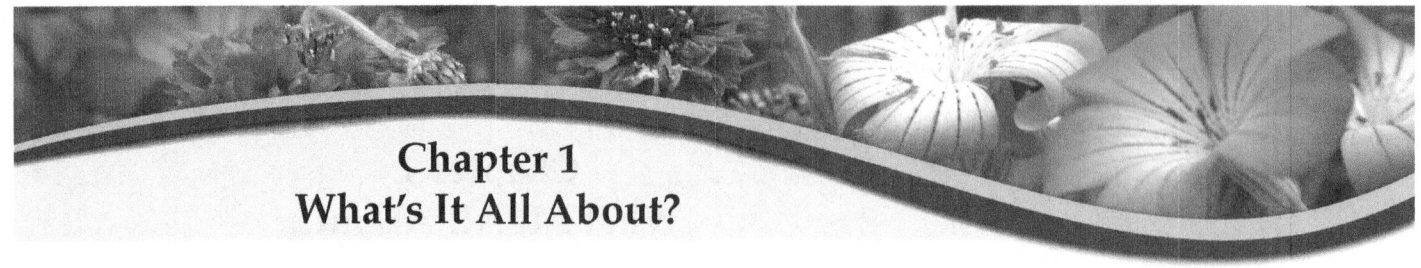

**Chapter 1
What's It All About?**

 # Putting it Into Practice

Pain vs. Suffering

Suffering is a concept not often well understood in Western culture. Pain is not the same thing as suffering, although suffering can and often does accompany pain. When a crises, such as a terminal diagnosis, comes, its effect on our life is not dependent on whether it is a major or minor loss, but how profoundly the loss affects our world.

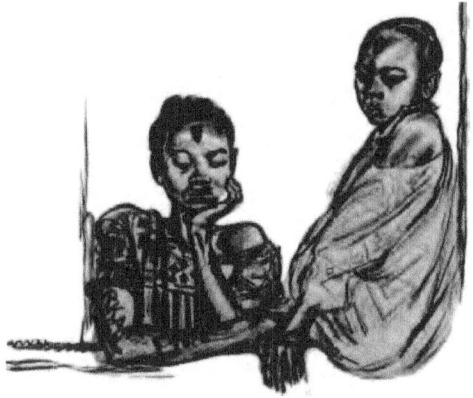

> Think of the most painful experience you've had in your life. How did the pain of that experience affect you? Draw a picture in the space below that depicts the pain.

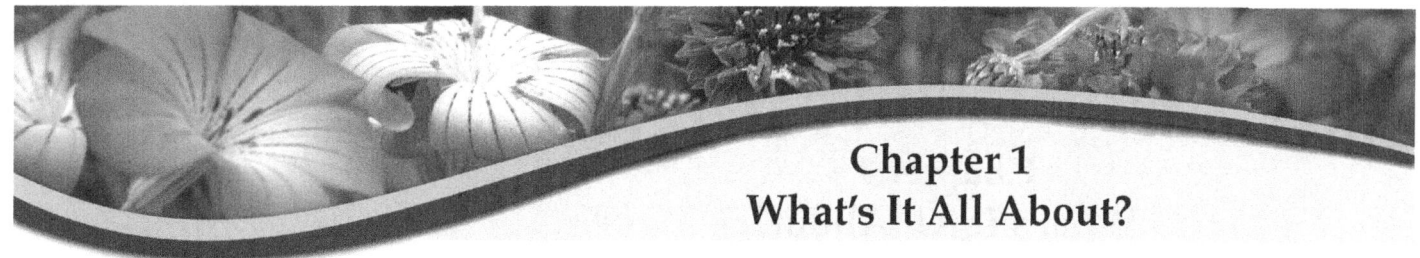

Chapter 1
What's It All About?

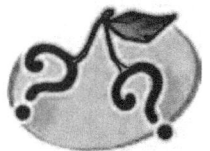 **What is the difference between pain and suffering?**

When a loss is profound, **suffering** can keep the person stuck in what feels like a revolving door of pain. **Suffering** is **pain** in search of meaning.

- Suffering is a reaction to pain when there seems to be no purpose

It might seem that a person responding to a terminal diagnosis and facing the loss of everything they hold dear would surely be suffering because of the pain of this tragic turn of events. But it isn't the **pain itself** that causes the suffering. It is the sense that there is no **purpose** to the pain that brings about the suffering.

This is true of physical as well as emotional and spiritual pain. There are many examples of painful circumstances that are endured with courage when the person perceives that there is meaning to the pain, such as in childbirth or when undergoing uncomfortable treatments that have a definite goal for healing in the body.

The primary task of the grief process is to examine the loss from every angle; from anger, to bargaining, to sadness, until the purpose is brought to light and the pain is given perspective in the person's heart and mind.

- Pain can be endured when it has meaning

One of the best gifts we can offer to our patients or loved ones who are suffering from the pain of loss in the face of a terminal diagnosis and the progression of the disease process at end of life is to give them our loving presence and the opportunity to grieve. Providing a listening ear lets the person know they are **visible**. Staying attentive to signs of physical discomfort and keeping symptoms controlled lets them know they are **safe** to let to of the fear and do the grief work at hand.

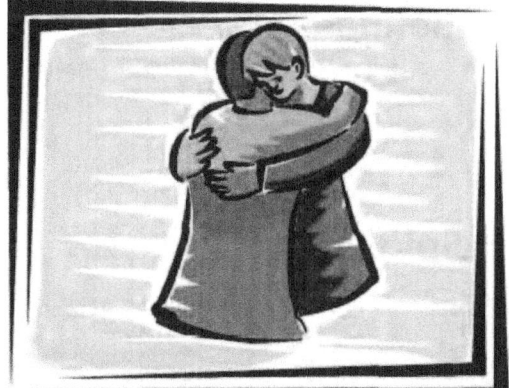

Processing the grief is the only way to find meaning in what is happening to them. Providing the space in which the patient can do this is, bar none, the most important thing you can do for them.

Putting it Into Practice

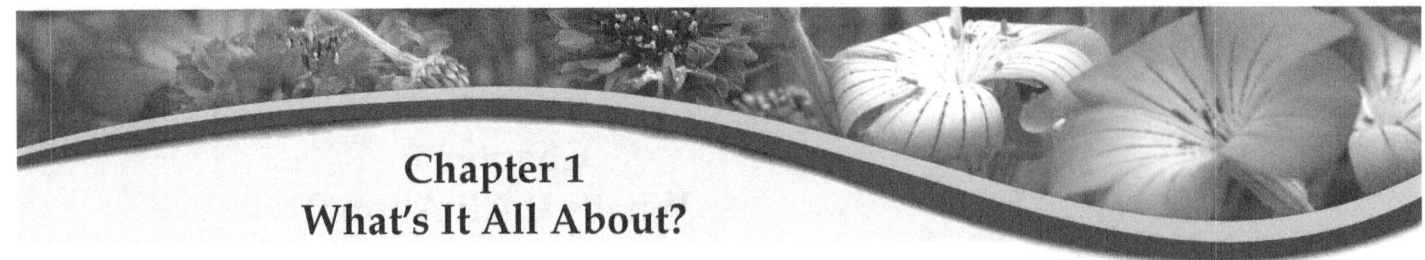

Chapter 1
What's It All About?

Intensifiers of Pain

Write about the ways in which each of the following can make it difficult to find meaning in an experience and thus intensify pain. How do you think these emotions could affect your patient's ability to process his or her grief? How have they affected you in yours?

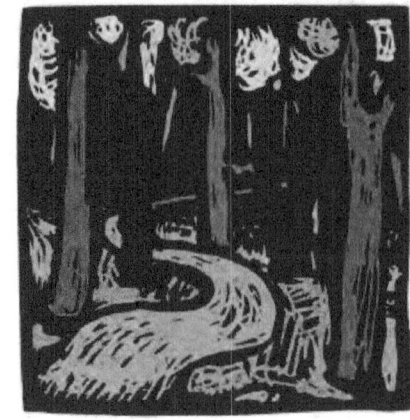

- **Fear**

- **Anger**

- **Guilt**

- **Loneliness**

- **Helplessness**

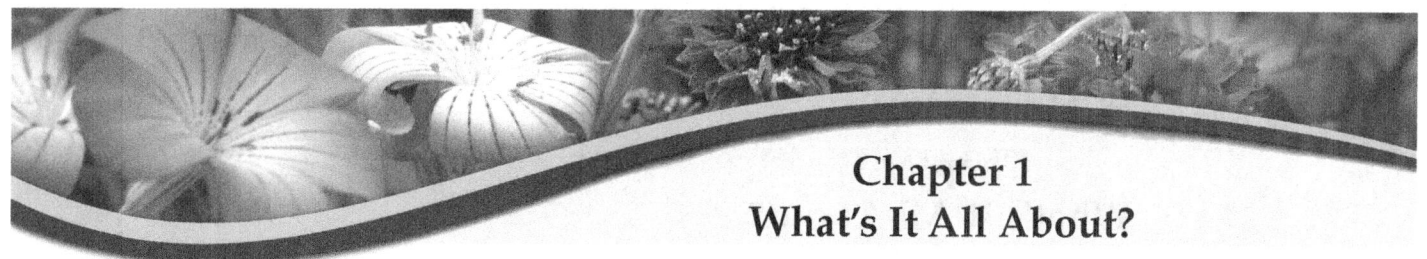

Chapter 1
What's It All About?

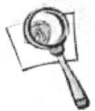 # A Closer Look

Let's focus in a little closer on the care team. Drawing from the information given on the DVD, describe the role of each of the following members of the team:

Patient and Family

Patient's Physician

Medical Director

Volunteer

Nurses (hospice and facility)

CNAs (hospice and facility)

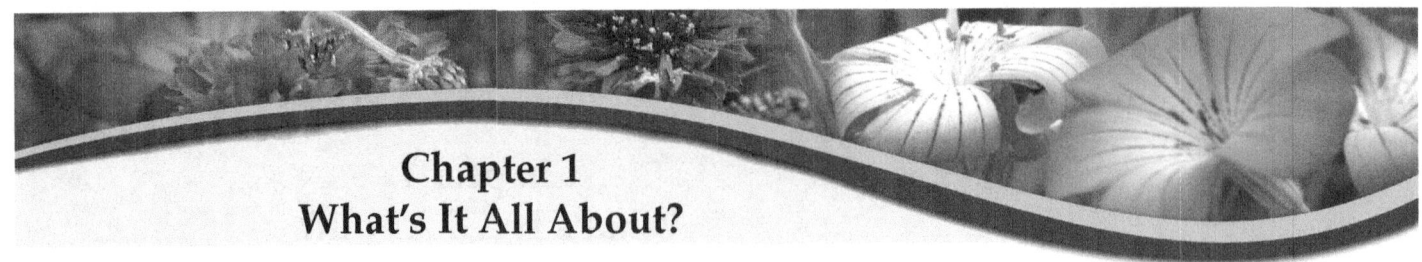

Chapter 1
What's It All About?

Privately hired or volunteer family caregivers

Social workers (hospice and facility)

Chaplain

Speech therapist

Occupational Therapist

Physical Therapist

Dietician

Pharmacist

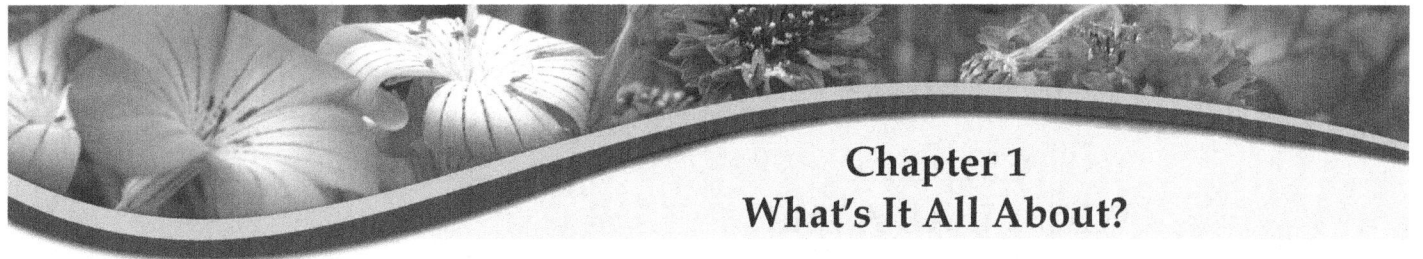

Chapter 1
What's It All About?

Write about what the following statement means to you:

> *"We may choose to live our dying instead of just enduring it... We have not lost the ability to choose how we live our dying, simply because we are dying."*
>
> Hospice of New Orleans

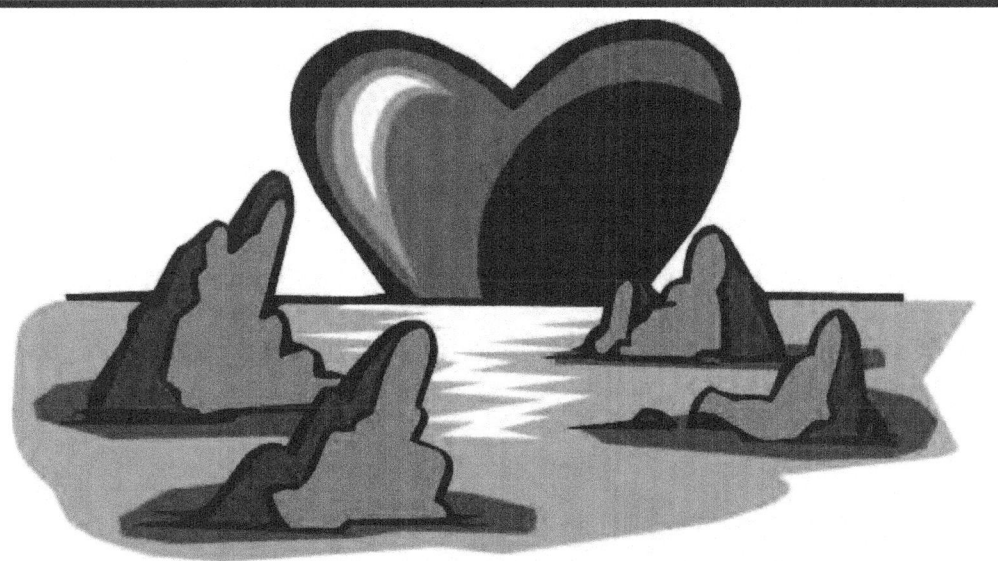

A Closer Look

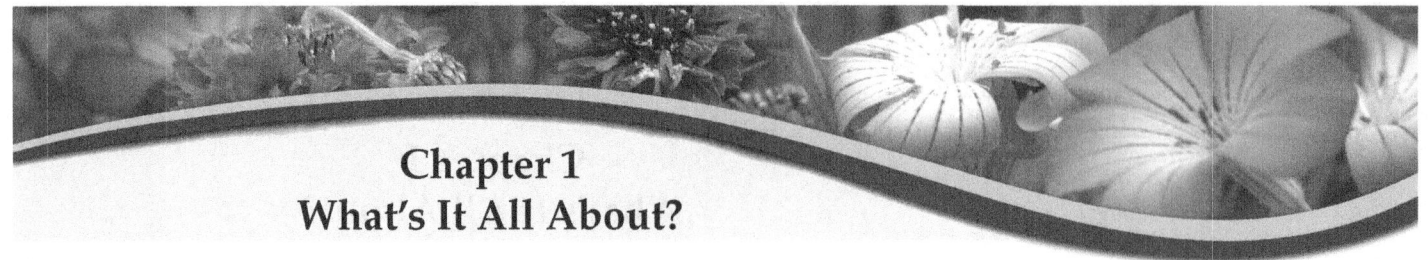

Chapter 1
What's It All About?

How you, as a volunteer, fit in

Welcome to the beginning of your journey toward becoming a hospice volunteer! You have chosen a unique and wonderful field in which to offer your special gifts. Many people say that hospice workers are born to do this work, and in many ways that is true. There is a certain type of person that is attracted to the work of caring for the dying. Do you fit the "mold"?

As a hospice volunteer, it is essential that you be a caring, emotionally mature, committed person who is comfortable talking about death and dying. If that is the kind of person you are, you will probably find that you gain a sense of satisfaction from making a difference in people's lives and glean valuable insights from relationships with patients and their families and from working with the hospice team. Frequently, supporting someone through the dying process can heighten your own sense of spiritual values and help you focus in on those things that matter most in life.

Here are some questions to ask yourself about the volunteer role:

- Am I comfortable with the concept of death and dying?

- Am I comfortable to be alone with someone who is dying?

- What if a patient or loved ones start trying to convince me of their views on politics or religion?

- Can I refrain from trying to convince them of mine?

- Am I capable of dealing with the tears and/or stress of patients or their loved ones without taking them on as my own?

- Am I capable of not taking it personally if a patient is rude or they display inappropriate behavior?

- Am I capable of setting my personal feelings and/or preconceived ideas aside and supporting the patient and family in the ways they need?

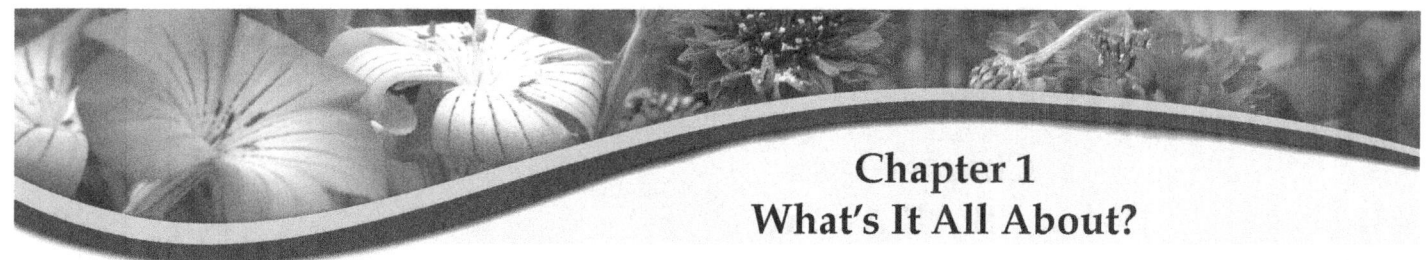

Chapter 1
What's It All About?

Now that you have all this knowledge about the hospice concept, what does it mean to you as a hospice volunteer? We'll be answering that question in a lot more detail in the next chapter, but let's look at some of the basics now.

Hospice volunteers have been a vital part of the hospice concept since the very beginning of the program. Many hospices started with an all volunteer staff. In most hospices today, volunteer time makes up about 5-10% of the total hours spent by the team in providing patient care. In some hospices, especially in countries other than the U.S., that percentage is much higher. Of all the hospice team member's time, the volunteer's is considered the most valuable in terms of all-around benefit to the patient.

Role blurring (when one discipline takes on some of the characteristics of the other disciplines) is a common occurrence in hospice. Although the primary focus of nursing is to control pain and symptoms in the hospice patient, the nurse may be called upon to offer spiritual care or emotional support as the situation demands. The same holds true for many of the other disciplines.

The volunteer position, however, is the one that calls for the most balance of all the areas in hospice. You, as a volunteer, will have the opportunity to provide physical, emotional, and spiritual support (within your scope of practice, of course). You also save money for your hospice by providing care on a volunteer basis. The work you do for hospice creates good will in the community, too, and there is no way to fully measure that.

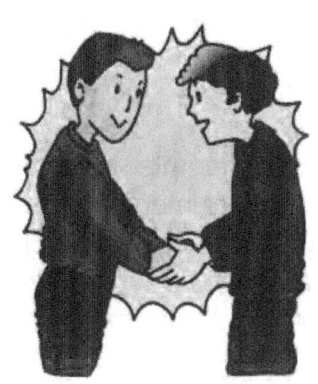

Some questions you may be asking...

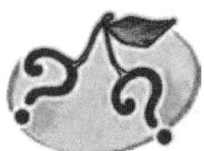 **How will I, as a volunteer, be assigned to a hospice family?**

When a patient is first placed on hospice services, the admitting nurse offers volunteer services to the family. Some patients and families want a volunteer and some don't. Your immediate supervisor, the hospice volunteer coordinator, also attends every IDT (interdisciplinary team) meeting and networks with other team members to determine which hospice families want and need a volunteer that may have initially felt they didn't need one.

A Closer Look

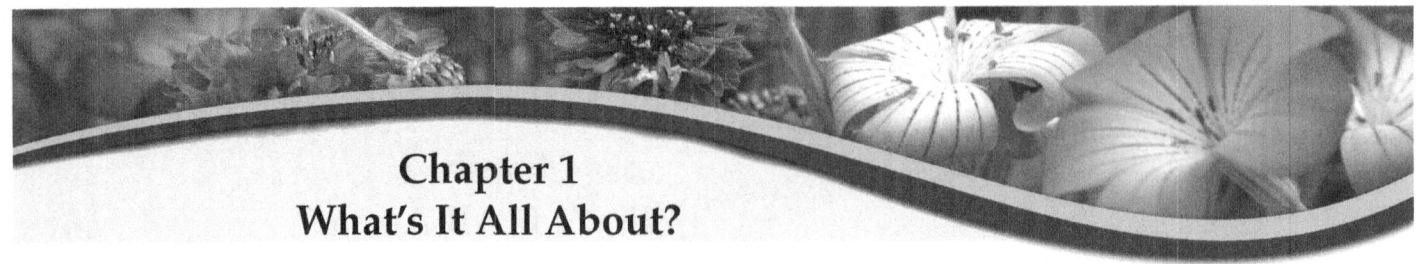

Chapter 1
What's It All About?

When the need for a volunteer has been determined, the volunteer coordinator reviews the files of all active volunteers, looking for a volunteer with similar or complementary interests, personality, background, and geographical area to the patient's. Once the match has been made, the coordinator approaches the volunteer to see if he/she is interested in accepting this particular assignment. If the answer is "yes", the volunteer coordinator makes a visit to the family with the prospective volunteer to introduce them to each other and give them a chance to "size each other up". If either the hospice family or the volunteer is uncomfortable with the other, another volunteer is assigned.

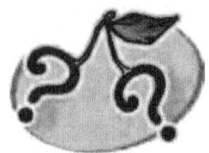 **Will I be expected to give medications, do dressing changes or give enemas?**

The only time a volunteer may be asked to do any kind of treatment to a hospice patient is if the volunteer is a licensed professional and that treatment is within his/her scope of practice. For example, a licensed massage therapist, who is acting as hospice volunteer, would be authorized to perform myofascial release treatments on a hospice patient for a comfort measure (with the physician's approval.)

Another example would be a registered nurse who is volunteering for hospice and inserts a catheter or administers medications. Volunteers who are certified nursing assistants may give baths and do other personal care tasks that require more extensive education than can be provided in a volunteer training session. Your volunteer coordinator will be alert to matching your professional capabilities with the needs of hospice families on services.

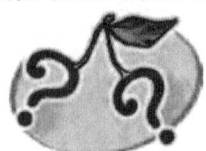 **How much time will I be expected to give to my hospice family?**

Most hospices ask for a commitment of 3-4 hours/week from each active volunteer. Of course, family vacations, times of illness or "respite", as well as other commitments may sometimes prevent the volunteer from being able to give that block of time. Many volunteers find that a two-hour visit with the hospice family twice a week is usually adequate.

A Closer Look

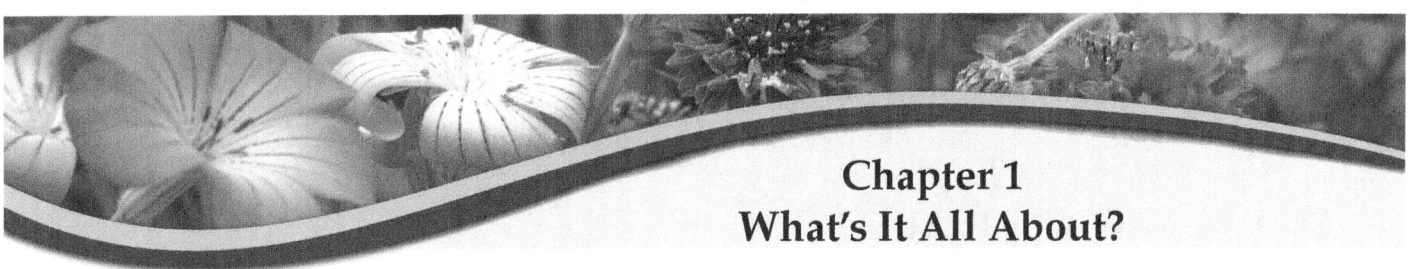

Chapter 1
What's It All About?

From your current knowledge of hospice, and remembering the story of the Alps Traveler on the DVD, take a few minutes to write out a paragraph outlining your view of the hospice philosophy and how you see yourself fitting in as part of the hospice team. Don't worry about specific tasks and responsibilities. We'll cover those in the next chapter.

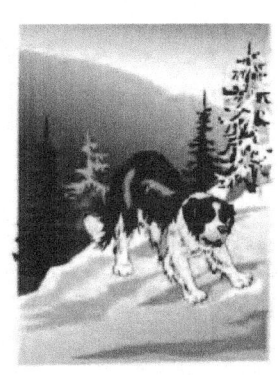

A Closer Look

Chapter 1
What's It All About?

Volunteers can play a significant role in reducing the effects of suffering in hospice patients. In the face of physical pain, the patient's emotional pain can sometimes be overlooked. You, as a volunteer, are on the front lines with the patient and family. If you recognize any of the pain intensifiers listed, such as fear, anger, guilt, loneliness, or a sense of helplessness, occurring with your patient or family, be prepared to report this to your volunteer coordinator.

This is important information for the team in providing care that takes the whole person's needs into consideration. That's the purpose and the beauty of the hospice team.

The team, functioning together as an "adopted extended family" to provide emotional, spiritual, and expert physical support to the patient, relies heavily on the volunteer as one of the most important members of the team.

There are several possible reasons for this:

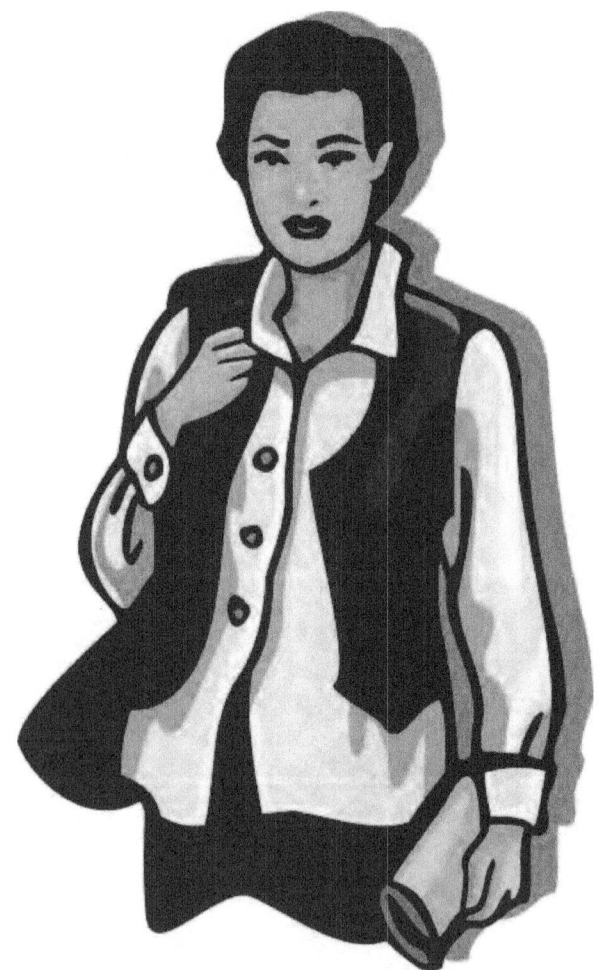

A. One volunteer is usually assigned to a particular family, so that volunteer has a closer relationship with the family than team members who share the responsibilities.

B. The volunteer is usually the only member of the team who is not receiving any pay for his/her contact with the patient and family, so the family knows the volunteer is there for no other reason than to help.

C. The volunteer provides support in the widest range of areas important to the hospice patient, offering emotional, physical, and often spiritual support as needed.

A Closer Look

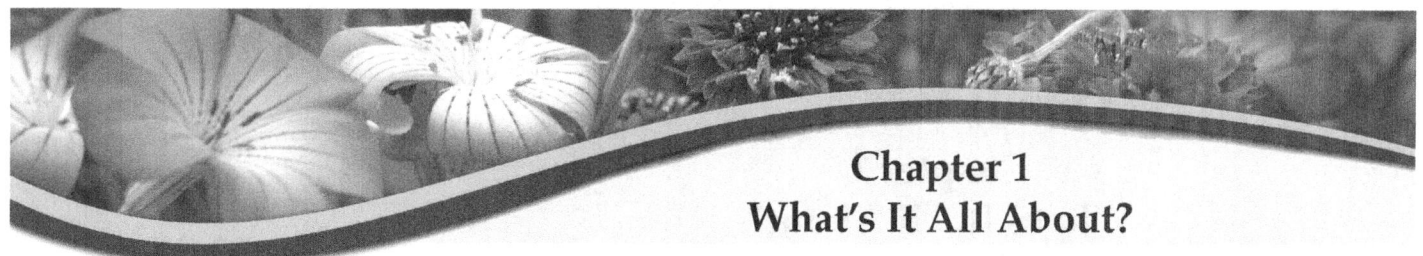

Chapter 1
What's It All About?

Orientation Policies and Procedures

If you haven't already covered the necessary paperwork your organization requires, this might be a good time during your first chapter to look over the packet of forms that are unique to your agency. You should have:

1. A volunteer agreement

2. A current volunteer job description

3. A volunteer bill of rights

4. Your agency's volunteer policy

5. A patient bill of rights

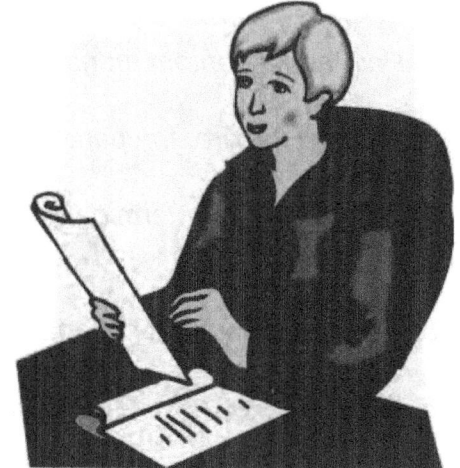

6. Copies of all the initial paperwork that the team uses to put a patient onto hospice services

7. An advance directive and a copy of your agency's policy concerning advance directives

8. Copies of the paperwork that your agency requires you, as a volunteer to fill out

If you have any questions about how to fill out the required paperwork, ask your volunteer coordinator or hospice supervisor. Paperwork varies from agency to agency, but the goals of service are surprisingly similar from Alaska to Florida, and from Maine to Hawaii.

The more you become familiar with the goals and philosophy of your agency, the better you will be able to represent your hospice to your patients and their families and to your community.

A Closer Look

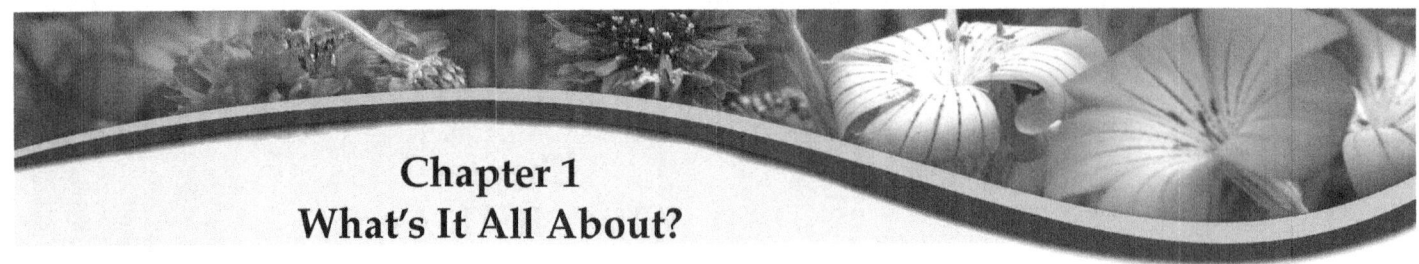

Chapter 1
What's It All About?

 *Skill Check*

T F 1. All that is necessary for good hospice care is an educated nursing staff.

T F 2. Pain and symptom management are key aspects of a hospice care program.

T F 3. In hospice care, the patient and the family are the focus of care.

T F 4. Taking care of a terminally ill person at home is a terrible strain on the family and therefore is usually not recommended.

T F 5. The spiritual and emotional needs of hospice patients are met only by the chaplain.

T F 6. Volunteers are essential to carrying out the professional work of the other team members.

T F 7. Patients who are admitted to hospice do not know they are dying.

T F 8. Hospice volunteers must come to grips with their own mortality.

T F 9. Someone on the hospice team is available to the hospice family 24 hours a day, seven days a week, should unexpected problems arise.

T F 10. A hospice care program is not concerned with the social needs of patients.

11. Identify 10 basic components of a hospice program (i.e. services offered).

Chapter 1
What's It All About?

12. Describe the hospice concept, its goals and its philosophy of care.

13. Identify the purpose of the hospice interdisciplinary team.

14. List the members of the hospice team and describe their individual functions.

15. What is the "core team", who is on it, and what are its functions?

16. In your own words what is the difference between pain and suffering?

Skill Check

Chapter 2
What Can I Do?

2. What Can I Do?
Activities and Interventions

"Just the facts, please..."

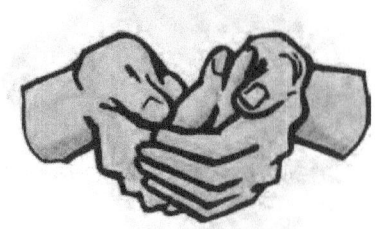

In centuries past and currently in some cultures, the extended family was and is a way of life. The popular phrase "it takes a village to raise a child" could be expanded to include the dying. It does, indeed, take an extended family to attend to the needs of a dying person.

In our mobile society, few extended families stay in close contact, much less live close enough to share the tasks of caring for a terminally ill family member. Often, a beleaguered spouse or adult child struggles alone, going for weeks and months without adequate sleep or any kind of emotional support at all.

This inherent lack of support spawned the hospice concept and created a climate in which it continues to thrive. Hospice becomes, to the terminally ill and their immediate families, an extended family system.

That is why the team approach to care at end of life works so well. The care team, including, as we saw in the last chapter, the physicians, nurses, therapists, personal caregivers, dietician, volunteer, chaplain and others, become this "village" to surround the patient and family with support and expertise to help them navigate the challenging path they must travel.

In this chapter, we will look at some of the practical ways to help as we provide care for a dying person. What does a dying person need?

Common fears of caregivers when working with the terminally ill, are:

"What if I say the wrong thing?"

"Will I know what to do?"

"What if their needs become overwhelming to me?"

By the time you are asked to care for a dying person, you will have completed many hours of training. As you relate to your patient with an attitude of openness and receptivity, he or she will let you know what they need. You, then, in turn, will let them know what you can offer. It all unfolds naturally.

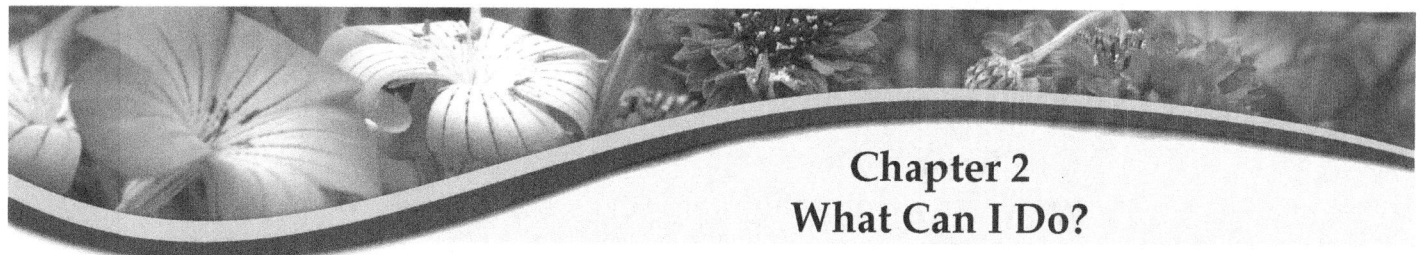

Chapter 2
What Can I Do?

Guidelines for Caring for a Dying Person

1. Be Genuine.

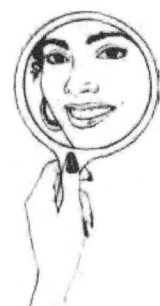

It's important to be yourself when working with the dying person and his or her family. People who are ill appreciate being treated "normally" because it reassures them that their illness has not made them different from others in the ways that count. Being yourself will put them at ease and give them the message that they can be themselves too, and that they are seen and heard as a fellow human being that matters.

2. Be Respectful.

Many of the people who will be in your care are from an older generation in which first names are reserved for close friends and family members. Never assume that you can call a patient or their family member by their first name if you haven't checked with them first and received permission to do so. A simple, "What would you prefer that I call you?" is appropriate.

Nicknames like "honey", "sweetie", or "sugar" are overly familiar and unprofessional. Using a louder voice than normal and a sing-song tone as if to a young child is demeaning and thus disrespectful. Don't assume that your patient is hard of hearing unless you ask them and they tell you that they need you to speak up.

3. Be Dependable.

To people in crisis, whose lives are in upheaval because of the devastating impact of a terminal illness in the family, it is essential to know that they can count on someone or something. Know your limitations and never offer more than you can deliver. A person with a serious illness often has little variety and few distractions in his/her life, so each outside contact is very important. A visit that may seem be a minor part of your week may be the whole focus of your patient's.

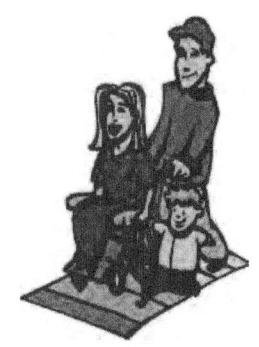

"Just the facts, please..."

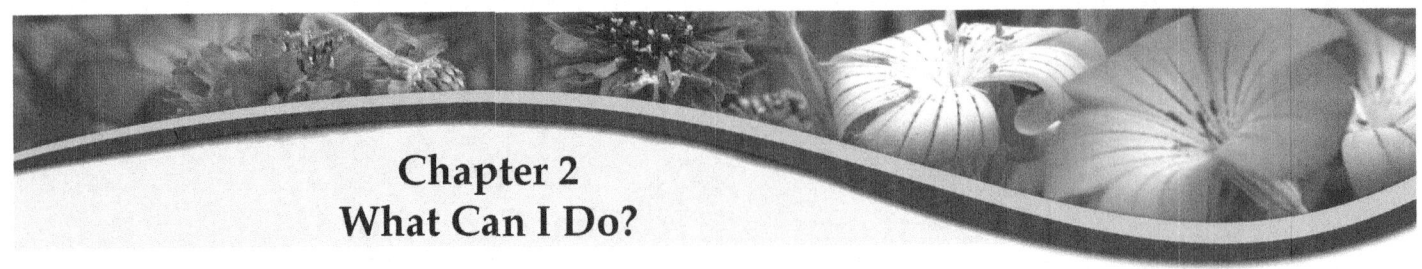

Chapter 2
What Can I Do?

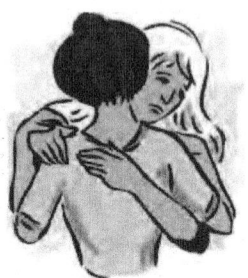

4. Be sensitive to the patient/family needs for physical contact.

Some people like to touch and be touched. Others don't. It's important to be able to read the cues of others to be sure you are, indeed, offering the kind of comfort that meets their needs. Most people respond positively to a hand on the arm or across the shoulders as a gesture that says, "I'm here and I care." Be open and do what feels right in the situation. Your comfort or discomfort will communicate itself, so be yourself.

5. Take initiative.

At the beginning of your relationship, your patient and family will usually look to you to set the pattern of the interaction. Regular phone contacts and brief visits to see how things are going will serve to break the ice. Don't assume that just because the patient or family hasn't contacted you that they don't need anything. Remember the heavy wooden door in the Alps Traveler story? It's hard to reach out for help, even if you need it, when things are so overwhelming.

On the other hand, be alert for clues that you may not be needed at that particular time. Don't prolong a conversation if you find you are doing most of the talking. Be careful not to push. Families may be afraid not to comply with your wishes, afraid of alienating you and the rest of the care team. When offering choices, give all the options equal billing so you aren't influencing their decision. Don't be afraid to show your feelings. If you feel sad, show it. In this way you will act as a role model to the family, demonstrating that nothing terrible happens when you experience your emotions.

6. Meet your patient's family where they are.

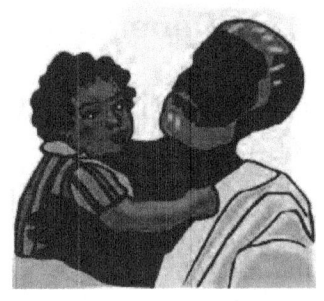

It is absolutely crucial that all caregivers tune in to the values and life patterns of terminal patients and their families and meet them there. Regardless of how you might disagree personally with their belief system or patterns of relating to one another, it is never appropriate to give unsolicited advice. Each family's life patterns have been formed over the years and are rooted in a history of which you have not been a part. Your job is to work non-judgmentally within the structure, not to try to change it.

"Just the facts, please..."

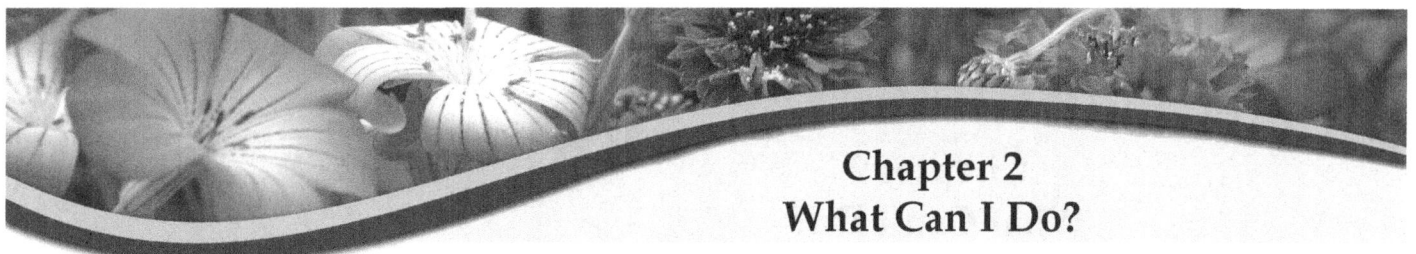

Chapter 2
What Can I Do?

7. Keep all interactions with your patients and their families strictly confidential.

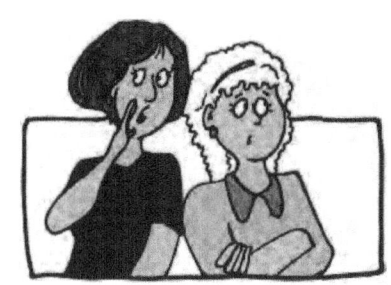

Any reference made concerning a patient or family member should by made only to another team member in the context of providing care. If information shared with you by a family member is of extreme confidentiality, it shouldn't be shared with the whole team in a group meeting, but should be divulged only to your supervisor, who will then make the decision regarding who to tell. Don't promise a patient or family member that you "won't tell anyone" something that they share with you. It is important to keep open the option of reporting sensitive information to the appropriate team members as needed.

HIPAA means "Zippa Your Lippa"

HIPAA laws regulate certain pieces of information that can't be shared without the patient's written permission and the ways that information can and can't be stored, retrieved, and transmitted. Knowing these laws is important and could cost you your job if you disregard them.

Confidentiality breaches occur when:

Any information about the patient and family is given to anyone else outside the family without written permission from the person involved (care team members can share information with each other only if it is necessary to provide care to the patient.)

Information given to a care team member is given to a family member without the client's express permission.

A conversation about the patient and family occurs between team members in a setting where it can be overheard (such as in an elevator, a doctor's office, or on the telephone.)

"Just the facts, please..."

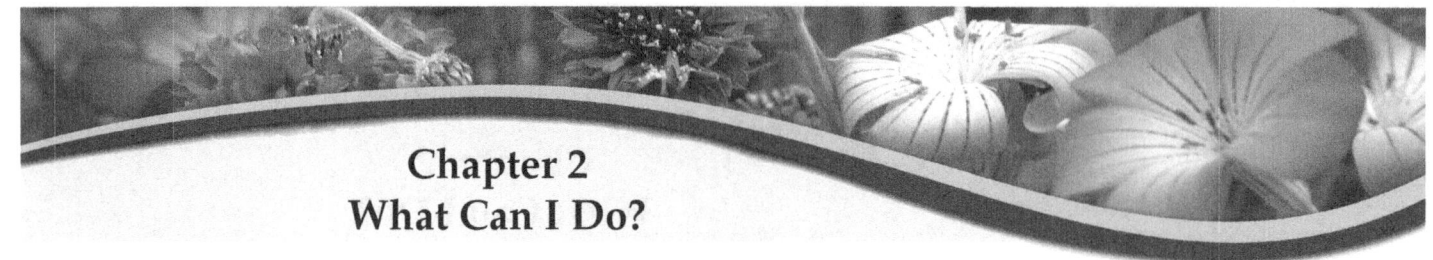

Chapter 2
What Can I Do?

Ways to Achieve a Healthy "Distance" in a Patient Care Context

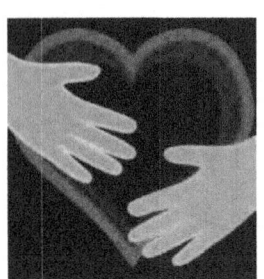

Practicing the art of distancing may seem contradictory to all we've learned about having an open, loving, caring relationship with your patient and family, but it's not. Healthy distancing doesn't prevent closeness, it makes true closeness safe for you and for the family you're working with.

Make a choice to leave the hospice family's problems at their doorstep when you leave their home or leave the facility.

This doesn't mean you don't care about them, but ruminating over them during your time away from them won't solve anything and it will keep you tied to them in unhealthy ways.

Don't talk about your personal problems.

Sharing information about your family and events in your life is a positive way to allow your hospice family to know who you are as an individual and thus increase rapport with them. Talking about personal problems, however, changes the dynamics of the situation, pulling you in to an emotional place where you may not be able to maintain objectivity and your hospice family may feel they have to take care of you at the expense of the emotional support they need.

Be alert for any signs that you might be developing a sense of possessiveness with your patient and family.

Ask yourself how you feel when members of the family express appreciation for another team member. Examine your responses when suggestions given by another team member are given higher credence than your suggestions are. If, at any point, you find yourself struggling with feelings of resentment toward other members of the team who are involved in "your" families care, find someone safe to share your feelings with. Explore the possibility that deeper issues might be involved.

Chapter 2
What Can I Do?

 *At the Heart of the Matter*

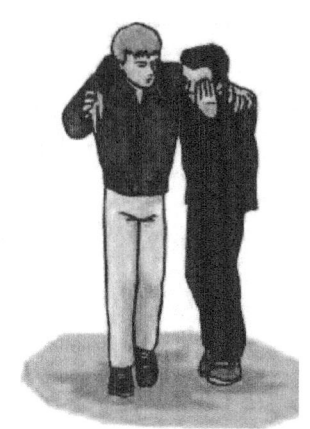

Some questions to ask yourself:

What are my most prominent strengths when I interact with others? In what areas do I feel I may need more development of my "people skills"?

Do I have a network of "safe others" with whom I can explore new ways to grow in my people skills? Who are they?

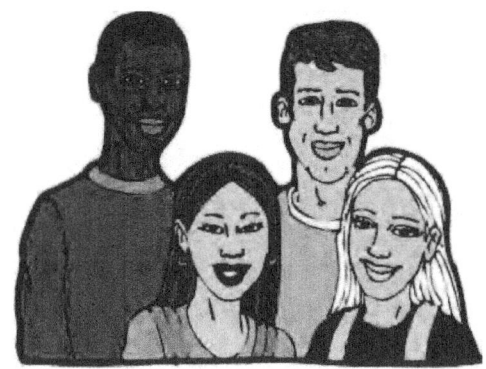

What steps can I take to develop one or expand the one I have?

At the Heart of the Matter

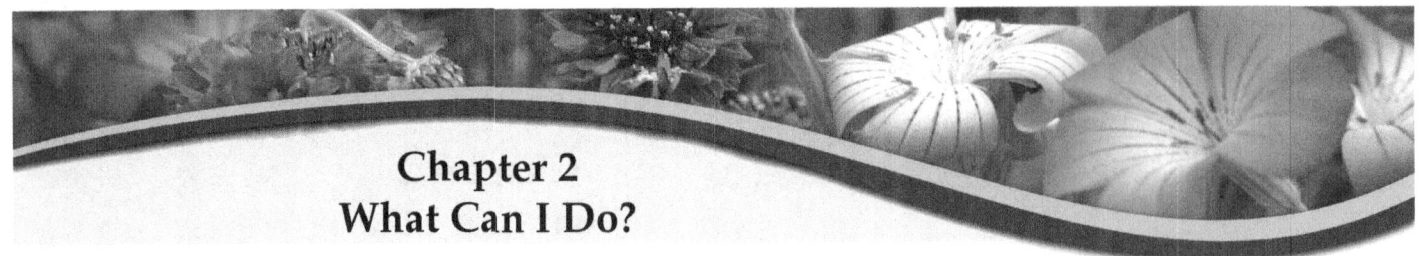

Chapter 2
What Can I Do?

A Bill of Rights for a Dying Person (Author Unknown)

Even though the goals of treatment may have changed, I, as a person with a terminal illness, have the right:

- *To be treated as a living human being until I die*
- *To maintain a sense of hopefulness, however changing the focus of that hope might be*
- *To be cared for by people who can maintain a sense of hopefulness as they interact with me*
- *To be able to express my feelings about my approaching death in my own way and in my own time*
- *To be part of the decision making process about my care*
- *To be dealt with honestly and openly*
- *To have my pain and symptoms controlled so I can use my energy for the tasks of preparing for the end of my life*
- *To have my privacy protected*
- *To have my individuality respected and my decisions honored, even if you don't personally agree with them*
- *To have access to the care I need without any partiality, no matter what religion, culture, race, sex or sexual preference, age, disability, or ability to pay for services I have*
- *To know that you are sensitive to my needs and are skilled and knowledgeable about my care*
- *To know that you want to be present with me and help me to face my death*
- *To die with peace and dignity*
- *Not to die alone*
- *To have help and support for my family in accepting and grieving my death after I'm gone*

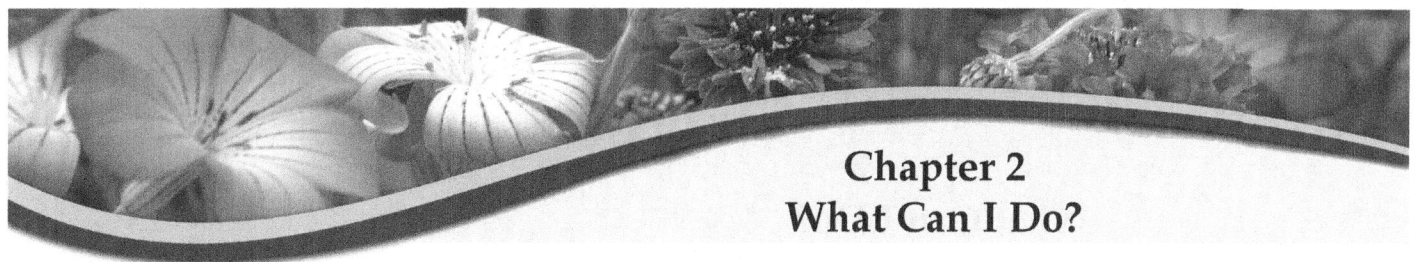

Chapter 2
What Can I Do?

I Am Your Patient and I Have Dementia

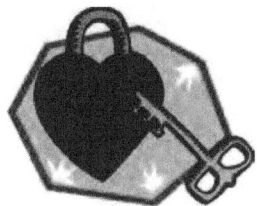

- Remember, I am a person with a history full of interesting experiences.

- Find out who I have been in my lifetime. You might be surprised at how much I have accomplished and how much I am loved by those who have known me.

- Dementia may have taken away my ability to connect to those things, but they are still there, deep in my heart.

- You can connect with me, even though I may at first seem unreachable to you, if you are willing to try.

- The only way you will really hear my heart is to grow quiet and listen to me with yours. My words may be scrambled but they are trying to tell you something. Listen for the pattern. I'm trying to tell you something.

- Touch me. Gently. With respect and love and tenderness. I am losing everything dear to me. Don't take away my chances for meaningful human touch, too. I need it as much as I need air and food and water.

- Talk to me with respect. Use adult language and use my name. It is demeaning to me to treat me like I'm a small child and call me "Honey" or "Sweetie". I may have been the president of a prestigious college or a gifted artist in my day. Honor who I am, even though you might not be able to see it on the outside now.

- I am still me. I am still in here. In this body that won't cooperate with me. In this mind that has forgotten so much of what has been important to me. Find me. Care for me well. Someday you may be in this place, too. And I hope that, in that day, you will have someone willing to see who you really are, too.

At the Heart of the Matter

Chapter 2
What Can I Do?

What to Expect if Your Patient has Alzheimer's Disease

There are three stages in the progression of Alzheimer's Disease, one of many forms of dementia. Alzheimer's Disease is a disease of the nervous system in which small plaques form in the brain and cause "disconnects" in the neural pathways. As their disease progresses, memory is lost and the person eventually can't take care of him or herself.

Stage One

- Short term memory loss begins to occur
- The person becomes disoriented to time
- Concentration becomes more difficult and attention span decreases
- Interest in work, leisure activities, dressing, etc. wanes
- Mood swings start to occur, with anxiety, depression, and agitation increasing
- Rude, ill-mannered, blaming behavior happens

Stage Two

- Disorientation increases
- May forget family and friends as memory loss becomes more pronounced
- Struggles with finding the right word or following directions
- Loses ability to read, write, and do math and speech becomes slurred
- Begins to be incontinent of bladder and bowel
- Difficulty sleeping, restless pacing and wandering ("Sundowners")
- Lack of control of impulses, with swearing, yelling, rude behavior increasing

Stage Three

- Total disorientation to person, place, and time
- Completely incontinent
- Unable to speak or communicate except for screaming or groaning
- Bed bound and totally dependent on caregivers to provide for needs
- Increased sleep problems
- Seizures, coma, and death

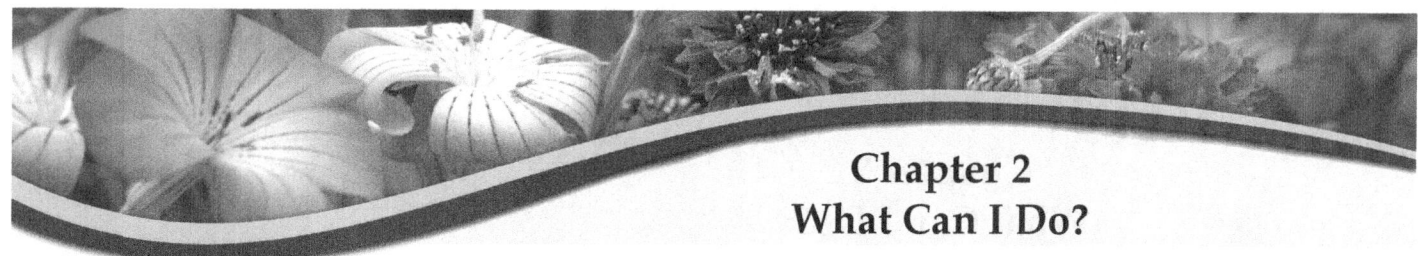

Chapter 2
What Can I Do?

Caring For Someone with Alzheimer's Disease

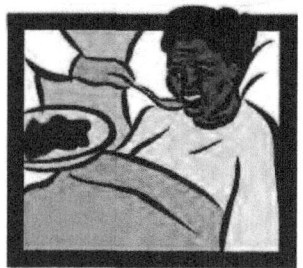

Your hospice patient may have Alzheimer's Disease along with another terminal diagnosis, such as cancer or end stage heart disease, or the Alzheimer's itself may be the primary diagnosis. Either way, there are special considerations to keep in mind when providing care for someone with this disease. Remember that the family will be dealing with an added dimension of loss and in active grief even before the patient dies. This is their loved one and they have been losing them memory by memory for awhile now. They deserve a lot of support in the process.

Here are some principles and practical strategies to keep in mind when caring for a patient with Alzheimer's that is still responding and active:

- If your patient insults you or accuses you of things you didn't do, remember that it isn't really them talking, but the disease. Look past the behavior to the person.
- Provide as much security and comfort as you can. Think of how frightening it must be to be unable to perform simple tasks for yourself. Be patient and understanding.
- Take each day as it comes. What your patient could do yesterday, he or she might not be able to do today. And each person is different. Don't make judgments or have expectations.
- Work with family members to learn as much as you can about what comforts and soothes the patient. They may have been a musician in their day and love the sound of classical music. Music often reaches a person with dementia when nothing else will.
- Promote independence for as long as you can. This goes a long way toward maintaining the patient's dignity and self-esteem. Assist them with grooming to help them look their best.
- Make the physical environment as safe as possible with pictures to identify rooms, stairs and windows marked with brightly colored tape, and rugs that could be tripped over removed from the area where the patient might walk.
- If an Alzheimer's patient engages in violent behavior, step out of reach and stay calm. Remove the triggers and attempt to redirect the patient to a soothing activity. Reduce noise and distractions that might agitate them. Be gentle and reassuring.

At the Heart of the Matter

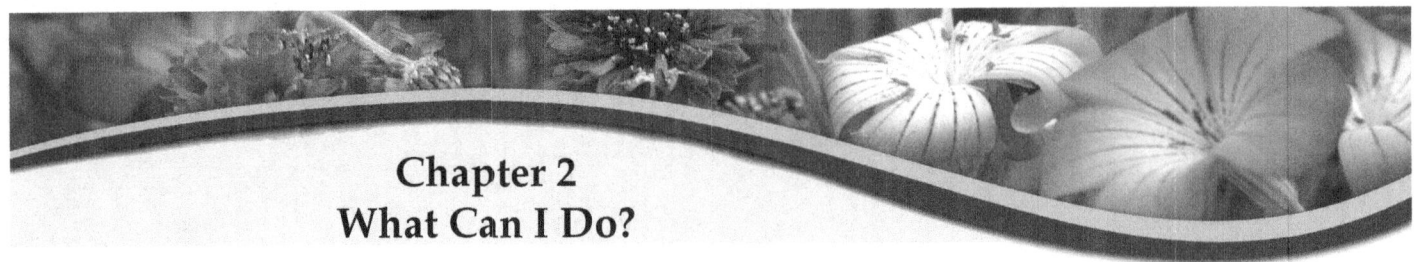

Chapter 2
What Can I Do?

How do you feel about caring for patients with dementia, such as Alzheimer's Disease?

Have you had a family member or friend develop this disease?

If so, how has this impacted you and your family?

Discuss the implications of the phrase, "I am still in here" from "I Am Your Patient and I Have Dementia..." on page 31.

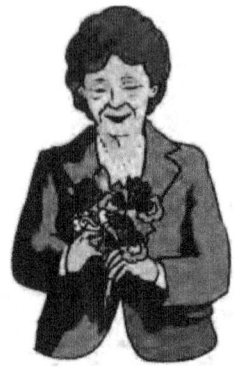

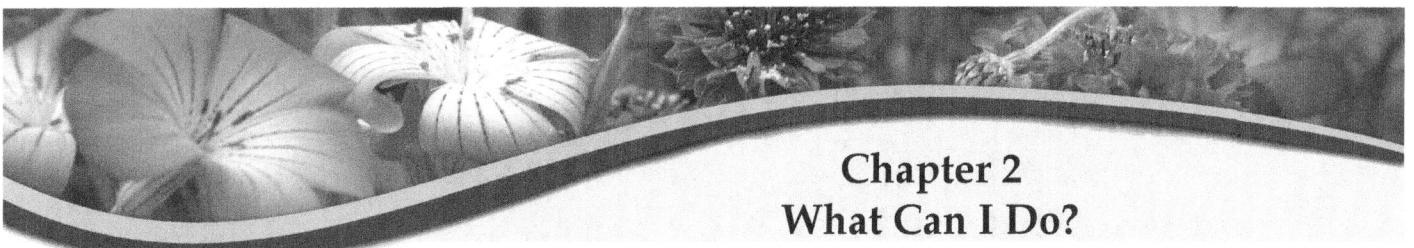

Chapter 2
What Can I Do?

Some Additional Tips for Caring for a Patient with Dementia

- Even though the patient may be unconscious and not responding, talk to them anyway.

- Introduce yourself each time you approach them, saying something like, "It's Jane Smith, Mrs. Winters. I'm here to sit with you for awhile."

- Always let the patient know what you are doing before you do it.

- Speak gently and soothingly, without condescension. Use your voice to smooth out any negative energy around the patient. (Try it, it really works!)

- Remember that with a dementia patient, they may be living in past memories. Take cues from the family members or from the patient themselves as to how to address them. If they are, in their mind, eight years old, they may want to be called by whatever name they were familiar with back then. If you call her Mrs. Smith, she may not know who you are talking to. Familiarity is important to dementia patients and in this case, using a more informal name would not be disrespectful.

- Trying to explain to a dementia patient what a volunteer is may be an uphill battle and cause more confusion than it clears up. Simply say, "Hi. I'm Jane Smith, and I'm a friend of (say the name of a family member)." The mood swings, personality changes and behavioral issues that present with a patient's Alzheimer's disease can be difficult enough for family members. This is a progressive brain disease, and short term memory can be greatly affected while their long term memory stays intact. Thus, a patient may not recognize an adult child or family member. This can be hurtful to the family member. Offer support and acknowledgment of how painful this can be.

- You may see your Alzheimer's patient getting medications under the tongue or in the sides of their cheeks. This method of administration is used when someone can't swallow. It prevents choking and is readily absorbed by the body.

- Amazingly enough, even though they can't remember family members or simple day to day activities, Alzheimer's patients often will retain the ability to sing. Instead of asking a question, try singing it. Sometimes this works like magic and the person will sing the answer back to you. Family members love to see this when it happens.

At the Heart of the Matter

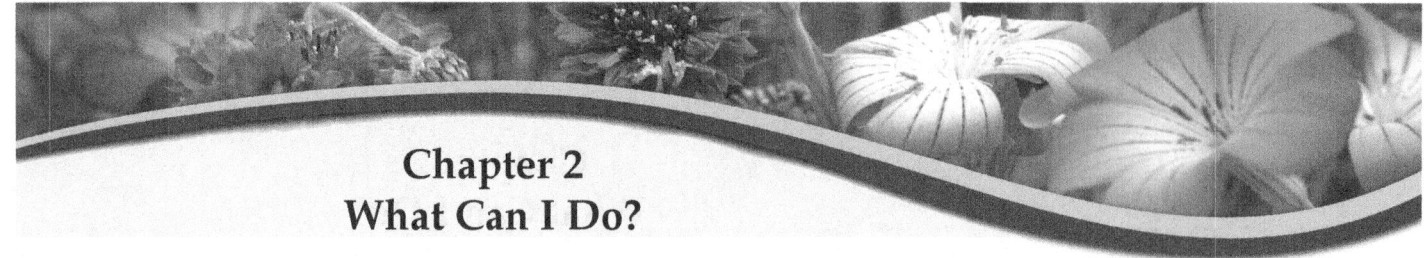

Chapter 2
What Can I Do?

Interacting with an Alzheimer's Patient

- Keep your facial expressions kind and sympathetic.

- Use lots of friendly eye contact and gentle touch.

- Use short sentences and easy to understand words.

- Say the person's name at the beginning of each sentence.

- Maintain a calm demeanor, even if the patient gets agitated. Do not respond in kind. Instead, redirect them into another activity.

- Don't quiz them about the recent past, instead ask questions about the distant past, tapping into their long term memory.

- Be as accommodating as possible, avoiding any kind of control.

- Watch for non-verbal cues in body language and facial expression. You can learn a lot about what's going on with the patient from these cues.

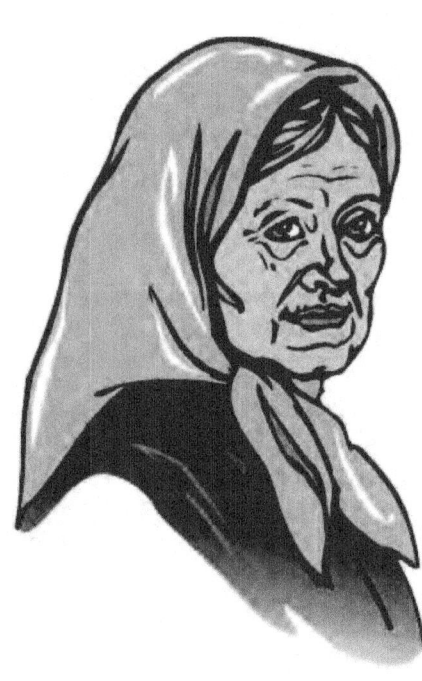

- Be creative! If the patient is wandering out of their room and safety is an issue, try putting a simple piece of tape or hanging a blanket in the doorway. Often, the patient won't remember that it's a door because it will look different and won't try to go through it.

- If your patient is supposed to be in bed but is trying to get up, don't restrain them. Call for a family member or a staff member to help.

- Patient's who revert back to their past as their disease progresses, may go back to a native language (if their first language is not English). The language barrier that this can create may be frightening to the patient and frustrating for family members. If you know the language they are speaking, use it to talk to them. If you don't, try to learn at least a few words. This can be very comforting to the patient.

At the Heart of the Matter

Chapter 2
What Can I Do?

Supporting the loved ones of an Alzheimer's Patient

- Give the family chances to grieve aloud with you about what is happening to their loved one. This is a role reversal and it can be very hard on adult children to see their parent decline in this way.

- Do lots of explaining and reassuring of the family. The more information you can give them about why their loved one is behaving the way they are, the more the family will feel that they have some kind of handle on things. Knowledge is personal power.

- Your calm, steady, respectful presence as you interact with the patient can be hugely reassuring to the family and build trust that their loved one is being seen as the valuable person that they are.

Interacting with Facility Staff

- **Introduce yourself to each member of your patient's care team.**

- **Let the facility staff know how long you will be with the patient each time you visit. This helps them plan their tasks around having you there to relieve them. Make sure you let them know when you leave.**

- **Always explain your scope of practice as a volunteer so the staff doesn't think you can do more with the patient than you actually can.**

- **Honor the facility staff's history with the patient and his or her care. Be super tactful when making any suggestions so as not to insinuate that they haven't been doing a good job. You want a collaborative relationship with the staff, not an antagonistic one.**

- **Don't assume that all the members of the facility staff know about the process of death and dying. They may not at all. You are receiving a specialized immersion in the principles of end of life care. Not all medical professionals have had this opportunity.**

- **If it is toward the end of the patient's dying process, offer the facility staff "alone time" with the patient. If they have been close to the patient, they need a chance to say their goodbyes too.**

- **Keep the staff updated on any changes you see in the patient.**

- **Give a report when you leave the facility and thank the staff for their help and for their care of the patient.**

At the Heart of the Matter

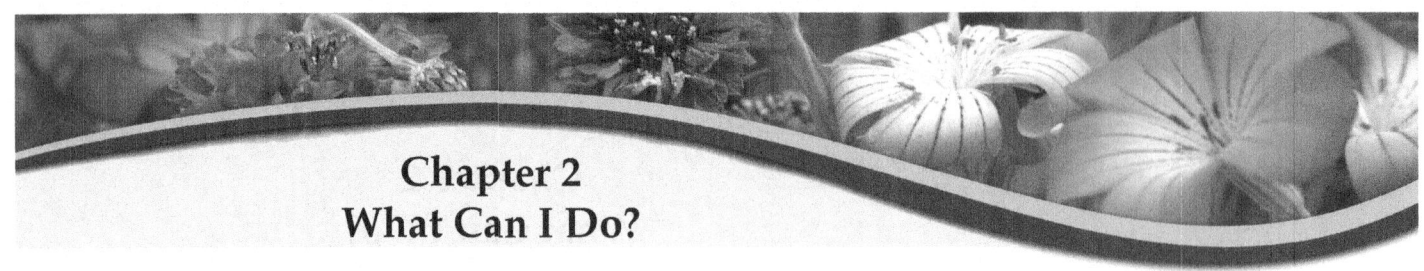

**Chapter 2
What Can I Do?**

There's a Lot You Can Do!
Providing Support to an Unresponsive Patient

Caregivers often find it frustrating to provide emotional support to someone who can't respond due to dementia, end stage disease, or severe stroke. What can you do to connect with someone who can't respond to you in words or gestures? Plenty!

- Center yourself before you enter the room to make certain you are emotionally available to connect with your unresponsive patient. Leave your personal stress and baggage outside, where you can pick it up later (or not!)
- Be sensitive to the environment. Provide soft music and low lighting.
- Be aware of the temperature of the room.
- Keep strong odors away (perfume or cologne, strong smelling foods, etc.)
- Talk to the patient even if they don't respond. Speak in a soothing, low-toned voice. Hearing is the last sense to go, so always assume the patient can hear you, even if he or she can't let you know.
- Don't talk *about* them in their presence, but talk to them. A person in end of life that is in the unresponsive stage is withdrawing bit by bit from this life. Be sensitive to this and keep your conversation with them immediate and meaningful.
- Don't chatter about outside matters that don't concern them. Picture a woman in labor, focusing on the task at hand. Your voice is connecting you into this patient's narrowing world, but you don't want it to be a jarring distraction.
- Touch gently. Watch your patient's body language and vital signs to see if the touch you are providing is soothing or stressful. Some people don't respond well to touch, if they have been the recipients of unsafe touch in the past. If their brow furrows or if they flinch instead of relaxing and becoming more serene, try moving your hands inches away from their skin in a smoothing motion, as if caressing away the stress.
- Avoid putting your hands on the top of their head or over their shoulders or on top of their hands. This may seem oppressive to them. Instead, cradling their arms or hands from underneath is a gesture of support.

At the Heart of the Matter

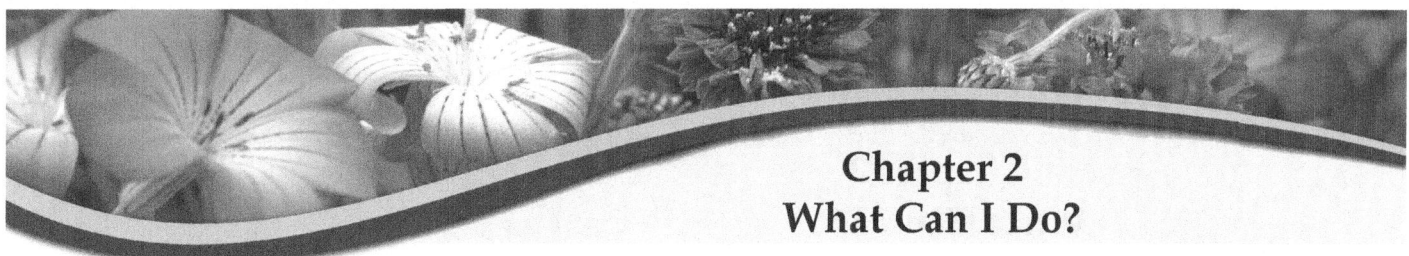

**Chapter 2
What Can I Do?**

 # Putting it Into Practice

Providing Care for A Patient Who Needs Help Transferring

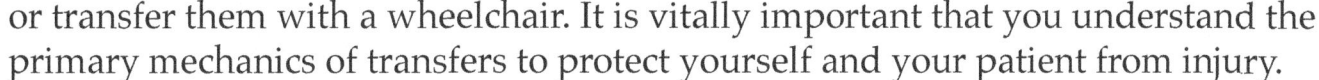

Whether you are visiting a patient in his or her home or providing care in a facility, there will surely come a time when you will need to help the patient in and out of bed or transfer them with a wheelchair. It is vitally important that you understand the primary mechanics of transfers to protect yourself and your patient from injury.

Here are a few of the basics:

Take Care of That BACK!!!

No matter what tasks you are performing with or for your patient, good body mechanics are something that you can't afford to overlook. Some of the general principles of body mechanics are:

- Maintain your own fitness and flexibility to prevent injuries.
- Plan your movements in advance, assessing whether it is safe for you do this task
- Keep your back in a balanced position, trying to work from the mid-ranges of your joints.
- When turning, pivot your feet, not your back.
- Change positions frequently.
- When standing, use a wide base of support, with your feet slightly staggered.
- When sitting, look for a chair with lumbar support and make sure your feet can rest flat on the floor.
- When reaching, decrease strain at your spine by getting as close as you can to your work. Adjust your stool height or leg position.
- Lift with your legs, not your back.
- Keep items close to your body when lifting or carrying.

Putting it Into Practice

Chapter 2
What Can I Do?

Wheelchair Preparation

1. Position the wheelchair at a 45-degree angle to the transfer surface.

2. Remove the armrest closest to the transfer surface.

3. Remove the footrest closest to the transfer surface.

4. Swing the other footrest out of the way.

5. **LOCK the BRAKE!**

Positioning the Patient in the Wheelchair

Remember:

- Always start with the brakes on.
- Place front casters in a safe position.
- Place the patient's feet on the foot rests.

Positioning the patient farther back in the wheelchair

1. Standing in front of the patient, position yourself as if you were doing a standing pivot transfer.

2. Instead of putting your knees on both sides of the patient's knees, butt your knees up against the front of the patient's knees.

3. Have the patient loosely grasp around your neck and, with your arms around the patient's lower back, lean the patient forward.

4. Rock the patient forward to un-weight their buttocks, then push back on their knee.

Putting it Into Practice

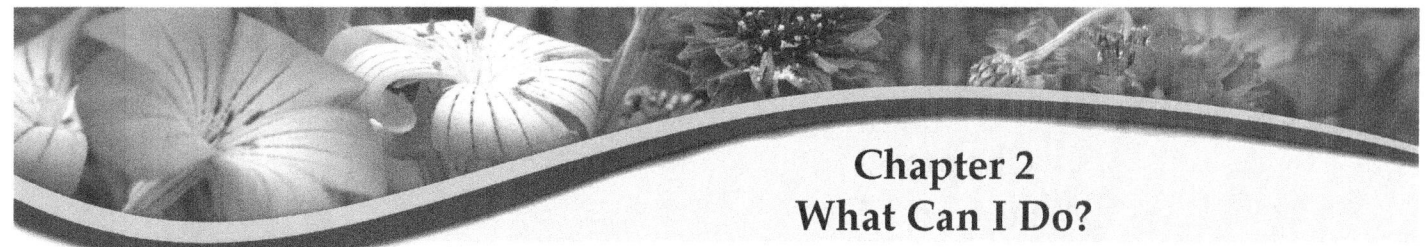

Chapter 2
What Can I Do?

Centering the patient in the wheelchair

1. Stand in front of the patient with your center of gravity stable and knees slightly bent.
2. Hold on for support under the patient's arm that is away from the direction you want the patient to move.
3. Lean the patient's body away from the direction you will be moving them.
4. Place your hand well under the buttocks on the side you will be moving.
5. Count aloud and after count of three, move the patient's buttocks to the center of the chair.

Standing Pivot Transfer

(Use this technique when the person is strong enough to stand up but needs help getting from the bed to the wheelchair.)

1. Prepare the wheelchair.
2. Assist the patient into a sitting position by having them lie on their side, then pivoting their legs around as you help them lift up the trunk of their body.)
3. Squat slightly, keeping your back straight, and place your knees on the outsides of their knees.
4. Place both of your arms around the patient's back and gently assist them to a standing position.
5. Pivot them 45-degrees until they are standing directly in front of the wheelchair.
6. Ease the patient into the chair and replace the armrest and footrest.

Car Transfer

1. Open the car door fully.
2. Move the front seat back as far as possible.
3. Pull the wheelchair up at a 45-degree angle to the car and remove the footrest and armrest on the side closest to the car (if they are removeable).

Putting it Into Practice

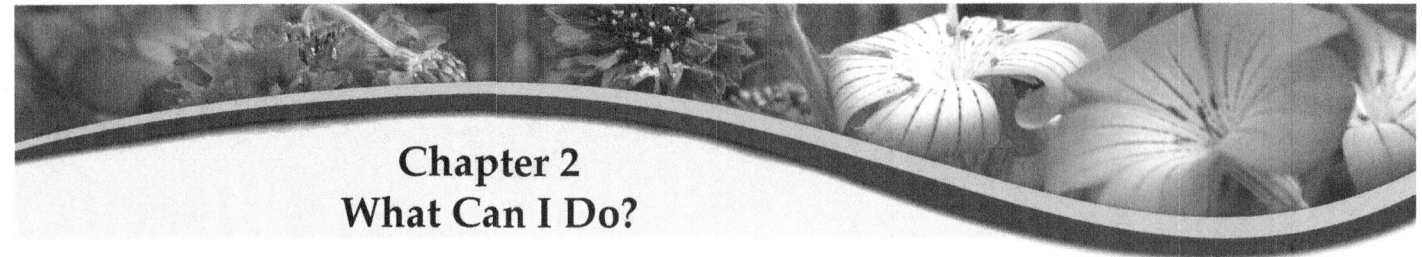

Chapter 2
What Can I Do?

4. Lock the brakes.

5. Assist the patient to a standing position with your knees on the outsides of their knees.

6. Pivot the patient into the car, adapting the movements to the tight space and making certain the patient's head doesn't bump on the door frame.

7. You may find that standing slightly to the side of the patient and assisting from over them, rather than around, makes the transfer easier.

Toilet Transfer

1. Prepare the wheelchair.

2. Unfasten any clothing necessary.

3. Use the standing pivot transfer, lowering the clothing as the patient reaches the position just in front of the commode.

4. Have the patient use the toilet safety frame for additional support while lowering to the commode.

Tub Transfer

1. Make sure there is a non-slip surface in the tub or shower.

2. Prepare the wheelchair.

3. Position the shower bench in the tub/shower.

4. Do the standing pivot transfer from the wheelchair to the end of the shower bench that is protruding over the edge of the tub.

5. Lift the patient's feet into the tub one at a time, guarding for loss of balance when lifting their legs.

6. Dry the patient and the floor completely before returning to wheelchair.

Putting it Into Practice

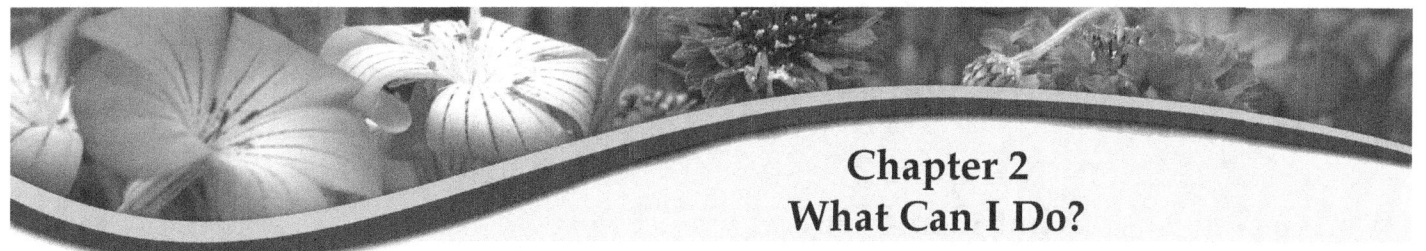

Chapter 2
What Can I Do?

Positioning a Patient in Bed

Remember before starting any move:

1. Put the bed brakes on.

2. Adjust the bed to the correct height (about hip height if standing, about mid-thigh height of knee on bed, so that the supporting knee is flexed.)

3. Always put the bed rail down on the side you're working.

4. Make sure that the turning sheet is correctly placed under the patient's hips.

5. Explain to the patient what you're going to do.

When doing a move:

1. Count out loud when you move the patient. Say "1-2-3 lift".

2. Use the momentum of your entire body (not just your arms) to shift any weight.

3. If the patient is heavy, rock the patient in the direction you want to move him/her on each count.

4. Whenever moving a patient, support them under their shoulder blades - do not pull on their shoulders.

Some important information on using turning sheets

1. Using a turning sheet reduces friction on patient's skin.

2. Using a turning sheet improves body mechanics by allowing your arms to stay much closer to your body, thus putting less strain on your shoulders, back, and wrists.

3. A turning sheet should be positioned from the patient's mid-thigh to shoulder.

4. You can use a draw sheet, a folded bed sheet, sheep skin, or a diaper changing pad with the plastic side down for a turning sheet.

Putting it Into Practice

Chapter 2
What Can I Do?

Moving a Patient Up in the Bed (using a turning sheet)

1. Stand at the head of the bed, facing the foot, and place one knee on the bed in line with the patient's head.

2. Grasp the turning sheet under both sides of the patient's shoulders.

3. Have the patient tuck his chin down onto his chest and bend his knees.

4. Count 1-2-3 and shift weight from your knee to your leg, pulling the patient's head and shoulders up onto your thigh.

Pulling a Patient to the Side Lying Position

1. Stand, facing the side of the bed, and place one knee on the bed.

2. Lean over the patient and grasp the patient's far shoulder and hip.

3. Have the patient tuck his chin and cross his arms on his chest, and cross his far leg (knee bent) over his near leg.

4. On count, shift your body weight from the knee that is on the bed to the other leg.

Pushing a Patient into a Side Lying Position

1. Facing the bed, place one knee up on the bed.

2. Place your hands on the patient's shoulder and hip that is nearest you.

3. Have the patient tuck his chin and cross his arms on his chest.

4. Help the patient bend his near leg and cross it over his far leg.

5. On count, shift your body weight from your leg to your knee that is on the bed.

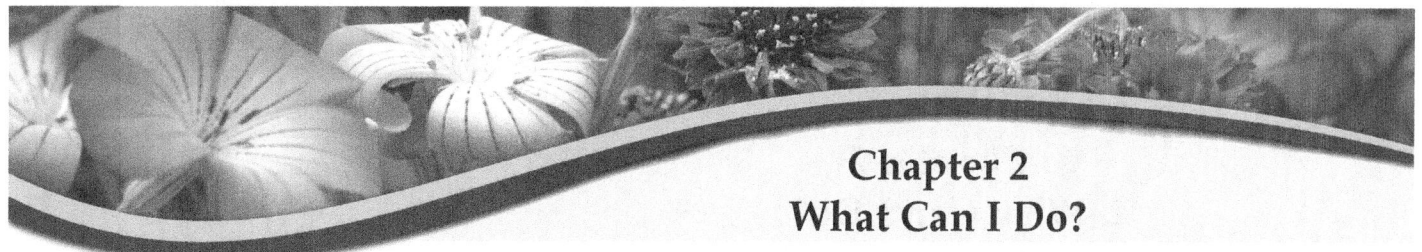

Chapter 2
What Can I Do?

Using Pillows to Support Limbs in the Side Lying Position

1. Make sure the patient is in good body alignment in the bed.
2. Place a pillow under their head and neck.
3. Place a pillow lengthwise behind the patient's back.
4. Position the top leg with the knee flexed in front of bottom leg with the hip in proper alignment.
5. Support the upper leg with a pillow.
6. Place a pillow lengthwise under the upper arm.
7. Be careful not to cover the patient's face with the pillow.

Range of Motion

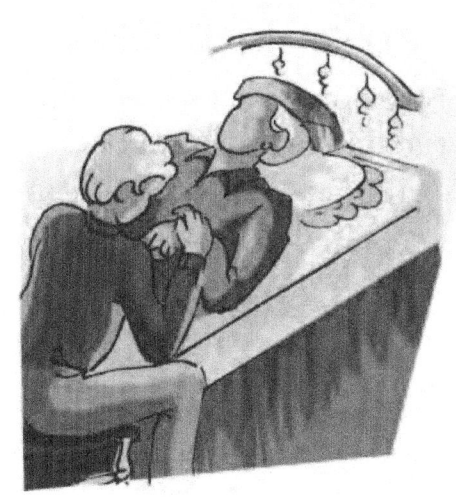

Moving the joints in the direction they are meant to, without putting any undue strain on them, is amazingly relaxing and comforting to someone who is in bed a lot. If you haven't been trained in doing range of motion, be sure to have a nurse supervise you the first time you do it. It is a comfort measure, not a treatment, so anyone can do it if they know how and are delegated to do it.

1. Position your patient on their back and lined up comfortably on the bed.
2. Support each joint by placing one hand under it while doing range of motion on it with the other hand.
3. While supporting the limb, move the joint gently, slowly, and smoothly through the range of motion. Stop if pain occurs. Watch for non-verbal signs of discomfort in the patient (furrowed brow, increase in pace of breathing, groan or sharp intake of breath, etc.)

Putting it Into Practice

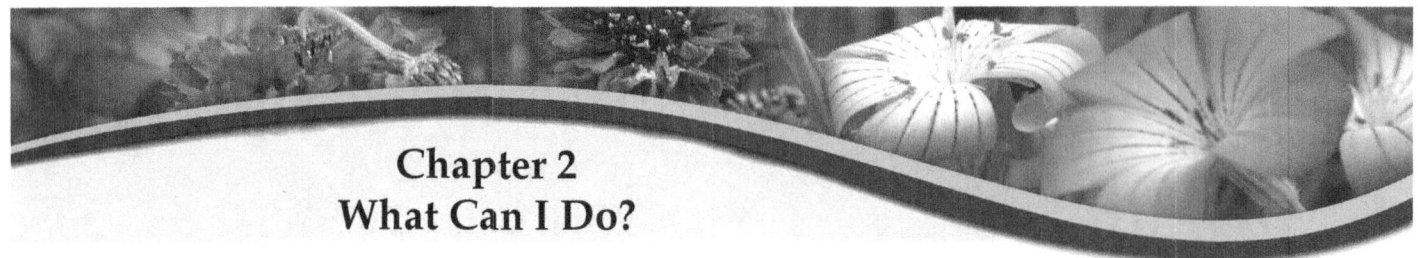

Chapter 2
What Can I Do?

4. **Shoulder joint**: grasp wrist with one hand and elbow with the other.

A) Flexion/Extension: Raise the patient's straightened arm, keeping it close to the body, toward the ceiling, back toward the head of the bed, then return to flat position.

B) Abduction/Adduction: Move the patient's straightened arm away from their side, then return the arm to the patient's side.

C) Rotation: Place the patient's flexed elbow outward at the patient's shoulder level. Rotate the forearm toward the head of the bed and then down toward the hip.

5. **Elbow Joint**: Grasp the wrist with one hand and the elbow with the other.

A) Flexion/Extension: Bend the arm at the elbow, so the hand touches the shoulder on the same side. Straighten the arm.

B) Pronation/Supination: Move the forearm so the palm faces downward and then upward.

6. **Wrist Joint**: Grasp the wrist with one hand and the patient's fingers with the other.

A) Flexion/Extension/Hyperextension: Move the hand downward, straighten the wrist, move the hand back.

B) Abduction/Adduction: Turn the hand toward the little finger, turn the hand toward the thumb.

7. **Thumb Joint**: Hold the patient's hand with one hand and the client's thumb with the other.

A) Flexion/Extension: Bend the thumb into the hand then move the thumb out to the side of the fingers.

B) Abduction/Adduction: Move the thumb out from the inner part of the index finger then move the thumb back.

C) Opposition: Move the thumb so that it touches the tip of each finger in turn, opening the hand fully between each touch.

8. **Finger Joints**: Hold the patient's hand with one of your hands and the patient's fingers with the other.

A) Flexion/Extension: Make a fist with the patient's hand, then straighten the fist by extending the fingers one at a time.

Putting it Into Practice

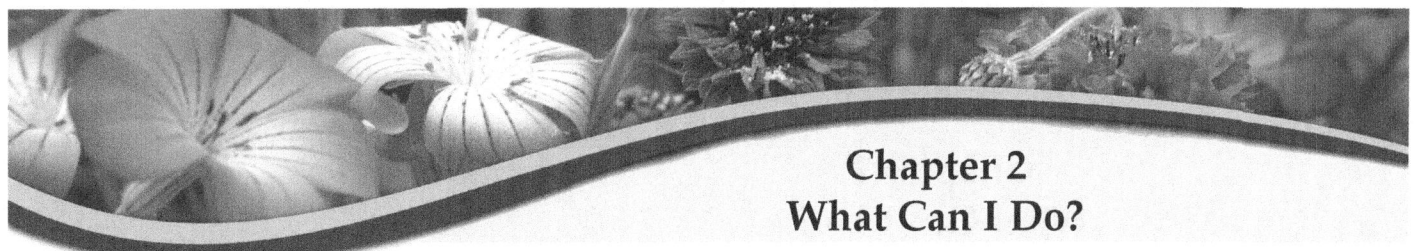

Chapter 2
What Can I Do?

B) Abduction/Adduction: Spread each of the patient's fingers and thumb apart, then bring the thumb and finger together again, one at a time.

9. **Hip Joint**: Place one hand under the patient's bent knee and one hand under the ankle.

A) Flexion/Extension: Raise the leg as you bend the patient's knee and move it toward their head, then straighten it back out again.

B) Abduction/Adduction: Swing the leg out away from the body, keeping it straight, then back toward the body again.

C) Internal rotation/External rotation: Roll the leg inward, then roll it outward.

10. **Knee Joint**: Put one hand under the patient's bent knee and the other under the patient's ankle, with their foot flat on the bed.

A) Flexion/Extension: Bring the lower leg up so the knee is straight, then bring it back down so the foot is on the bed again.

11. **Ankle Joint**: Keep the patient's foot close to the bed. Put one hand under the ankle and grasp the patient's foot with your other hand.

A) Dorsiflexion/Plantar flexion: Push the top part of the foot back toward the head of the bed with your hand over the toes, then point the foot back downward with toes pointing toward your chest.

B) Supination/Pronation: Turn the inside of the patient's foot inward toward the body, then turn the sole of the foot outward away from the body.

C) Rotation: rotate the ankle in circles.

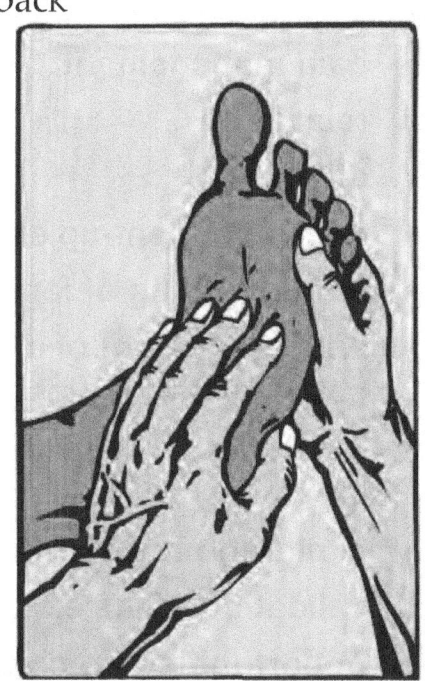

12. **Toe Joints**: Put one hand under the patient's foot and the other on top of their foot over their toes.

A) Flexion/Extension: Curl toes downward and under, then straighten them out.

B) Abduction/Adduction: Spread the toes apart, one by one, then bring the toes back together.

Putting it Into Practice

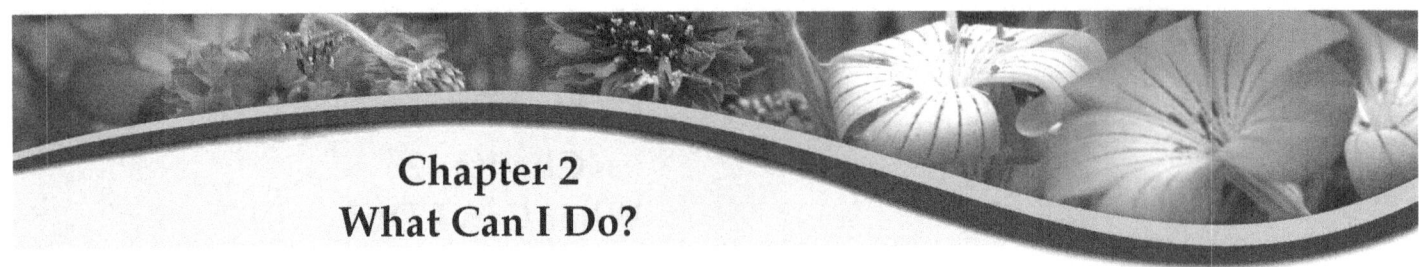

**Chapter 2
What Can I Do?**

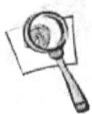 # A Closer Look

More and more, music therapy is becoming an important part of care at end of life. There seems to be a surge in awareness of the valuable part music can play in relaxation and peaceful transition for the dying patient.

Music therapy's purpose is to address the physical, emotional, and spiritual needs of the patient. It's considered a non-invasive treatment that, although ideally administered by a board certified music thanatologist, can be administered by other care team members under the direction of a music therapist or occupational therapist.

For more information about music therapy, contact:

The American Music Therapy Association, 8455 Colesville, Ste. 1000, Silver Springs, MD 20910. www.musictherapy.org. Phone (301) 589-3300.

Some of the benefits of music therapy include:

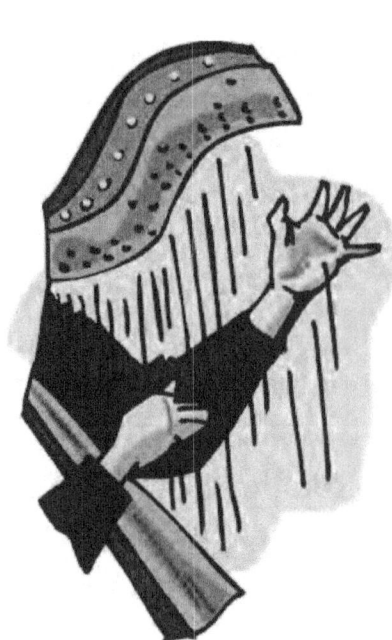

- **pain management**
- **relaxation**
- **diversion**
- **release of pent-up emotions**
- **strengthening of family bonds**
- **encouragement of choices and decision making on patient's part (helps patient maintain control)**
- **resolution of past conflicts through reminiscence and life review**
- **exploration of spiritual values**
- **validation of life experiences**
- **opportunities for creative expression**

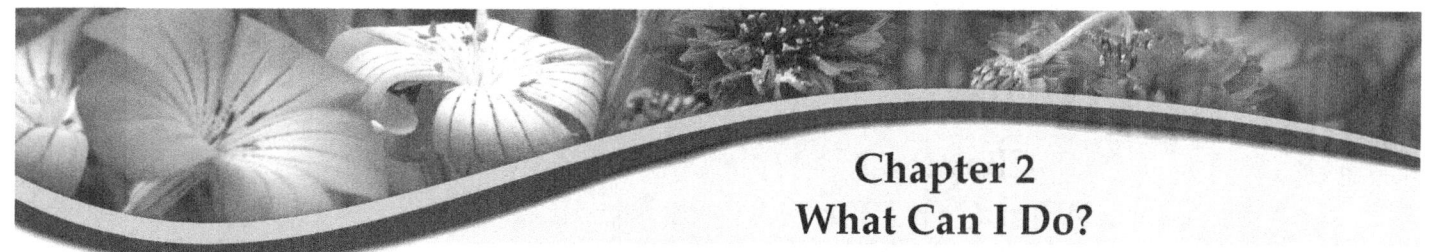

Chapter 2
What Can I Do?

Music for Better Health and Well-being
Suggested selections from
"The Healing Energies of Music" by H.A. Lingerman

Music to energize the physical body
1. Sousa - Stars and Stripes Forever
2. Elgar - Pomp and Circumstance, No. 1
3. Rossini - William Tell
4. Epic Soundtracks (e.g. Star Wars)

Strong music to air out anger
1. Tchaikovsky - Symphony No. 5 (last movement)
2. Wagner - Ride of the Valkyries
3. Poulenc - Concerto for Organ, Timpani, and Strings
4. Ginastera - Estancia

Music for Depression and Fear
1. Dvorak - Slavonic Dances
2. Handel - Water music
3. Grofe - Grand Canyon Suite
4. Handel - Choruses from Messiah

Music for Meditation and Prayer
1. John Michael Talbot - Come to the Quiet
2. J.S. Bach - Toccata and Fugue (orchestral version)
3. Humperdinck - Children's Prayer (from Hansel and Gretel)
4. Paul Horn - Inside the Taj Mahal

Music for Strength and Courage
1. Battle Hymn of the Republic
2. Copeland - A Lincoln Portrait
3. R. Strauss - Sunrise (from Also Sprach Zarathustra)
4. Beethoven - Piano Concerto No. 5 (Emperor)

A Closer Look

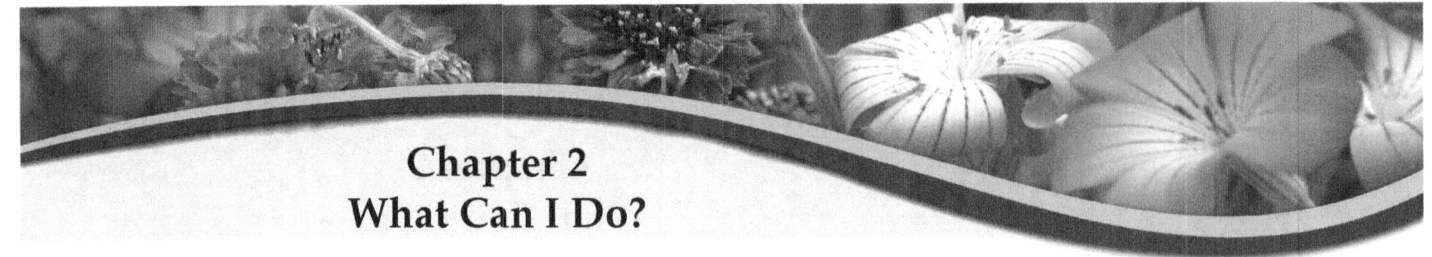

Chapter 2
What Can I Do?

Music to Relieve Boredom
1. Liszt - Hungarian Rhapsodies
2. Respighi - Pines of Rome
3. Rimsky-Korsakov - Scheherazade
4. F.J. Haydn - Trumpet Concerto

Music for Clear Thinking
1. Handel - Water Music
2. Psalms of David (sung by Kings College Choir)
3. Tibetan Bells
4. J.S. Brandenburg Concertos

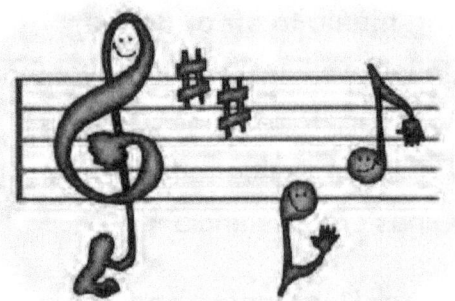

Music for Love and Devotion
1. Soundtrack - Somewhere in Time
2. J.S. Bach - Jesu Joy of Man's Desiring
3. Rachmaninoff - Love Theme
4. Pavarotti - O Sole Mio

Special Classical Musical Selections for Relaxation

J.S. Bach   Air on a G String
                Cello Suites
                Jesu, Joy of Man's Desiring
                Sheep May Safely Graze

Barber   Adagio for Strings

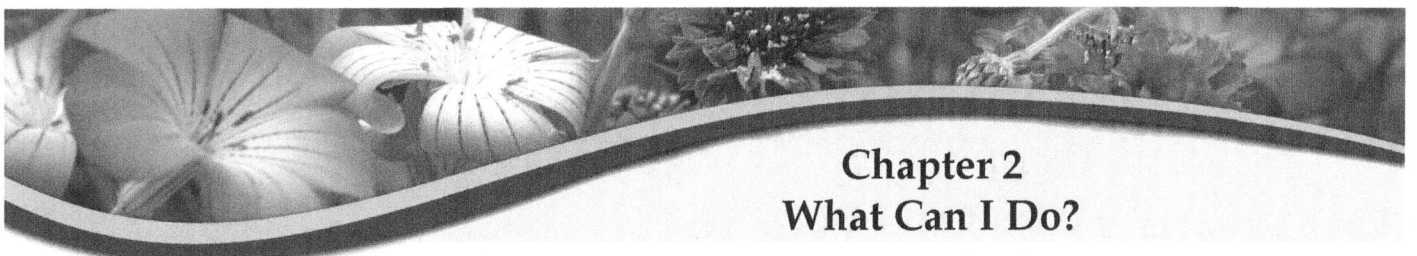

Chapter 2
What Can I Do?

Beethoven	Piano Concerto No. 3 (Second Movement)
	Piano Concerto No. 5 (Second Movement)
	Piano Sonatas
	Symphony No. 9 (Third Movement)
Brahms	Violin Concerto (Second Movement)
Chopin	The Meditative Chopin by Roy Eaton
Debussy	Claire de Lune
Dvorak	Cello Concerto (Second Movement)
	Symphony No. 9, "New World" (Second Movement)
Franck	Panis Angelicas
	Symphony in D Minor
	Violin Sonata (First Movement)
Mahler	Symphony No. 4 (Third Movement)
	Symphony No. 7 (Second Movement)
Massenet	Meditation from Thais
Pachelbel	Canon in D
Rachmaninoff	Piano Concertos No's. 2 and 3
Schubert	Ave Maria
Vivaldi	The Four Seasons

A Closer Look

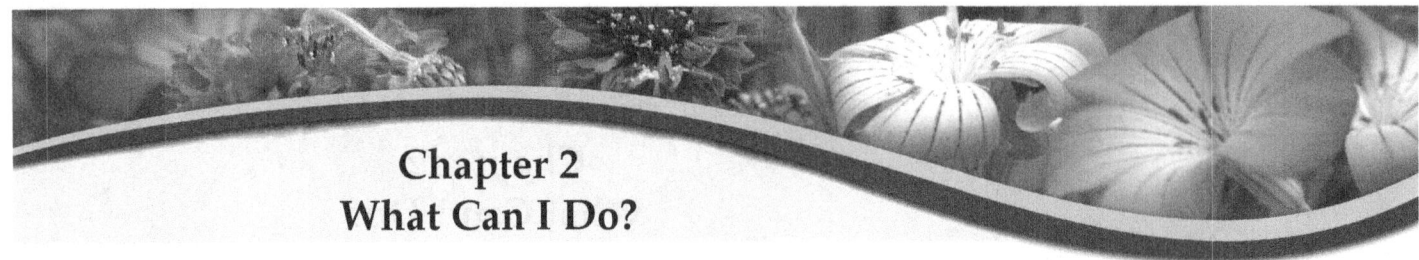

Chapter 2
What Can I Do?

Tips for Relaxing to Music

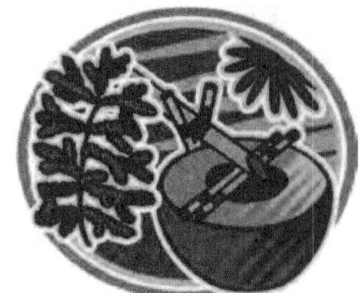

1. Try to stay awake for the whole tape.

2. Get comfortable- lying on your back, sitting in a chair, whatever allows you to completely relax.

3. Make sure you are warm and feel protected and safe - cover yourself with a blanket if necessary.

4. Choose a time that you will not be interrupted - unplug the phone and put a "Do Not Disturb" sign on the door.

5. Dress in loose, non-constricting clothing.

6. Be aware of your breathing as the air moves gently in and out of your lungs.

7. Don't try too hard to relax, just let yourself go - free yourself of tension and any criticism of yourself or others.

8. View your time spent relaxing to music as your special time that you deserve to take to strengthen yourself and heal inside.

Chapter 2
What Can I Do?

Animals as Volunteers

A hospice chaplain I know once spoke with me about his experiences with hospice families in crisis. Providing spiritual care to the dying and their families is challenging, he said, and I agreed. At this time of high intensity and emotional crisis in the family, the focus is most often on physical care and relief of physical symptoms. I asked him how he got past that, how he built trust and encouraged sharing on a deeper level.

"I brought my rabbit with me," he said, flashing a bright smile.

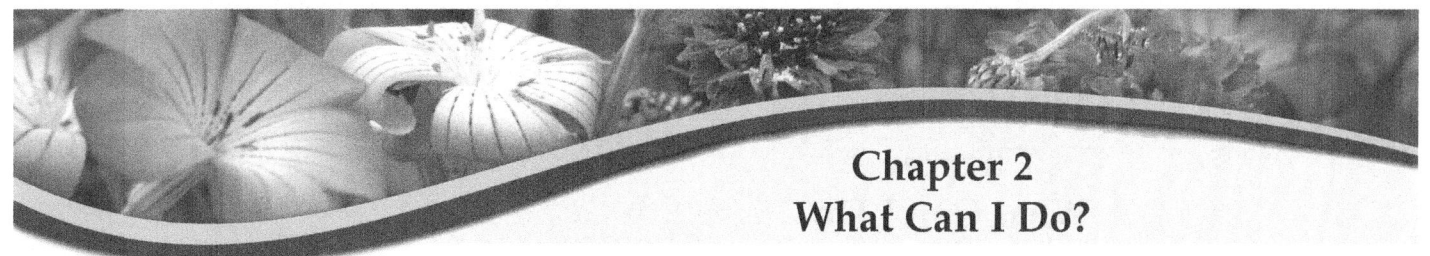

Once he convinced me he was serious, he told me experience after experience in which, as soon as he entered the room with his fluffy white lop-eared rabbit, defenses dropped like rocks and eager arms reached out to hold the friendly creature. The rabbit sensed his mission and held perfectly still while patients and family members stroked his silky fur and marveled at his beautiful ears.

"It was an easy transition from there," he told me. "It's amazing how much people will open up while they are holding and stroking an animal. There is something that happens on a deeply primal level with this kind of close contact. When a loving creature asks for nothing beyond gentle touch, it opens the person's heart up. It's almost miraculous."

Using animals as therapy has become much more popular in recent years. Bringing animals into nursing homes has been shown to boost the residents' moods and enhance social interaction. Animals provide a constant source of comfort, something safe to focus attention on, and draw the person out in a positive way. Animals have been proven to increase life span in the elderly and help dental patients relax more with better outcomes for their treatments.

A Closer Look

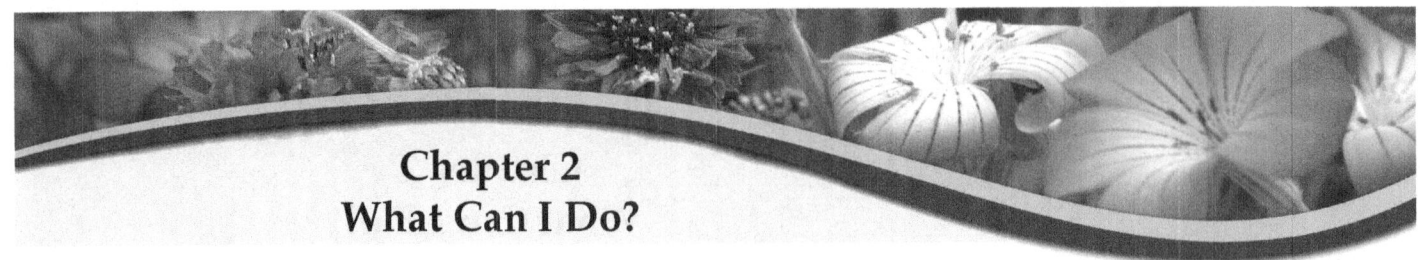

Chapter 2
What Can I Do?

The Delta Society (www.deltasociety.org), an organization that specializes in animal therapy, suggests the following benefits of using animals as volunteers (My paraphrase. Visit the website for more complete detail on this topic):

Eliciting empathy
This is true across the board, but especially in children, who see pets as peers. With animals, everything is direct and clear; their body language is consistent. Human interactions are more complex and not as direct. Children can read an animal's body language and feel safe with them.

Pulling the focus out from self to the outside world
People with mental illness or a low self-concept tend to be inner-focused. Animals can pull their attention away from themselves and their problems and help them think and talk about something else that is still in the emotional realm and relational, but not so threatening.

Providing something to nurture
We all have a deep need to love and be loved. An animal provides for both of these needs. While we are petting and providing loving connection to a pet, we are also receiving nurturing.

Opening up a channel of communication
A place where an animal hangs out feels safer. This can open up a way for a resistant person to relax and share their feelings more easily.

Providing unconditional acceptance
An animal's acceptance is complete. They don't play games. They don't care what you look like or even what you say to them. They just accept you as you are. This is very healing.

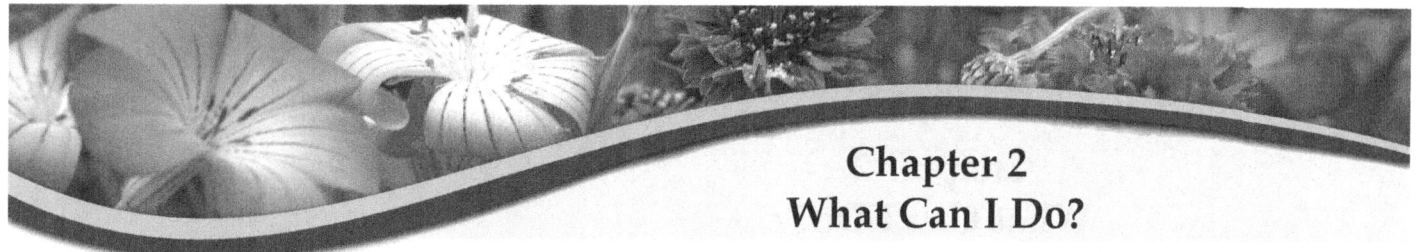

Chapter 2
What Can I Do?

Offering a source of entertainment

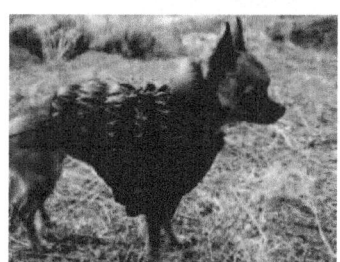

There is a lot of value in distraction. And animals are a guaranteed source of it. I had a three pound Chihuahua who wore a tiny down coat when I walked her in the wintertime. No one who passed me on the street could resist the urge to stop and watch her and laugh. I have often thought that if our value on earth were measured in the number of smiles we generate in others, little Mia would be the Queen of the world.

Increasing socialization

People laugh and interact more with each other in the presence of an animal than they would ordinarily do. In care facilities, staff interacts with the residents more and families report that they can talk more easily with the patient when an animal is present.

Providing mental stimulation

When folks in an institutional setting interact with an animal, often the story telling starts. They recall memories of happier times, and they tend to laugh and share these memories with others around them. This is excellent mental stimulation and decreases the sense of isolation and alienation that can happen in a care setting.

Giving the opportunity for touch

Touch is crucial for the well-being of our mind and spirit. We all need it, but some people's unsettling past may not allow them to fully trust even safe, close people to meet their touch needs. They may have experienced a history of abuse and have a difficult time trusting enough to allow themselves to be touched by another human being. Touching an animal is safe and non-threatening and gives the person the chance to cuddle and hug and feel close to another creature in a very healing way.

A Closer Look

Chapter 2
What Can I Do?

Providing physiological benefits

Just watching a goldfish swimming in a bowl has been shown to lower a person's blood pressure and heart rate. One study demonstrated that a dog's heart rate tends to be slower than his human master's, but when the two connect, the dog's heart rate rises and the human's lowers until they achieve a new rate that matches each other's. Could this be why many people swear that their dog is their best friend?

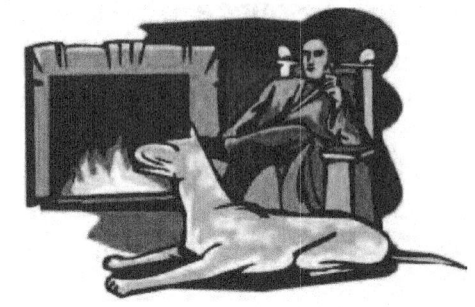

Enhancing spirituality

As my chaplain friend discovered, many people experience a deeper sense of meaning and purpose and a sense of oneness with nature (and thus with the universe) when they are with a pet. Animals can play an important role in teaching spiritual lessons.

This is especially true with equine therapy, in which horses are used to help children and adults who have experienced broken trust due to a history of abuse find healing through connection with a horse. Many great books are available on this subject. Some of my favorites are:

Chosen by a Horse by Susan Richards
Hope Rising by Kim Meeder
and **Horses Don't Lie** by Chris Irwin

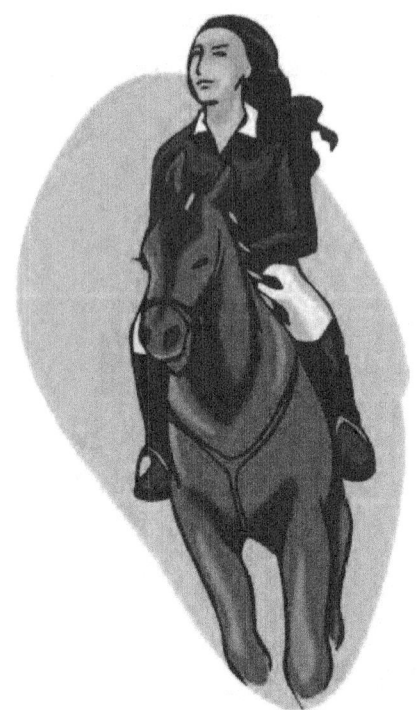

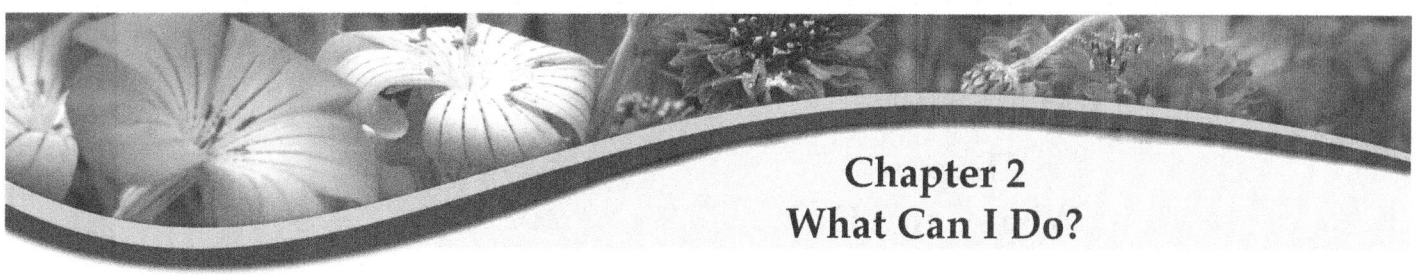

**Chapter 2
What Can I Do?**

Hugs

Are practically perfect:

they are

low energy consumption,

high energy yield,

no monthly payments,

non-fattening,

inflation-proof,

no pesticides,

no preservatives,

non-taxable,

non-polluting,

and, of course, fully returnable.

Author Unknown

Chapter 2
What Can I Do?

Hands-on Patient Care

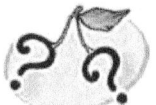 **What if the hospice family asks more of me than I can give?**

This is a perfect time to have a heart-to-heart talk with your volunteer coordinator. Some mutually agreed upon boundaries may need to be set, kindly but firmly, with the hospice family. As you work with hospice you will find that family systems vary considerably and some are more challenging for the hospice team to deal with than others. (We'll talk more about family systems in the next chapter.)

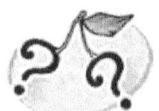 **Should I give my phone number to the hospice family I'm assigned to?**

First, check your agency's policy on this one. If there isn't one, use your own discretion. Many volunteers do choose to give their phone numbers to their hospice families. It's comforting to the family to know they can reach you to talk whenever the need arises. Before you hand over the number, think it over carefully and ask yourself: Is it really okay with me to get called in the middle of the night or on a weekend?

What if they don't like me?

The first visit as a volunteer with a hospice family is usually hard. "What if they don't like me?", "Will I know what to do?", and "What if I say the wrong thing?" are very common "first visit" fears, even for veteran volunteers. It helps to remember at these times that you've been selected to serve as a hospice team member because people experienced in the field believe you can do it. Just plunge right in, trusting your training and your instincts, and as you relate to your assigned hospice family, let them know what you can offer and you will discover what they need. Trust that your relationship with the patient and family will develop naturally.

Chapter 2
What Can I Do?

Guidelines for Meeting Your Patient and Family for the First Time

Whether your hospice patient is at home with loved ones or in a facility, the basic approach is the same. Your primary goal in this first meeting are to protect the privacy of the patient and to help the patient and family feel supported and safe.

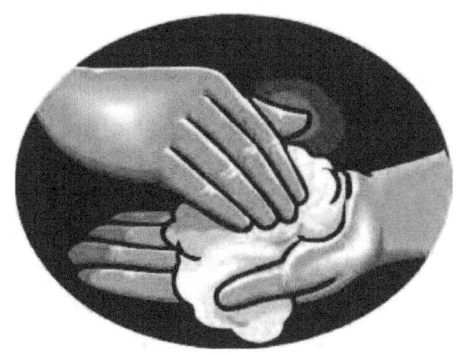

- *Before anything else*, **disinfect your hands**. Carry a bottle of hand sanitizer with you and use it before you even touch the door handle to enter the facility or the patient's home.
- **Cover your badge**. It is not anyone else's business who is on hospice and your badge will shout the information to anyone you walk past on the way in to the patient's home or room. Once inside, it's good to uncover it for identification.
- **Be responsible for the energy that you bring**. Go in with openness and a calm, confident attitude. The family will pick up on that and mirror your energy.
- **Always knock**. Ask if you can come in, even if the patient is unresponsive or confused. This is common courtesy and says, "I respect you and your home."
- **Wash your hands.** Once you get into the home or patient's room in a facility, ask if you may use their sink to wash your hands. This isn't as awkward as it might seem and the fact that you are making the effort not to bring any germs from the outside to your patient sets up a sense of safety with you from the beginning.
- **Enter the patient's field of vision**.
- **Smile**. It's a universal sign of good will everyone understands.
- **Address the patient appropriately**. Mr. or Mrs. is the respectful greeting for any adult that you don't know. It's safe to start with this. If they want you to call them something less formal, they will let you know.
- **Kneel or sit down next to the patient**. It can be intimidating to "tower" over someone when you talk to them. Get down to eye level with them so you can maintain the best eye contact.

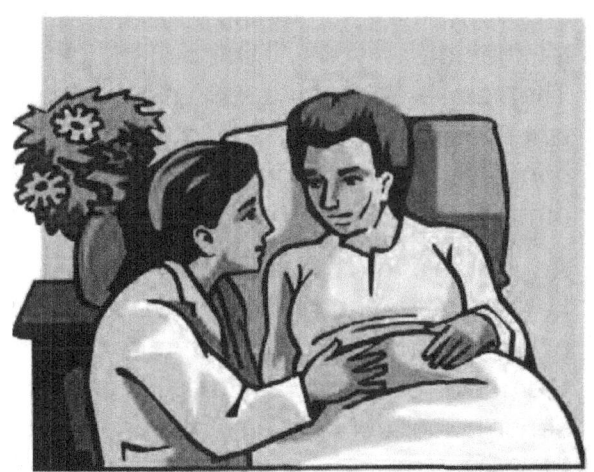

A Closer Look

Chapter 2
What Can I Do?

- **Speak clearly, in short sentences.** If you have a high voice or one that is pitched softly, lower your voice register to deeper tones. They are easier to hear. Speak distinctly without shouting. Ask your patient if he or she can hear you okay. Unless they are confused, they will tell you if they have a hearing problem and need you to crank up your volume.

- **Do not use the word "hospice".** It's possible the patient or a family member present doesn't know the person is on hospice. This is not to encourage deception, but rather to allow the family to communicate about hospice in their own way and time.

- **In the case of an unconscious patient, introduce yourself to the family members first.** Do this individually, going around the room, giving each person direct and friendly eye contact, and extending a hand for shaking. Personal introductions make each person feel seen and heard. It increases their trust in you right from the beginning.

- **Point out something positive.** It might be the way the nursing assistants positioned the patient or a vase of beautiful flowers that a family member brought. Be sincere. It will set a tone of hope.

- **Write your name somewhere easy to find.** Write "volunteer" on the paper and then post it somewhere easy to find, on a bulletin board or on the refrigerator, but be sure the family knows it is there. There will be so many other team members coming and going, it will be good for the patient and family to have a reminder of your name to refer back to.

- **Ask questions.** "How are you holding up?" "What has the doctor told you about how he's doing?" "What would be especially helpful for me to do for you right now?" Especially appreciated are the questions about the patient's life that allow the family to reminisce and tell favorite stories about the patient.

- **Answer questions as you can, but don't guess at the answers.** If it's something you don't know the answer to, tell the person you will find out and get back with them. Then make sure you do. Remembering to follow up on what you say you will do is a great trust builder. (And the converse is true. If you don't, they won't believe you in other areas either.)

- **As you are leaving, ask if it's okay if you come back.** Let the patient and family know when you are available or scheduled next and make sure that time works for them. Don't assume anything. This gives the family a sense of control over a small part what is happening to them.

60   **A Closer Look**

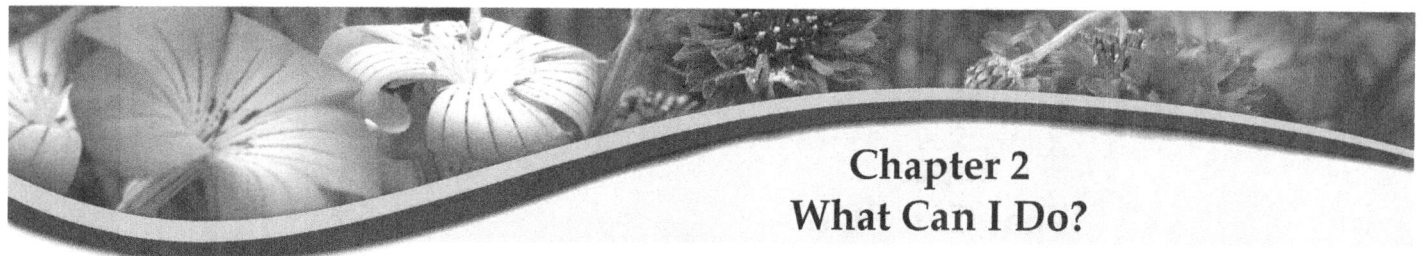

Chapter 2
What Can I Do?

More About HIPAA and a Patient's Right to Privacy

It's important in general to be sensitive to a patient's need for (and right to) privacy. Step out of the room when personal care is being provided and always make sure the curtain is drawn or the door is shut when you, yourself, are providing some kind of care to the patient (within your scope of practice, of course.)

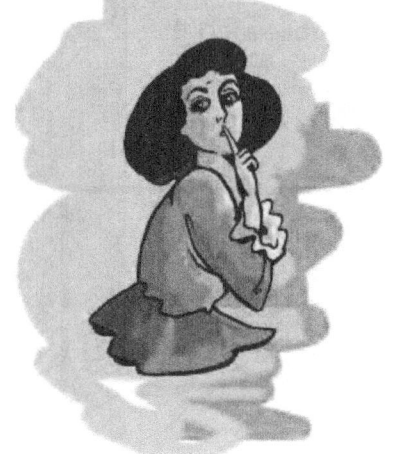

Remember that HIPAA laws apply even when a patient is actively dying. Not obeying these rules could have serious consequences for you and for your hospice. If family members or friends, who are not the designated health care representative for the patent, call or visit and want to know about the patient's condition, you cannot give them any information. Kindly respond that you will have the nurse or the caregiver talk with them. Even if they get angry and threaten you (as sometimes happens when emotions are high), respond kindly but firmly that you are not authorized to give out health information on the patient.

Calling 9-1-1

When should you call 9-1-1? In a word, **never**. Even if the patient is struggling or if they die, don't panic and dial 9-1-1. The EMTs who respond to your call have to start CPR. This could have disastrous consequences for the patient since they have specified that they wish not to have such measures done to them as a hospice patient.

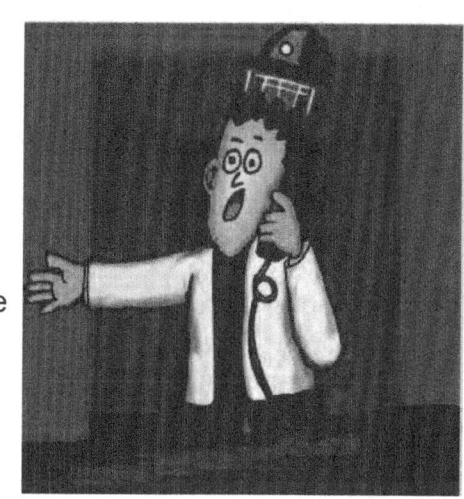

It's a good idea for all family members, the patient, and you, as the volunteer, to have the hospice number programmed into your cell phone as the emergency number. If anything happens to the patient or you are uncomfortable in any way with what is happening in the home, always call hospice.

Of course, this applies only to the hospice patient. If a family member or visitor chokes, collapses, complains of chest pain, or otherwise experiences a medical emergency, it is imperative to call for help immediately. Then follow up with a call to hospice to let them know what is happening and ask for back up.

A Closer Look

Chapter 2
What Can I Do?

As a group, study and practice the transfer techniques in the Putting it Into Practice section of Chapter 2. Remember to use good body mechanics. It helps to have three people in your group for practice. One will be the patient, one will be the person doing the transferring, and one will be reading the instructions and observing technique, giving feedback as needed.

One of the most important skills you will need to know is good hand washing technique. Review Renee demonstrating good hand washing on the DVD, then practice it yourself, following these guidelines:

1. Push your watch, if you wear one, up to the middle of your forearm or remove it.

2. Be sure you are standing far enough away from the sink that your clothes aren't touching it.

3. Turn on the water and adjust the temperature.

4. Wet your hands and wrists thoroughly. Keep your fingers pointed down.

5. Apply soap.

6. Lather all the surfaces of your hands, front and back and up as far as the area above your wrists. Rub your hands together vigorously, lacing your fingers together to get between them, and under a ring, if you are wearing one. Clean fingernails by scrubbing fingertips against the opposite palm.

7. Wash for at least 20 seconds. (This is long enough to sing the Happy Birthday song through twice.)

8. Rinse thoroughly under the running water, keeping your hands below your elbows and your fingers pointed down to keep the water from running back up onto the clean area.

9. Dry with a paper towel and discard it.

10. With another paper towel, turn off the faucet. Don't touch the sink.

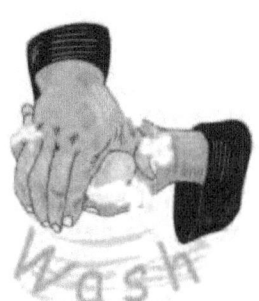

A Closer Look

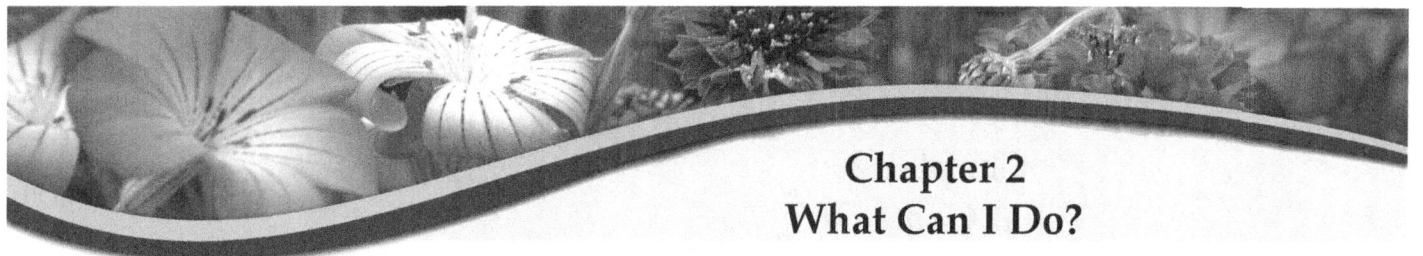

Chapter 2
What Can I Do?

Things You Can Do For Your Hospice Patient

Not sure what you can do when you get into your patient's home? Here's a list of 52 ways to help a hospice family. But don't limit yourself to this list! The possibilities are as endless as the variety of people who are admitted to hospice services. Each patient is a unique person with special needs. Let your imagination soar!

1. Walking
2. Fishing
3. Table games
4. Mending
5. Shop for food
6. Clothes to cleaners
7. Do laundry
8. Make phone calls
9. Talking books
10. Read their favorite book to them
11. Pray with them (only at patient request)
12. Write letters
13. Child care
14. Paint
15. Hook rugs
16. Do Pottery
17. Vacuum
18. Dust
19. Clean bathrooms
20. Shine shoes
21. Prepare food
22. Help with bedpan
23. Do minor repairs
24. Teach relaxation
25. Care for animals
26. Create a terrarium
27. Provide some time away for the family
28. Listen to music together
29. Pick up medication
30. Give a back rub
31. Remember special days
32. Watch TV with patient
33. Shop for personal items
34. Help with dressing
35. Walk the dog
36. Rake leaves
37. Plant flowers
38. Participate in life review
39. Watch videos
40. Arrange to watch a slide presentation
41. Set up a bird feeder
42. Help the patient to write experiences
43. Sing for patient or together
44. Look at old photos
45. Empty trash
46. Bring flowers from your yard
47. Do clerical work
48. Laugh with patient
49. Start an herb garden
50. Listen
51. Brush their hair (use only their own brush)
52. Put lotion on their hands (only use their own lotion since they may have allergies and need a special kind of lotion)

A Closer Look

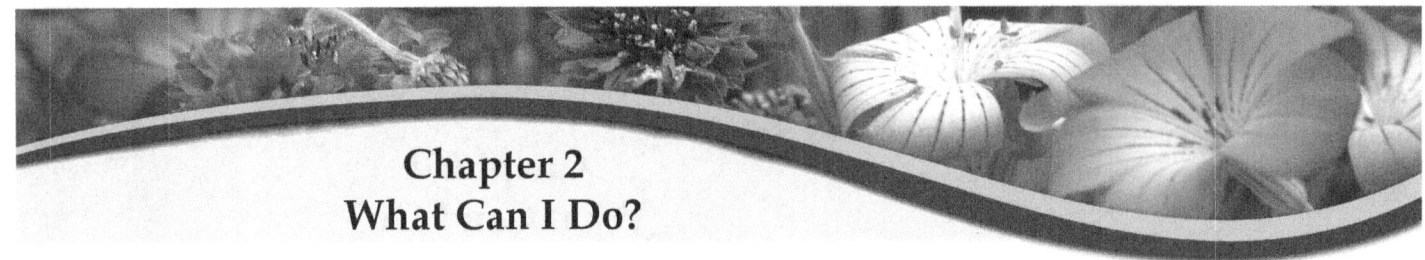

Chapter 2
What Can I Do?

Things to Avoid

- **Giving an estimate of how long you think the patient will live**
  There is no way we can know for sure when a patient will die. The process is highly individual. Sometimes it takes longer than we think and sometimes it may happen quickly and relatively unexpectedly. Patients often "choose" who they want to be with them at the time of death and may wait for a family member to arrive or die when everyone is gone but the family members he or she wants to be present.

- **Trying to convince patients or families of your religious or political views**
  It's important, for the patient and family to feel supported, that you meet them where they are. This means not sharing your political or religious views with them even if they ask you to engage a conversation about them. There are ways to graciously decline. Support them in talking about whatever they want and need to, but let them be where they are and make no attempt to change that through proselytizing.

- **Arguing**
  It isn't our job to straighten out the patient or family. They may be in denial about the dying process and where the patient actually is within the process. The patient may be confused about person, place, or time. Be gracious. Don't argue with them.

- **Generalizing**
  People, even from similar beliefs, backgrounds, ethnicities and cultures, are not necessarily on the same page in their beliefs or customs or needs. So, even though it helps to know something of their culture to know where to begin the conversation, don't assume that they will adhere to the cultural norms. Ask. Find out who this person is, as a unique human being.

- **Judging**
  You may (and probably will) encounter some tough situations in which the family system doesn't react the way yours would. Don't judge them. If you're struggling with something that really bothers you, bring it up to your Volunteer Coordinator or the nurse who sees the patient. You may need to take a break to work through why their issues are triggering you personally. (Usually we judge in others what we fear to face in ourselves.)

64   A Closer Look

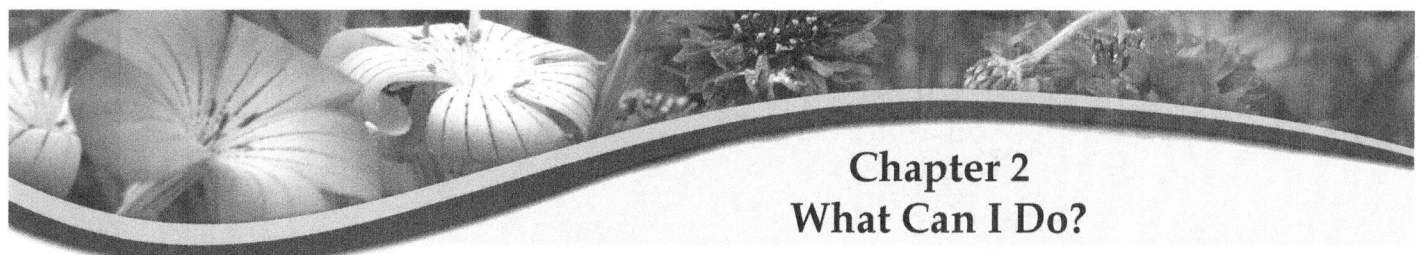

Chapter 2
What Can I Do?

- **Wearing too much cologne/perfume**
  It's best to wear none at all. Many people are chemically sensitive. Toward the end of life, the patient can become increasingly sensitive to smells and may be battling nausea besides. Be kind. Come to their home just smelling like you.

- **Use of euphemisms**
  Especially if children are involved. Death is a normal part of life and children (and adults) can handle the real words. Using euphemisms ("She's asleep") when talking to children can cause them to misunderstand and form ideas that can create anxieties surrounding the process of death and dying.

- **Promising confidentiality**
  Not a good idea. There are situations you might encounter in which you are obliged (sometimes by law!) to share certain information with your supervisor or other team members.

- **Making or receiving private phone calls**
  There is no place in your time with the patient and family for private phone calls. Talking on your cell phone or texting is very unprofessional and inappropriate while with your patient. Set your phone on vibrate so you can be reached if a hospice team member needs to get in touch with you or if it is an emergency. If it is personal, however, be sure it truly is an emergency, otherwise let it ring. If it is a call you must take, excuse yourself and step outside to take it.

- **Accepting gifts**
  Unless it's a thank you card or a jar of homemade jam, it is inappropriate to accept gifts from your patients or family members. If they feel they must give something, suggest that they give to their favorite charity in your name.

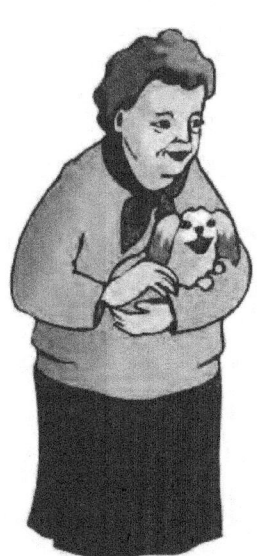

- **Depersonalizing the patient**
  Always keep in mind that you are with another human being, even if they are unconscious. Continue to talk to them and always refer to them by name when talking about them to family or other team members.

- **Problems with pets**
  If you are allergic to cats, dogs, birds, or other animals that might be in the patient's home, alert your Volunteer Coordinator of this immediately so you can be reassigned. Pets often pick up the emotions of the "alpha" male or female in the home, so be cautious. A pet with a gentle, non-confrontational history can suddenly bite if he thinks he is being threatened or thinks that his master is threatened. On the other hand, pets are very comforting to a family in stress. Pets are often some of the greatest soothers, moving in close (often up on the bed) to be present with the dying person.

A Closer Look

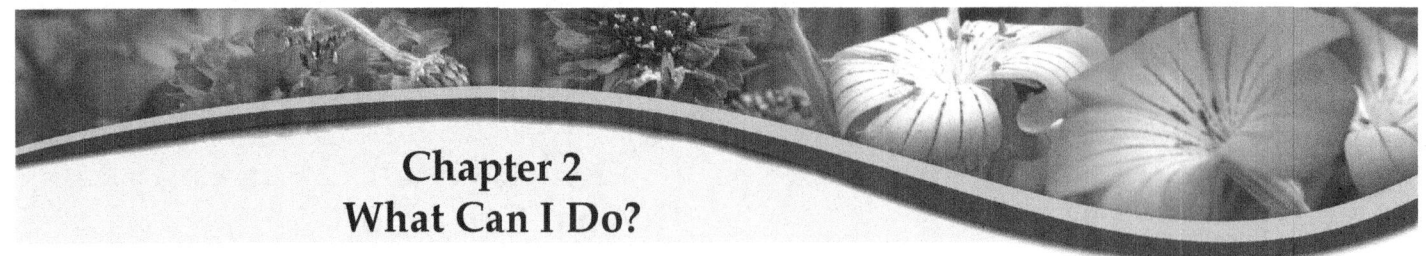

Chapter 2
What Can I Do?

 ## Skill Check

Complete the following sentences:

1. The most valuable skills a hospice volunteer can possess are

2. Confidentiality means

3. If a hospice family member tells the volunteer something of a highly sensitive nature, the volunteer should

4. Healthy distancing is accomplished by

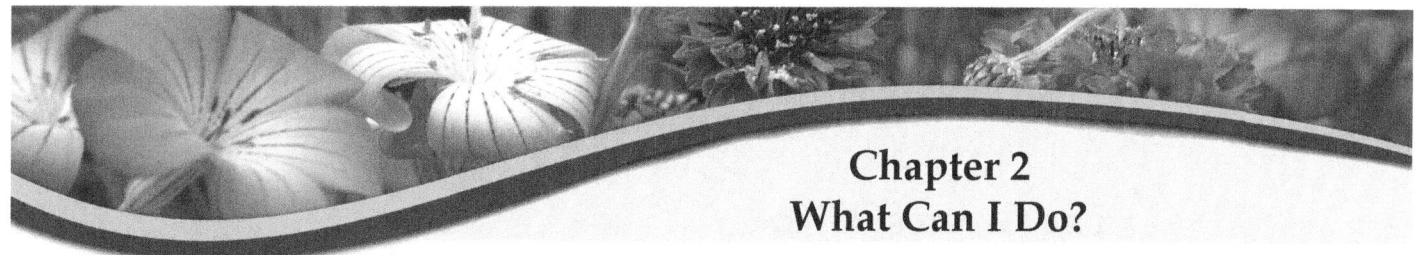

Chapter 2
What Can I Do?

5. List at least 20 activities that you could do as a hospice volunteer with your patient and/or family.

6. List 5 things you should avoid.

7. List 5 benefits of animal therapy.

8. List 3 goals of music therapy.

Skill Check

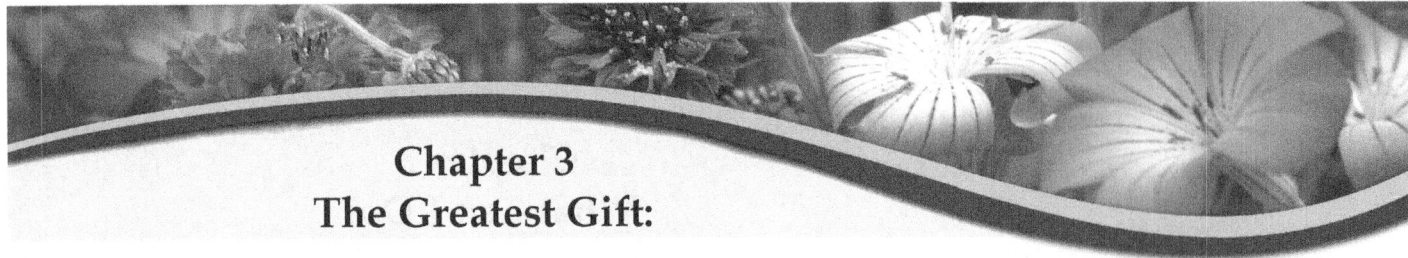

3. The Greatest Gift:

Learning to listen with love

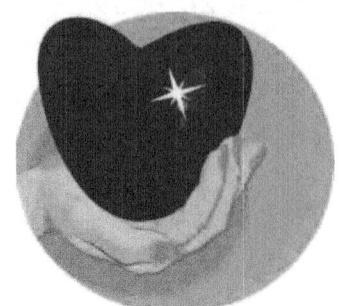

"Just the facts, please..."

Experts dealing in the area of death and dying have identified certain stages that people go through from the time they find out they are dying to the time they truly accept what's happening to them.

There are many variations on the theme, but the most widely used description of the stages of dying describes five basic stages: denial, anger, bargaining, depression, and, finally, acceptance.

It's important, when studying these stages, to remember that:

- All people are different. No one has exactly the same experience as anyone else. Each individual will experience the stages of dealing with his impending death in his own way.
- The family of the person who is dying will go through these stages of grief along with the terminally ill person.
- Although the stages of dying are given in a particular order, people who are going through them may jump from step to step at any time and in any order.
- One common thread persists throughout the stages and is crucial for the patient and family to be able to endure. That thread is HOPE. (Sometimes it may seem to the family that they are holding on to hope by a thread.) It is important for the care team to work with the patient in nurturing and protecting his hope.
- Understanding where a person is in relation to the stages of dying is not nearly as important as being there and sincerely listening and caring.

Listening from the heart, *really* listening without judgment or preconceived ideas, is truly the greatest gift we can give to our patients and their families. Long after they've forgotten anything we might have told them, they will remember that we were there with them and that we listened.

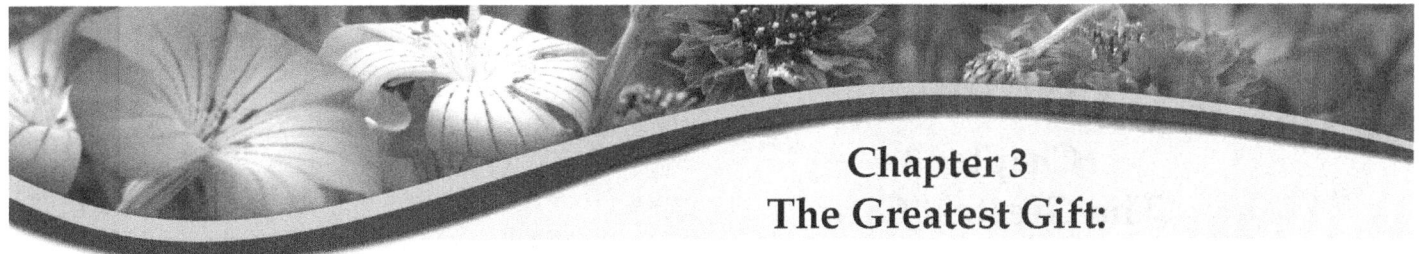

Chapter 3
The Greatest Gift:

Some questions you may be asking...

How will I know what stage of the dying process my patient is in?

You won't always know. And it won't really matter if you do or don't except to sometimes help you understand why they may be reacting in a certain way. For example, a dying patient who is suddenly very angry because you hung the dish towel on the "wrong" towel bar is probably in the anger stage. Your behavior may be the target of their anger, but it's not the reason.

The emotional stages of dying are as follows:

- ## Denial

This stage is often described as a state of "numbness". The patient may have heard the doctor's diagnosis of a terminal illness, but it isn't sinking in. The patient talks about the future as if nothing has changed. He may still discuss the details of his hunting trip with his buddies next fall or she may continue to make plans for celebrating next Christmas with her grandchildren.

Although this stage is very often the first reaction to the news of impending death, patients may slip back into denial at any time during the course of their illness when things get a little overwhelming for them. It's important not to impose our ideas on the patient concerning how to cope with the situation. Let him or her deny as much as needed. Expect a little bouncing from denial to acceptance and don't let it throw you.

- ## Anger

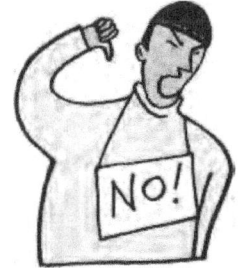

This is often the most difficult stage for us as care providers to deal with. When we do all we can to nurture and help someone, it's natural for us to want to receive gratitude and respect in return. To someone who has just emerged from denial of a terminal illness, however, and is beginning to feel the intense pain of the implications of that diagnosis, hospice workers may represent the very presence of their disease.

"Just the facts, please..."

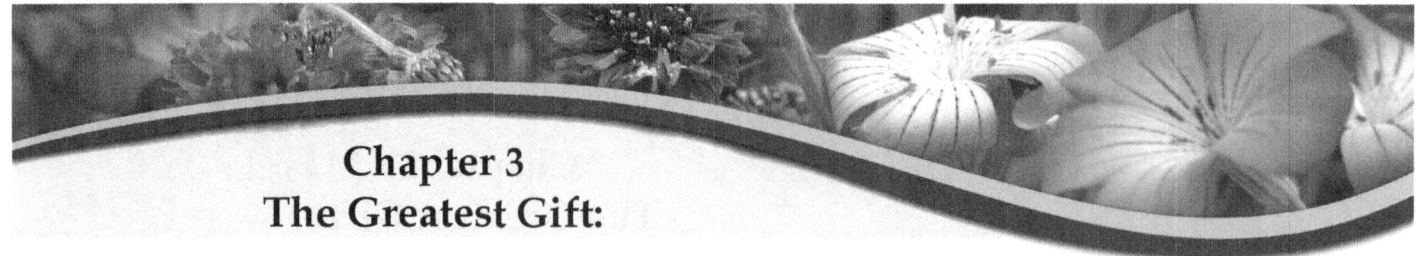

Chapter 3
The Greatest Gift:

Even if a hospice patient uses you as a target to vent feelings of anger, you can respond with love and understanding. Avoid arguing back. If you find yourself reacting defensively, you may want to examine your feelings about your own mortality.

- ## Bargaining

The bargaining that a dying person does is usually not aloud. Many times it is a promise - usually to God (whatever the person's understanding of "God" is). It may be an exchange, such as "If I act nice, maybe God will give me more time", or, "If I can just have one more chance at life, I'll do things differently".

It is often during this stage that unresolved spiritual issues from the past are addressed. The hospice chaplain can be of great benefit to the patient in helping to work through these issues. Unresolved guilt over past events can cause restlessness and increased physical pain, so it is important to let the patient know that spiritual assistance is available.

- ## Depression

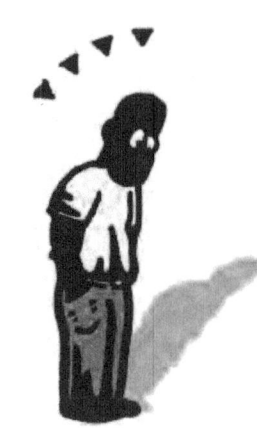

As the terminally ill person realizes the full extent of his loss, a sense of sadness may envelope him. This depression often deepens as he experiences role changes and faces physical changes that occur as his disease progresses. This stage is one of the hardest for family and friends to deal with, because the patient may withdraw into sadness, isolating himself from those around him. Hospice workers can help the family by modeling loving acceptance of the patient's need to express sorrow in his own way. Touch is often the best way to communicate this acceptance.

- ## Acceptance

This stage in the dying process should not be mistaken for happiness. A sense of peace prevails but it is often almost void of feelings. It is as if everything that needs to be done in preparation for death has been completed. There is no more bargaining, no more anger, no more fear.

The dying person may want only one or two chosen people to be with them at this time. This doesn't mean the others are unimportant, but simply that she has "taken care of business" with them and said her good-byes.

Chapter 3
The Greatest Gift:

It is during this time that family members may need help in "letting go" of their loved one. Just giving them permission to tell the patient good-bye can be helpful. Telling someone that it's okay to die can feel like abandonment to a family member that doesn't understand the dying process.

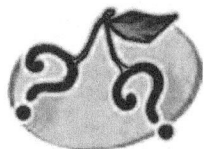 **Some families seem to communicate more openly about emotional issues than others. Are there any guidelines for talking with different families about the dying process?**

No and yes. Each family you work with will be a unique blend of its own cultural heritage and life experiences. No specific guidelines will prepare you to deal with the variety of attitudes and personalities that you might encounter.

It helps, however, to understand what kind of family structure you are working with, because some accept help easily, others not so easily, and some can't accept it at all.

Open Family System

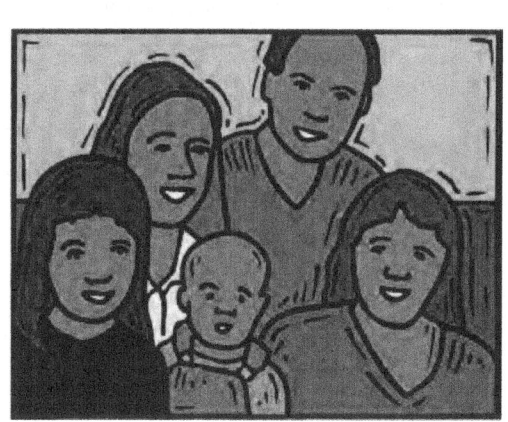

In an open family system, self-esteem of the individual family members is high. The family has few, if any, secrets. Communication is direct, clear, specific, and growth producing. It's okay to talk openly about feelings, be sad, or cry in front of other family members. It's okay to let children see adults show their emotions. It's okay to let times of crisis open up old hurts so they can be forgiven and set aside.

"Power" is equally distributed and there are clear, consistent boundaries in this type of family. There is closeness, yet individuals are given room to be themselves. There are shared values and an ability to tolerate change and make mistakes. Spirituality is valued and nurtured.

The open family is willing to receive validation from people outside the immediate family, so it welcomes outsiders' participation. Flexibility is encouraged and family members have full freedom to comment on everything that's happening.

"Just the facts, please..."

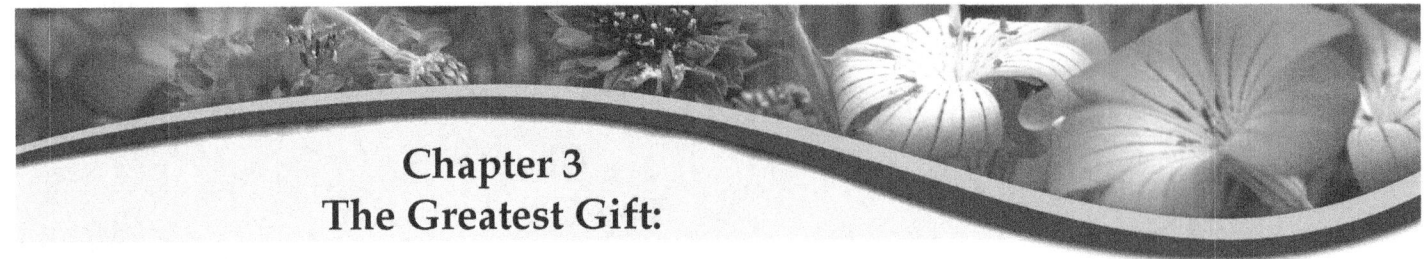

Chapter 3
The Greatest Gift:

The Closed Family System

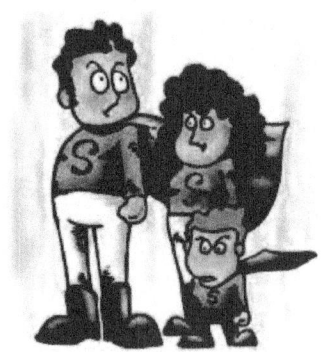

The rules are quite different in a closed family system. Here, there may be so many secrets you can never take for granted anything you experience with them. Family members who smile and tell you everything is okay may be hiding anger or fear that they are unable to express.

Individuals in the closed family system often have low self-esteem. Their communication tends to be indirect, unclear, and unspecific. There may be obvious incongruities between what they are saying and what their body language is telling you. Double messages and "double binds" are common. The ability to play and be spontaneous may be absent. There is often a high tolerance for inappropriate behavior, even physical, emotional, or sexual abuse.

Maintaining the established rules is very important to closed family systems. Children who don't agree with or support the rules generally leave. Family members are required to change their needs to conform to the rules, which may tell them:

1   Be strong and never cry in front of each other.
2   Never talk about anyone in the family who may be an embarrassment or mar the family image.
3   Someone is always to blame.
4   Crying and other emotional displays are a sign of weakness.
5   Love hurts and is supposed to be painful.
6   Love means not having to talk.

Closed family systems are often labeled as "dysfunctional", which simply means "living in pain".

A closed family system will have a much more difficult time accepting outside help because this means admitting that they can't solve their family "problems" alone. Often, these families will wait until they are in crisis to allow any intervention at all.

When you find yourself working within a closed family system, remember to do frequent reality checks with the members of the family to be sure what you are offering is what they want from you. Be prepared for rebuff. It won't be a personal affront, but simply a statement that they may not able to tolerate the level of involvement that you represent.

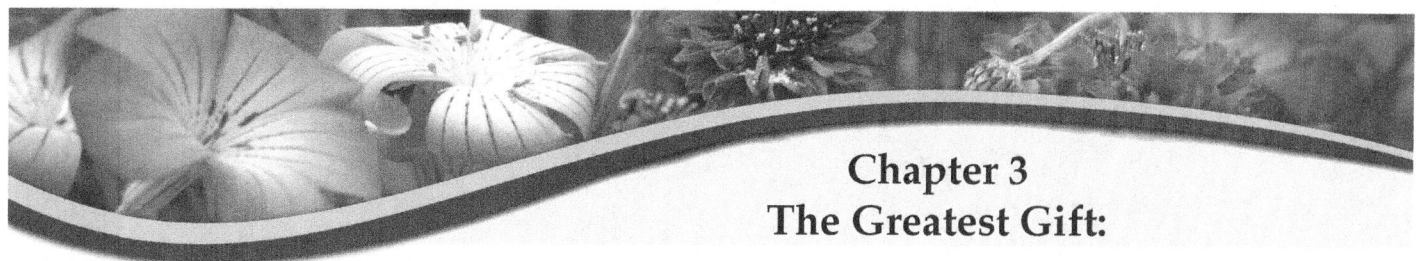

Chapter 3
The Greatest Gift:

 *At the Heart of the Matter*

Listen with your heart...

When I ask you to listen to me and you start giving advice,
you have not done what I asked.

When I ask you to listen to me and you begin to tell me why I shouldn't feel that way,
you are trampling on my feelings.

When I ask you to listen to me and you feel you have to do something to solve my problem,
you have failed me, strange as that may seem.

Listen! All I asked was that you listen, not talk or do- just hear me.

Advice is cheap.
A quarter will get you both Dear Abby and Billy Graham in the same newspaper.

And I can do for myself. I am not helpless.
Maybe discouraged and faltering, but not helpless.

When you do something for me that I can and need to do for myself,
you contribute to my fear and inadequacy.

But when you accept as a simple fact that I do feel what I feel, no matter how irrational,
then I can quit trying to convince you and can get about the business
of understanding what is behind this irrational feeling.

And when that's clear, the answers are obvious
and I don't need advice.

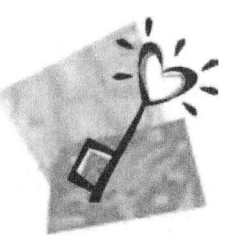

Author Unknown

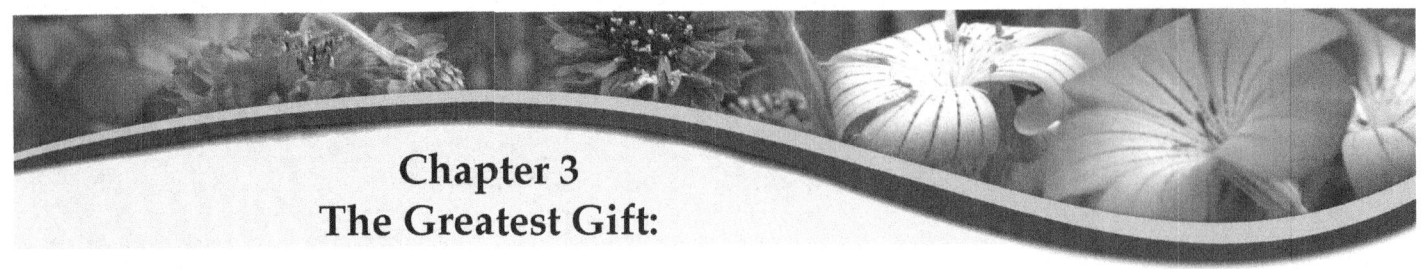

Chapter 3
The Greatest Gift:

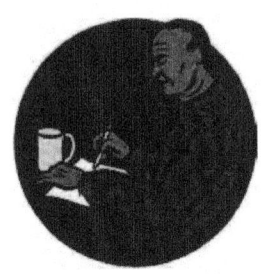

Write out your answers to the following questions about "The Lottery" on the DVD and discuss them as a group. (If you are studying these materials individually, your diagnosis is end stage lung cancer.)

1. *Imagine yourself really receiving the diagnosis that was written on your slip of paper. What would be your greatest fears? What would you be angry about?*

2. *What would be your deepest need right now with this new diagnosis?*

As you listen with an open heart to those whose lives have been turned upside down by a terminal diagnosis, chances are you'll frequently hear the words "I'm afraid..." What are the fears of the patient and family when a loved one is dying? Understanding them can help you listen with empathy.

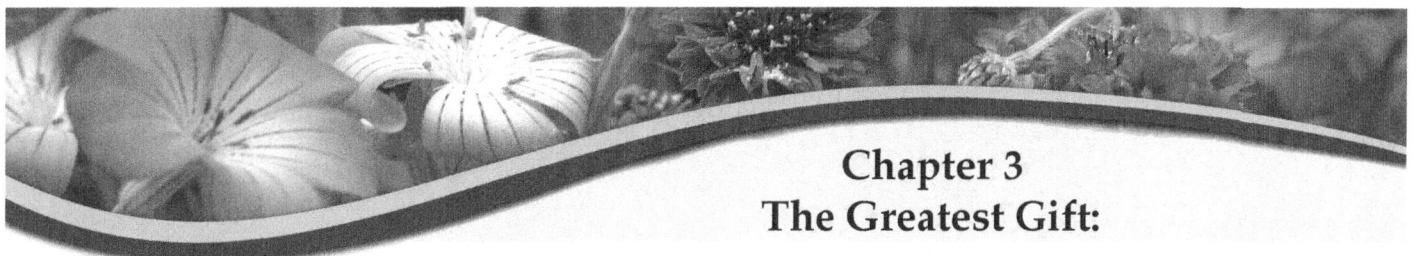

Chapter 3
The Greatest Gift:

The patient may fear:

- *Loss of relationships*

- *Loss of control*

- *Being a burden*

- *Pain*

- *Progression of the disease*

- *Disfigurement*

- *Rejection*

- *Loss of identity*

- *Invasion of privacy*

- *Stigma of disease*

- *Not knowing the truth*

- *Alienation from important others*

- *The dying process*

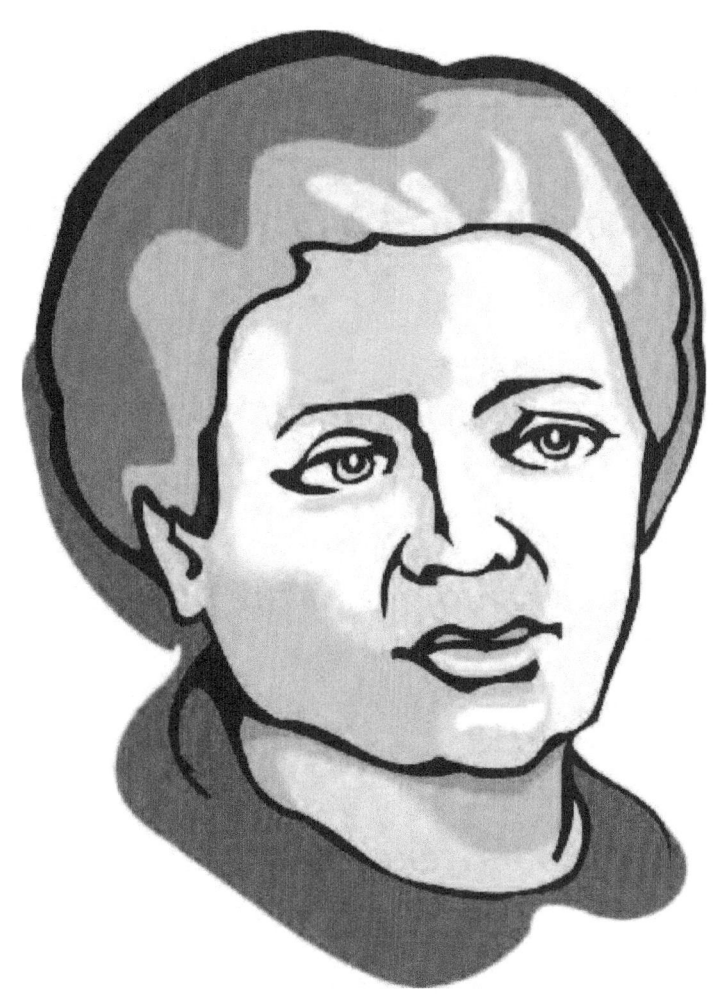

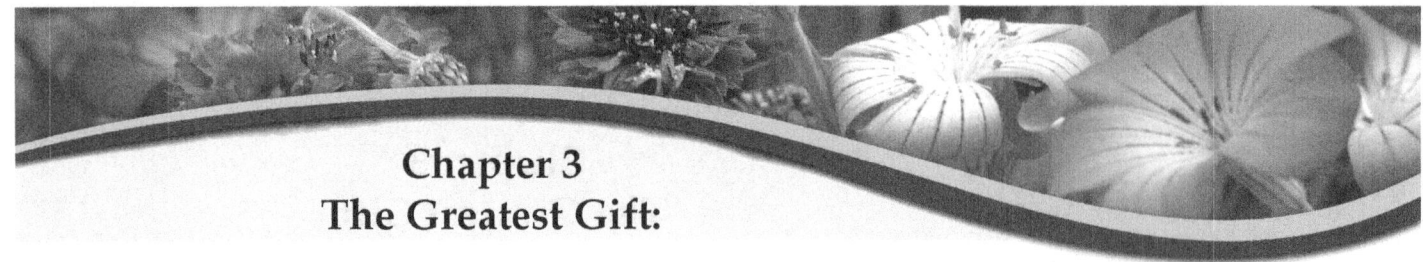

Chapter 3
The Greatest Gift:

The family may fear:

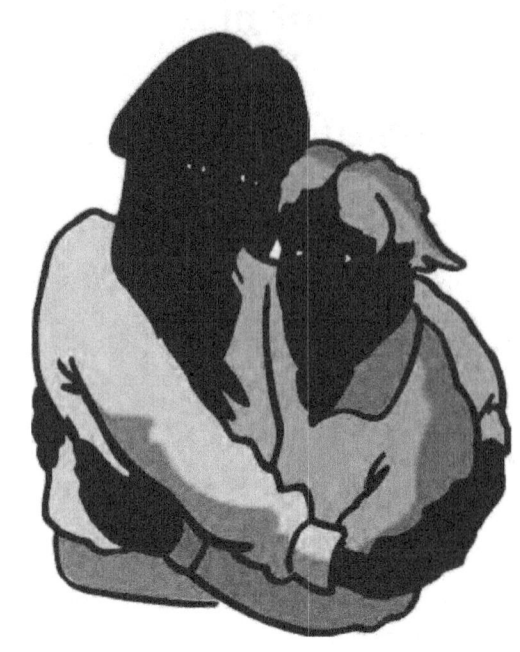

- *Unknown new role*

- *"Poor performance"- not being able to adequately care for the patient*

- *Loss of physical relationship with the patient*

- *Outside interference in family relationships*

- *Physical changes in the patient*

- *Uncertainty*

- *That the patient will "give up" when hospice becomes involved*

- *That the patient may not be valued*

- *Economic loss and guilt*

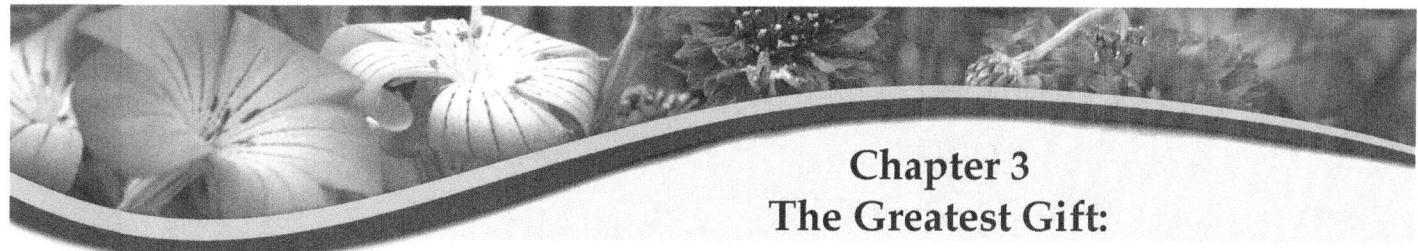

Chapter 3
The Greatest Gift:

Putting it Into Practice

Practical listening skills can serve us well in any area of our lives, but they are absolutely crucial to master when working with hospice patients and their families.

How to Listen to Others:

- **Stop talking and concentrate on what they are saying.** You can do this by actively focusing your attention on the words, ideas, and feelings expressed.
- **Empathize with them.** Try to put yourself in their place so you can better understand what they are trying to tell you.
- **Look at them.** Watch body language, expressions, eyes. These will communicate more to you than the actual words they are speaking.
- **Smile, nod, and respond appropriately.** Genuinely. These responses provide reinforcement. Be careful, though, not to overdo it.
- **Use clarifying statements and questions.** When you don't understand or when you need further clarification, ask for more information, but make sure your questions don't come out as a put-down.
- **Don't interrupt.** Give the person time to give the full message.
- **Set your own emotions aside.** Don't allow yourself to be distracted by your own worries, fears, or problems. Try not to get angry at what is being said as it may prevent you from understanding the meaning the other person is trying to convey.
- **Don't argue mentally.** Debating with the person in your mind while they are talking will prevent you from hearing what they are really saying.
- **Get rid of distractions.** If you can't keep your hands off your watch or resist fiddling with the pencil in your hand, move them out of your reach. Playing with these distractions will give the other person the message that you would rather be somewhere else.

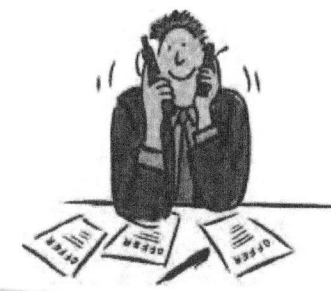

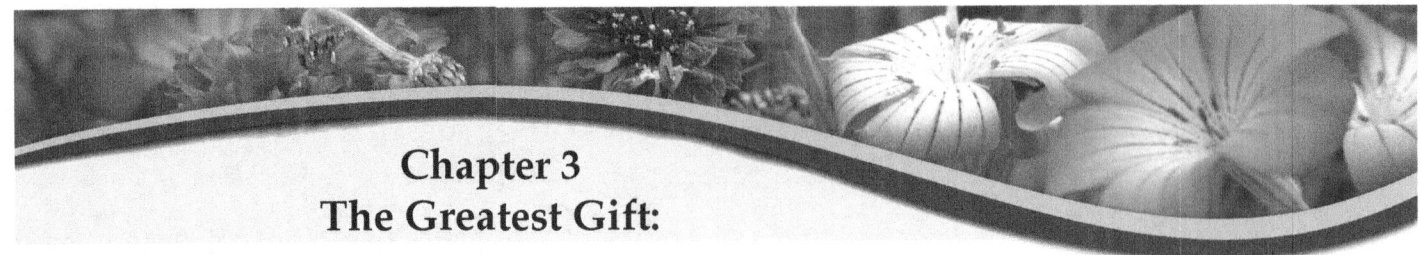

Chapter 3
The Greatest Gift:

How to Shut People Up:

- **Have a condescending attitude.** Say, "Tell me all about it, I can help you."
- **Negate their feelings.** Pat them on the hand as if you were their mother. Or say, "Don't worry", as if their concerns are unimportant and need not be explored further.
- **Blackmail them.** Clutch at your heart and tell them that what they are saying to you is giving you chest pains (or that it's making you cry and you hate to cry).
- **Interpret what they're saying.** Say, "You're angry because I remind you of your mother... (or your dog, or your ex-boyfriend.)"
- **Punish them.** When they tell you their feelings, especially if it involves something you said or did, say, "Oh, yeah? Well, let me tell you what you did."
- **Pretend to be stupid.** This technique works best when you're trying to avoid an uncomfortable subject. Look blankly at the person and say, "I'm sorry, I don't understand what you are talking about."
- **Pass the Buck.** Tell the person that it's not your problem.
- **Play lawyer.** Say, "When did I say that? I never said those words." Use your smoothest tone of voice.
- **Scold. Judge them.** Scowl and say, "You should be ashamed to feel like that" or "That was rude of you to say."
- **Act bored or absent-minded.** Jerk yourself back to the present after staring out of the window and say, "Oh, I'm sorry, I didn't hear you."
- **Turn the whole thing into a joke with a witty remark.**
- **Respond to what they are saying before they have a chance to express their feelings fully.**
- **Maintain a flat affect with no response at all to what they are saying.**
- **Address the content of what they are saying and ignore the emotion.**
- **Use clichés.** Say, "Everything will be all right" or "All's well that ends well."

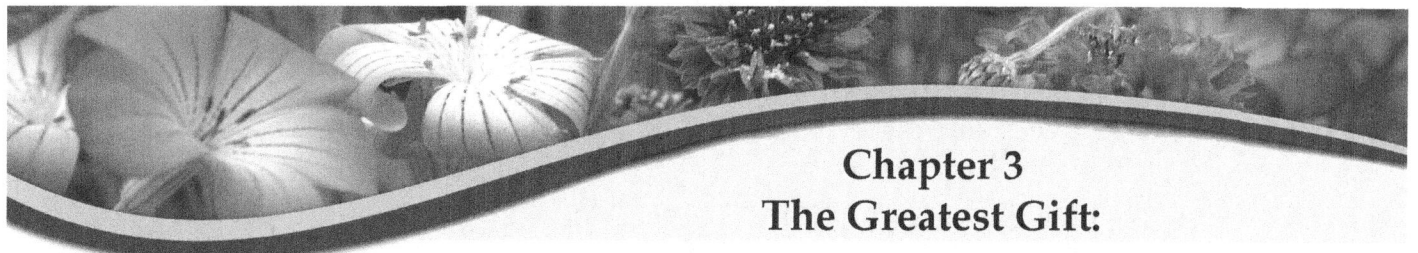

Chapter 3
The Greatest Gift:

The Best Techniques for Listening:

- **Encouragement.** Show interest and willingness to be involved in the conversation by saying things such as, "I'd like to hear more", or "Tell me about..." This gives the person permission to share.
- **Restatement.** Reword what the person is telling you and repeat it back to them in a slightly different way. This helps you clarify what you are hearing and helps the person speaking by allowing him to hear his thoughts reflected back to him.
- **Silence.** Just listen, all the while maintaining eye contact and demonstrating interest through body language.
- **Prompters.** Short phrases such as "I see", "Yes", and "Um-hm" help to encourage conversation without interrupting the speaker's train of thought.
- **Leading statements or questions.** This technique helps move the person on to additional thoughts or new areas to explore. It is very helpful in problem solving. If the person says to you, "I don't really know what to say to my husband about his illness" you can say, "What would you like to say to him?" The response to a question like this is usually a list of the options, which helps the person clarify their own thoughts and feelings.
- **Observations about non-verbal behavior.** If you notice the person you are listening to frowning or sighing, it may be helpful to mention these non-verbal behaviors. You could say, "You seem upset" or "This seems to really be bothering you." This allows the person to either verify or disagree with your observation, and at the same time clarify their own feelings.
- **Honesty.** This is especially important in hospice. Don't offer false hope or reassurance. At the same time, don't destroy hope.

Putting it Into Practice

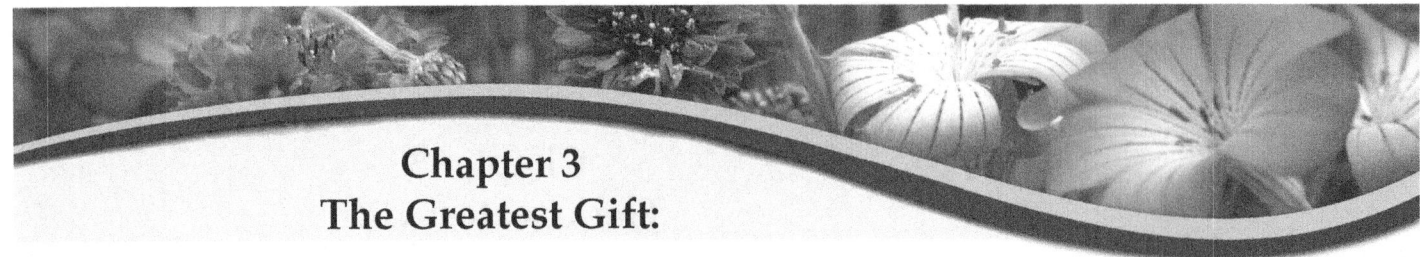

Chapter 3
The Greatest Gift:

More About Your Body Language

How we think and feel is communicated largely by non-verbal means: expressions, subtle movements, eye contact, etc. One of the most important aspects of good listening involves understanding these non-verbal cues and making sure we're giving a consistent message of respect and interest to the person we are listening to.

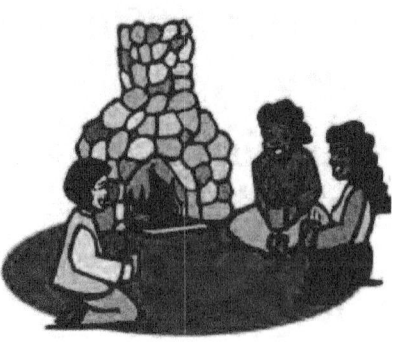

Eye Contact

Most eye behavior is so subtle that we are aware of it only on a subconscious or intuitive level. It is, however, one of the most potent elements in communication.

Think about some of the interactions you've had with others. Maintaining eye contact for even a few seconds longer than you ordinarily would, shifting your eyes away at just the time when you needed to maintain eye contact, refusing to make eye contact at all... Each of these subtle gestures, involving only a few tiny muscles in the eye, carried powerful messages to the person you were communicating with, even if no words at all were used.

Try an experiment. The next time you are having a conversation with someone that makes you feel accepted and liked, watch what they do with their eyes. You will probably notice that they look at you more than usual with each glance a little longer than ordinary. This kind of eye contact portrays interest in you as a person rather than just an interest in the topic being discussed.

Eye contact can be overdone. This would be interpreted as staring and could be considered intrusive. It can also be underdone and portray avoidance. Patterns of eye contact are also culturally related. If you are working with someone from another culture it would be wise to observe their interactions with family members to determine acceptable eye contact patterns.

The general rule of thumb, however, is to look at people just a few seconds longer than would be customary in a "professional" relationship. This will help communicate a caring, warm feeling to the person you are talking to.

Putting it Into Practice

Chapter 3
The Greatest Gift:

Body Positioning

The way we position ourselves when we talk to someone also communicates a great deal. In our culture, the basic attentive listening posture is to lean forward slightly, with an alert but relaxed attitude. Not bothering to turn toward the other person, or turning your back on them, can convey disinterest or rejection, while turning toward them transmits a message of attention and interest.

The physical distance between you and the person with whom you are communicating can also be meaningful in conveying a message. When you are in a situation in which you are listening to someone who is sharing their feelings with you, it's a good idea to follow their lead in how close to sit. Be sensitive to the amount of physical distance they may need to feel safe sharing with you. Make sure there are no desks or other objects between you and the other person to create an artificial barrier that would affect physical as well as emotional closeness.

Facial Expression

A flat affect or a facial expression that is not consistent with what is being said (such as smiling or frowning inappropriately) communicates inattentiveness. A smile or frown at the right place in the conversation, however, tells the speaker that you are listening carefully. Nodding at the right places helps to show understanding, too. When you listen with empathy to what is being shared with you, it's easier to match your facial expression to the feelings that are being conveyed by the other person and in this way, create a sense of closeness and caring.

Putting it Into Practice

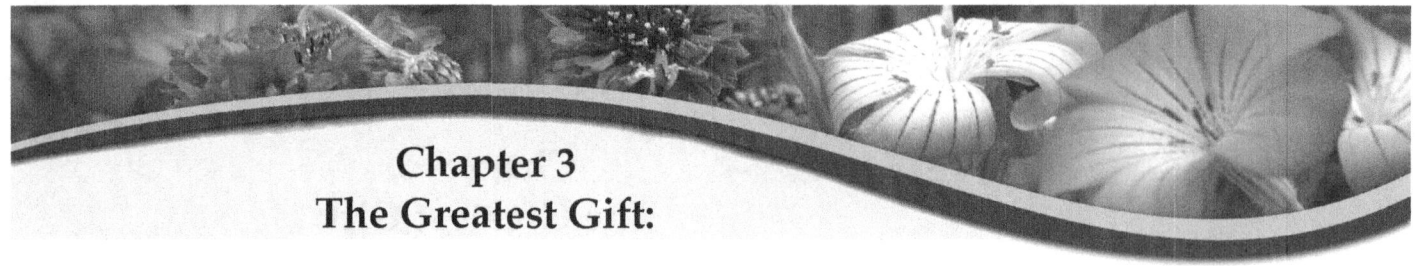

Chapter 3
The Greatest Gift:

Learning Activity

Divide into pairs and find a comfortable place to have a conversation. Choose which one of you will be the dying patient and which will be the listener. Applying the principles of good listening that we've just discussed, carry on a therapeutic interaction.

When your moderator calls time, switch places so that the "patient" becomes the "listener". (If you are working through this training series by yourself, have someone be your "patient" to allow you to practice listening.)

Here are some conversation starters for the "patient" to use:

- "My father is falling a lot. He's a military guy and I'm really afraid of what is going to happen to his self concept as he loses his independence. I've been losing sleep thinking about it"
- "My parents both died of cancer, two of my uncles died of cancer, my daughter just had surgery for cancer, and now they tell me I have it too."
- "I keep trying to talk to my kids about the fact that I'm dying, but they don't want to accept it. They keep trying to find something that will make me well."
- "I've always hated being around sick people, especially if they are dying. Now the doctor says I'm dying. I'm afraid to die."
- "Why is this happening to me? What have I done to deserve this? How could God do this to me after all I've done to serve Him?"
- "I've taken care of myself all my life. I never smoked or drank and now I have cancer. Why?"
- "I look so terrible. I hate looking in the mirror. My skin is so yellow and ugly."
- "I just retired six months ago. My wife and I had plans to travel and do all the things we didn't have time or money to do all these years. We even bought a motor home. Now the doctor says I have two months to live."
- "My husband has been very forgetful lately. I found his socks in the freezer last week. I took him to the doctor and he says it's Alzheimer's Disease. I don't know how I am going to be able to care for him. I'm so afraid. I don't know where to turn."

Putting it Into Practice

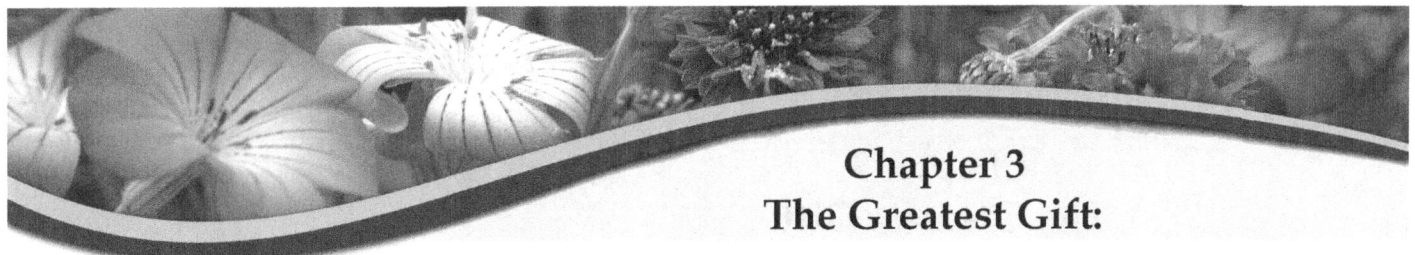

Chapter 3
The Greatest Gift:

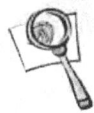
A Closer Look

The social worker and the volunteers are the members of the care team that probably do the most therapeutic listening. In addition to being a good listener, the social worker is responsible for:

- **Establishing a support network in the community to refer patients and their families to when the need arises**
- **Organizing and facilitating family meetings**
- **Assisting the family with funeral arrangements**
- **Providing guidance and direction to the team in how they can best emotionally support the patients and families**
- **Providing opportunities for care team members to get their own needs for emotional support and processing met**
- **Individual counseling with patients and family members who need specialized support**

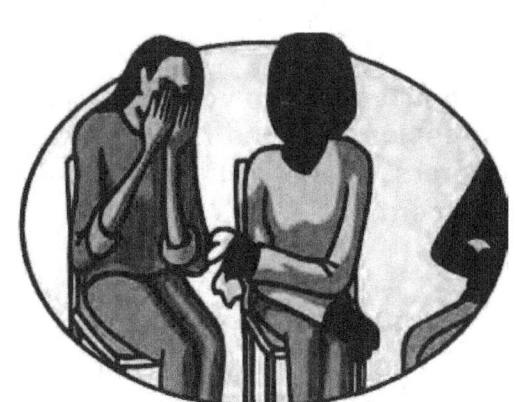

Ask a social worker to identify their biggest pet peeve in working with the terminally ill and they may likely tell you it's the use of clichés. Here are some of the worst offenders. I'm sure you can identify many more of your own! The bottom line is: there is no place in end of life care for clichés.

1. "I know just how you feel."

There is no way you can know "just" how someone else feels. Humans are like snowflakes, no two are exactly alike. And no two people's life experiences are exactly alike. This insensitive statement pulls the focus away from the sufferer and onto you. As a result, the hurting person may feel more alone than before he attempted to reach out to you.

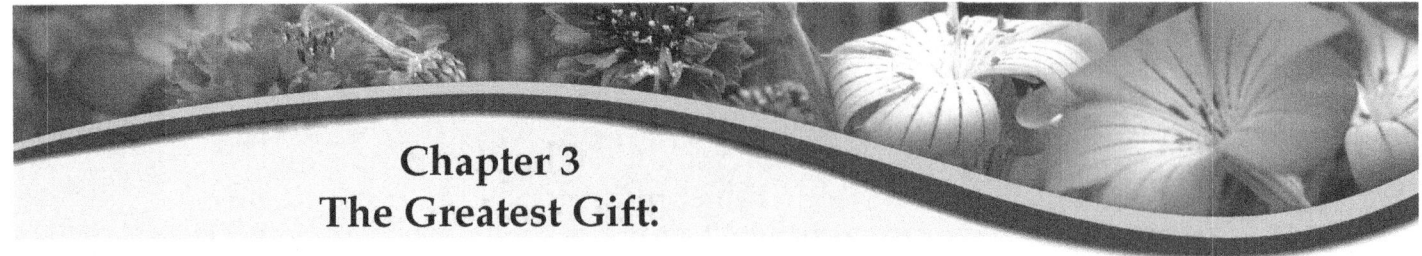

Chapter 3
The Greatest Gift:

2. "We are never given more than we can handle."

Inability to cope is not necessarily related to a lack of faith or strength. Sometimes the stresses of life can be too much to bear. That's why we have each other to offer support when pain is intense and feels overwhelming. This statement is actually a subtle criticism of the sufferer's coping skills, not the reassurance that some may think it is.

3. "It's God's will."

And just how can you be so sure of God's will? A statement like this could give the impression that God is a cruel, vicious force that doesn't care what happens to human sufferers. Even if you view God that way, it won't be helpful to your patient to make this statement.

4. "I'm sorry."

These words have become a socially acceptable way to respond to tragedy and death, but whom do they comfort? We may be sorry that people are hurting. Or we may be sorry that we've just been reminded that such terrible things could happen to us, too. But what is the sufferer supposed to say back? Thank you? That's okay? It's not okay! There just isn't an adequate response to those words and it's best not to use them.

5. "Call me if there is anything I can do."

These words are too general. They can almost be translated, "I don't really want to put myself on the line here, but I also don't want to feel like an insensitive putz, so I'm trying to make it appear that I am available to you."

People in crisis are usually feeling so overwhelmed that they don't even know themselves what they need. Specific direction, offered gently and with no strings attached, is the most helpful.

The best thing to say is, "I can do _____ and _____ for you if it would help you. Which day this week would work out for you?"

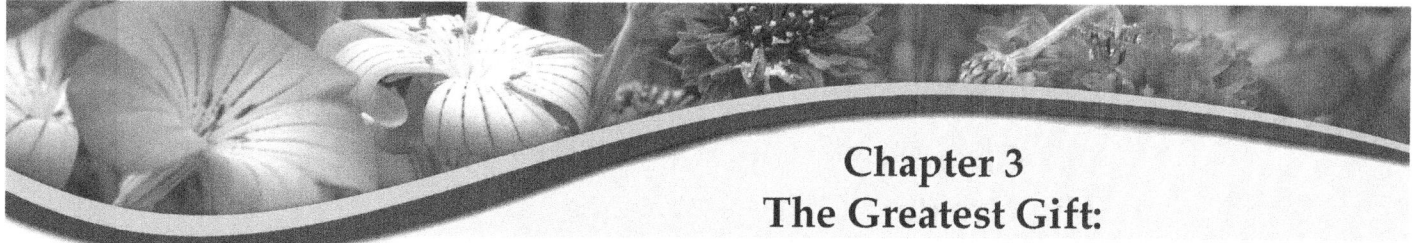

Chapter 3
The Greatest Gift:

6. "She lived a good, long life and it was her time to die."

There just isn't a good time to die. It doesn't matter whether someone is five or one hundred and five, it hurts when their life ends. This statement invalidates the very real feelings of grief and loss that the family feels when they lose a loved one, young or old.

7. "You must be strong for your children."

Actually, being "strong" for the children is more damaging to them than allowing them to see real grief being processed in a normal healthy way with tears, expressions of sorrow, and other displays of emotion. People who try to be "strong" often end up with ulcers and unresolved grief that cripples them for years.

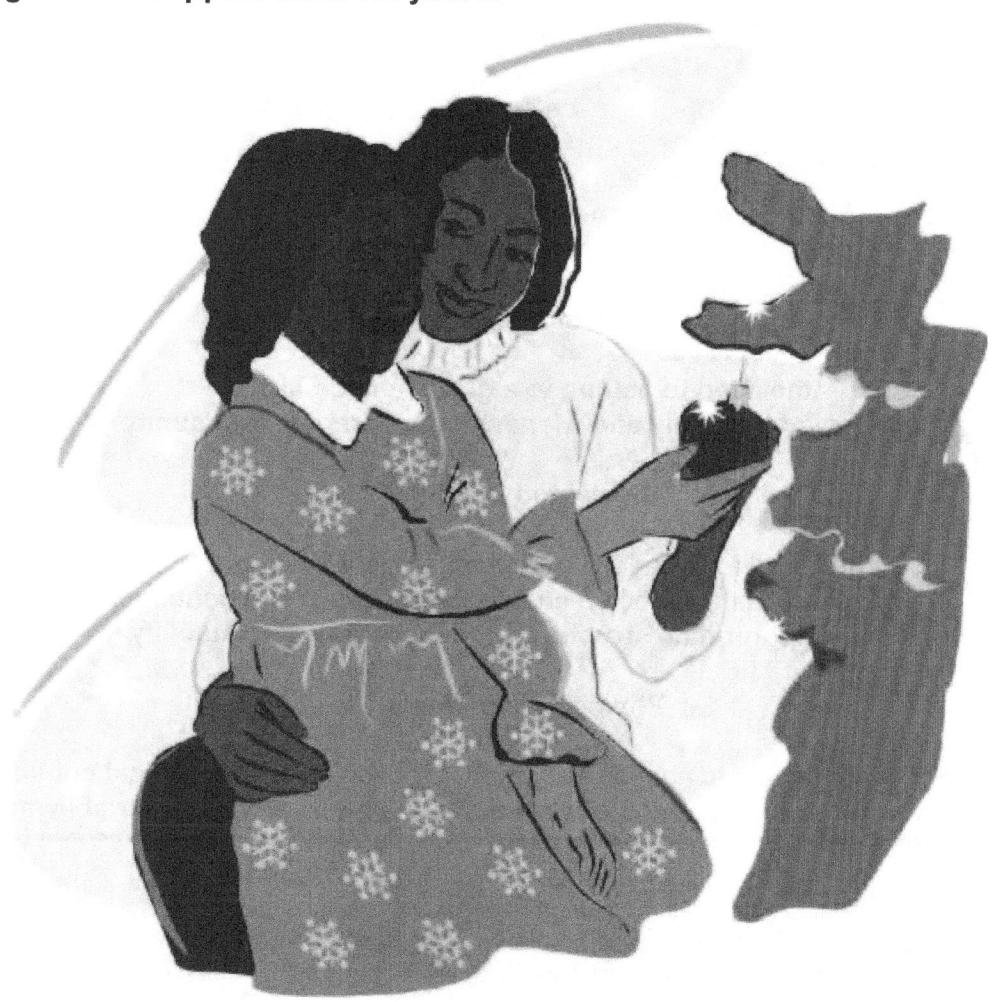

A Closer Look

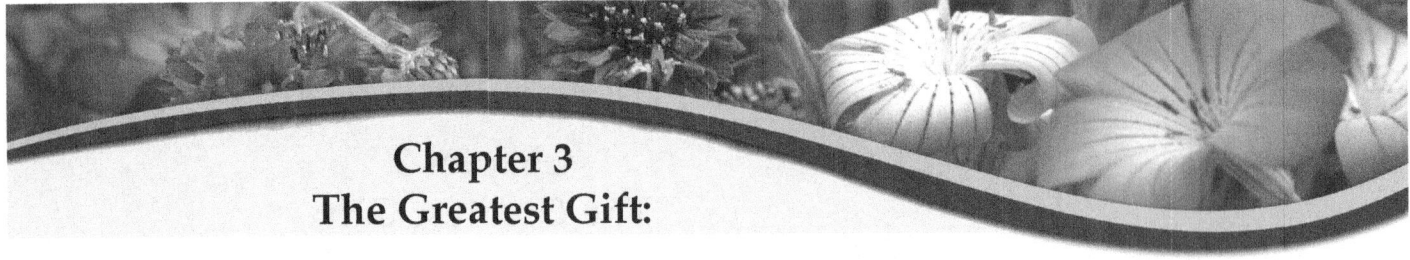

Chapter 3
The Greatest Gift:

Maslow's Hierarchy of Needs
(as it relates to end of life care)

Self-Actualization

the need to find meaning in existence and to know that life counted for something, to realize spiritual fulfillment

Esteem

the need to be respected, to respect oneself, to be competent to maintain personal integrity

Love and Belonging

the need to belong to a group and be liked to be loved by family and friends, to be part of a community

Safety and Security

the need for freedom from fear, anxiety, and chaos to maintain a balance between dependence and independence to have appropriate structure, limits, security, and stability

Physiological Needs

the need to have the basic necessities of life that lead to physiological comfort to have food, water, and air and to be free from pain and other uncomfortable stimuli

*note- The base of the pyramid holds up the entire structure. Unless the patient's basic needs are met, the higher levels of need will not be adequately met. Thus the hospice emphasis on making sure pain is controlled and the patient feels comfortable and safe before addressing "higher" issues such as meaning of life,

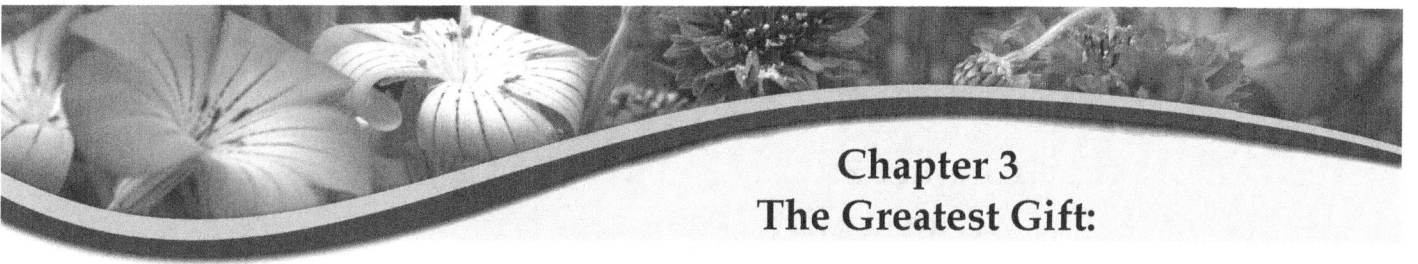

Chapter 3
The Greatest Gift:

I know you believe

you understand

what you think I said,

but I am not sure

you realize

that what you heard

is not what I meant.

Author Unknown

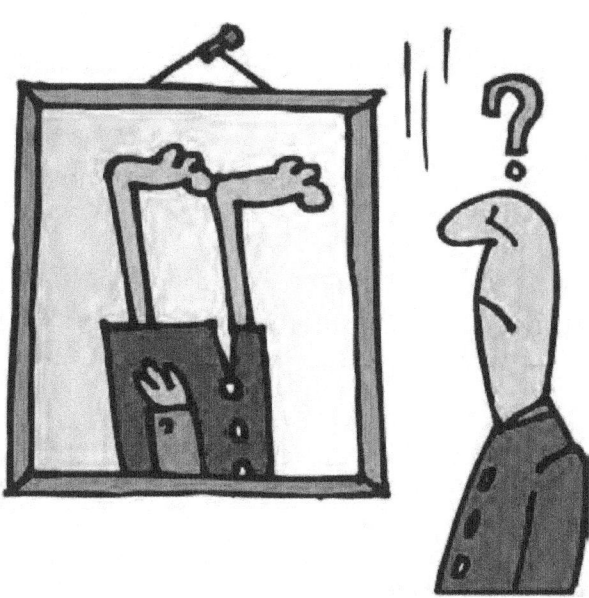

A Closer Look

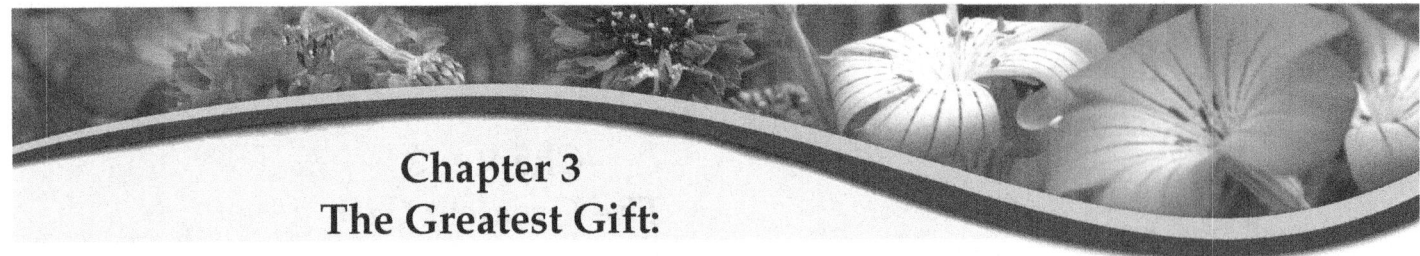

Chapter 3
The Greatest Gift:

The Gift of Mindfulness

Learning to listen well is truly a central value in the hospice concept and a crucial one for you as a volunteer. One of the most important aspects of listening, in fact the thing that makes true listening even possible, is the act of being present. And being present requires an attitude of ***mindfulness***.

How to be mindful.

- Do not allow yourself to be distracted by your phone, the clock, your watch, or anything else but what is happening in the room between you and your patient.

- Avoid using the word "should", which will take you immediately out of mindfulness and into judgment.

- Keep your body open. Don't cross your arms or legs. Keep hands unclenched.

- Be attentive to the patient's body language, too. Watch for frowning, crossed arms, refusal to make eye contact, fidgeting and other signs that something is bothering them.

- Make direct, but non-threatening eye contact with the patient and/or family members.

- Accept the patient where he or she is and don't push them to talk. If they want to sit in silence, sit with them comfortably and quietly.

- Avoid questions that start with the word "why." These tend to move you into a judgmental space.

- Listen attentively without interrupting.

- Respect the person's life journey and don't attempt to fix. Honor the patient's boundaries by just being present.

- Pay attention to your own boundaries and make sure they are honored as well.

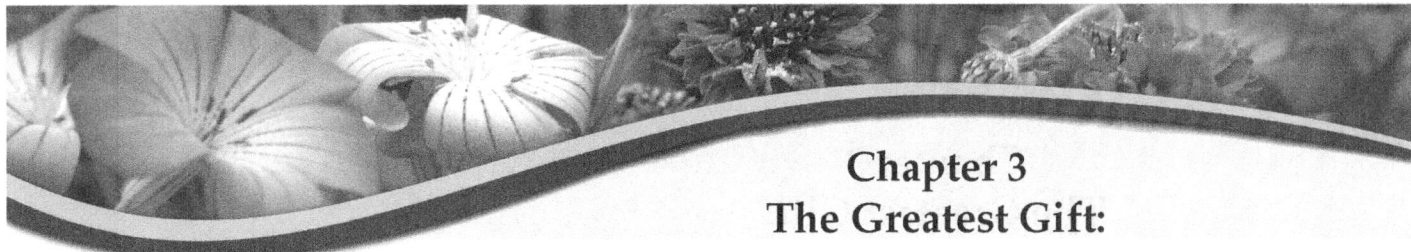

Chapter 3
The Greatest Gift:

Dealing with Family Members

It helps to understand family systems and what can influence a family's behavior when a loved one is dying. You will still, however, need to interact with them in a positive way. Here are some suggestions for better interactions with the family.

- Remember that each person is an individual, with their own emotions, during a very stressful time. There may be many things affecting their behavior and responses.

- Stay Switzerland! Never choose sides in a dispute between family members. Observe and report to your supervisor and other team members what you see, but stay out of it.

- Don't make judgments, even in your own mind. Stay patient and open-minded.

- Use tact and discernment in your conversations. Be aware of your impact. You represent hospice to the family. They will probably put a lot of weight on your opinions. Be careful how you use them.

- Make sure the family knows that hospice is there for them as much as it is for the patient, that their needs are important and that support is available to them.

- Remember that support is there for you, the volunteer, as well. You don't have to face a stressed out family by yourself. Call for help.

- Your supportive and stable presence can go a long way toward creating a calmer atmosphere with the family.

- Make sure each loved one has the time alone with the patient that they need. You are not there to interfere with family relationships, but to provide them the freedom to connect more deeply.

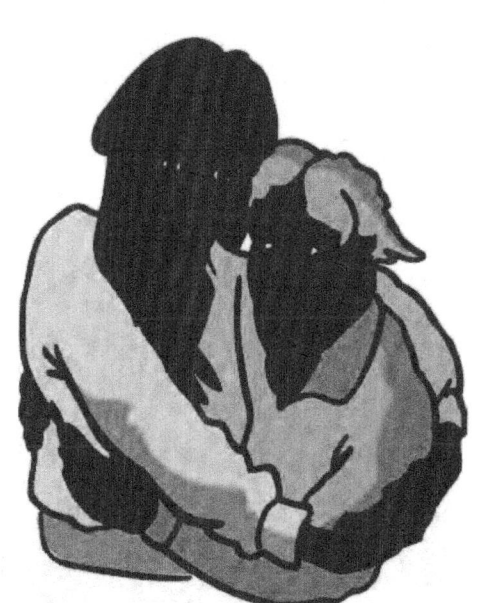

A Closer Look

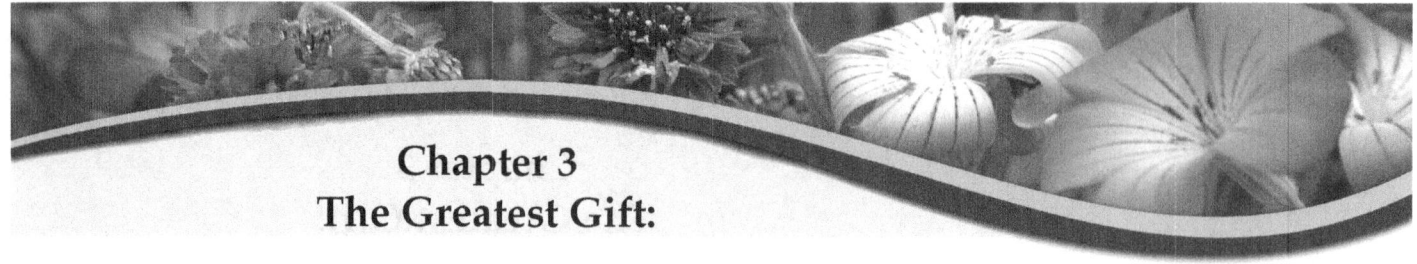

Chapter 3
The Greatest Gift:

- Answer questions and reassure the family about the dying process. They may ask the same questions over and over. Answer each time as patiently as if it were your first time to address it. Often, family members need to hear the same information repeated many times before their hearts can accept it.

- Encourage family members to take care of themselves. A nap, a walk, a trip to the mall or the hairdresser may be just what a beleaguered spouse or other family member needs to gain the energy to keep going. Affirm their efforts and let them know they are giving their loved one a priceless gift with their care.

- Reassure family members that it is okay to cry and express their sadness at losing their loved one.

- Let them know that people each grieve in their own way. You can say, "I know about grief, but I don't know about *your* grief."

- It's okay for you to be vulnerable, within your own boundaries. Sometimes family members will feel more free to open up with you when you are vulnerable with them.

- When you offer help, make it specific and concrete. Many of the older generation were raised to be very independent and not ask for things. So say, "I can make you a sandwich now if you'd like me to" or "I can stay with her now while she naps. Would you like to take a walk?"

- Give family members concrete tasks to do. There is so much that feels out of control about the situation, it often feels good to a family member to have something specific to do. It makes them feel useful and part of things.

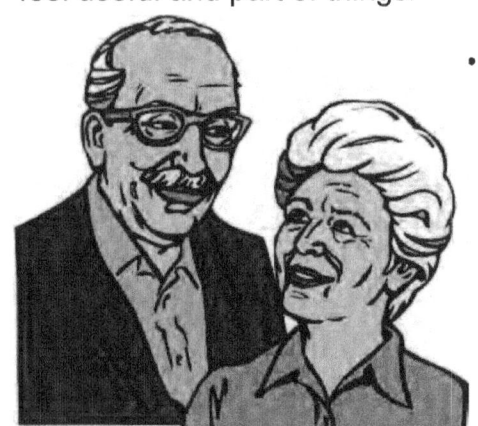

- If you have to leave the home or facility before a family member arrives, leave them a personal note to let them know how the patient is doing and asking them how they are. This is a great way to communicate concern and create a sense of connection and "teamwork" with the family. They will love you for it.

A Closer Look

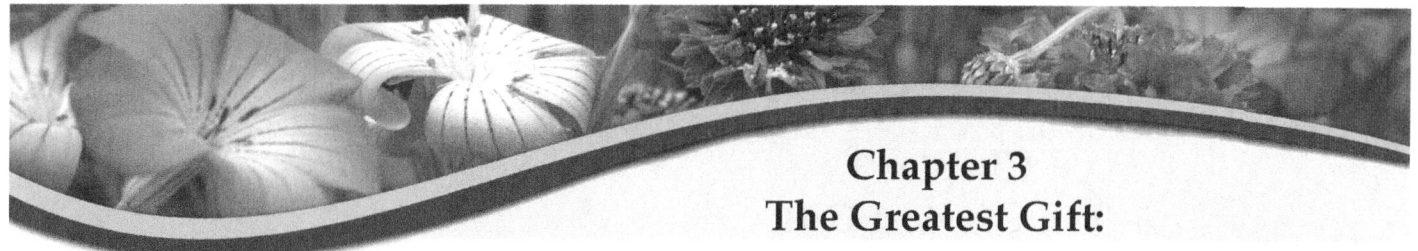

Chapter 3
The Greatest Gift:

The only way to provide the space for your patient and family to get down to the real issues that bring up fear for them is to listen with your heart. Mindfulness allows this to happen.

Sitting in Silence

We are a society obsessed with "doing something". Anything, just to be taking action. The greatest gift you can give your patient as a volunteer, however, is your presence. There is no more poignant and powerful way to communicate your pure presence with a person than to sit with them in silence.

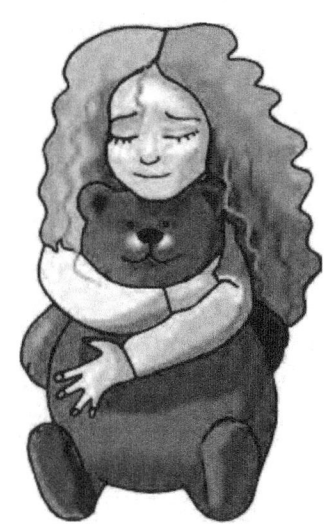

This "just sitting there" can be disconcerting for volunteers. However, this time in which the person receives total, undivided attention without having to say a word, without having to do anything but just be, is a profoundly sacred space. How rare to be fully accepted in the moment, allowed to be totally oneself, with no judgment or expectation of any kind by someone with no agenda, who doesn't want anything in return!

Divide into groups of two. Take turns sharing something painful from your past (or create something, if you don't have something you are comfortable sharing on that level right now.) As one person shares, the other listens mindfully, staying fully present. Then sit in silence together, with no agenda but to be present, for five minutes.

How did it feel to be silent for that long? What came up for you?

A Closer Look

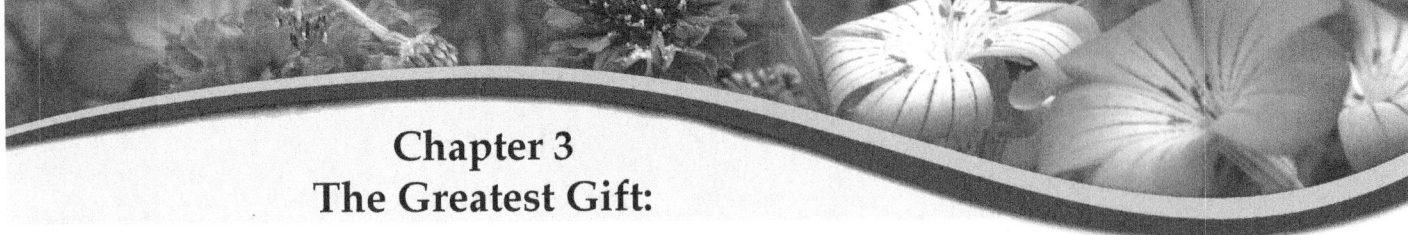

Chapter 3
The Greatest Gift:

Here are some ways to promote a mindful conversation:

- Do not interrupt them while they are sharing. Allow them to completely explore their thoughts without derailing them.

- Invite the other person to share more with short statements like: "Yes, go on.", "I see, tell me more."

- Nod thoughtfully, while encouraging them to think of different options. You aren't giving advice or telling them what to do. You are asking questions that help them find their own answers.

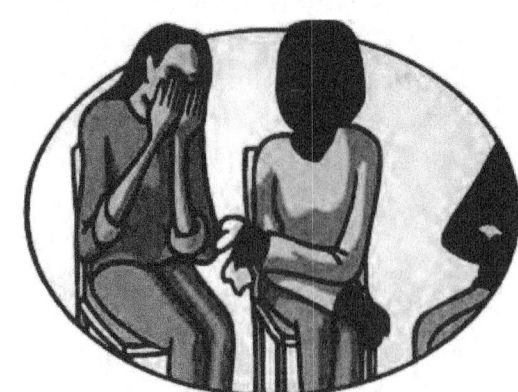

- "Have you thought about how to…?"

- "What would you need to make things more bearable?"

- "What would help you the most to achieve your goal?"

- "How can I help?'

- Restate what you hear the person saying: "I get the impression that this transition is difficult for you. Would that be a fair statement?"

- "The fact that your mother is not eating seems to concern you."

- Your nonverbal communication goes a long ways toward encouraging mindful conversation.

- Clear and direct, yet non-threatening, eye contact, a gentle touch or holding a hand support the impression that you care about the person and want to hear what it on their heart.

- An open posture communicates emotional availability.

- Allow for silence – it lets the person know that you are really listening and carefully considering their words.

Chapter 3
The Greatest Gift:

More reminders of statements and actions that can be communication barriers:

- Arguing. "I don't think you're right about that. This is how it really is. I know."
- Encouraging them to be angry, by saying, "Oh no! That's awful! How could they do such a thing!"
- Being dismissive. "Oh, I know you don't mean that. That's silly, don't say that."
- Using clichés: "He's with God now.", "At least she's out of pain.", "Be glad you had the time with him that you did."
- Making assumptions that your experience is the same as theirs. "I know just how you feel. That happened to me, too."
- Minimizing what is important to them by saying things like: "Don't worry, it'll be okay," or "Don't be ridiculous," or "That is silly," or "Oh, forget about that, who cares."
- Limiting options with negatives. "You should.." "He can't …." "You shouldn't…" These statements are expressions of judgment and feel closed and limiting to the hearer, shutting down communication.

Draw a picture in the box below that represents mindfulness to you.

A Closer Look

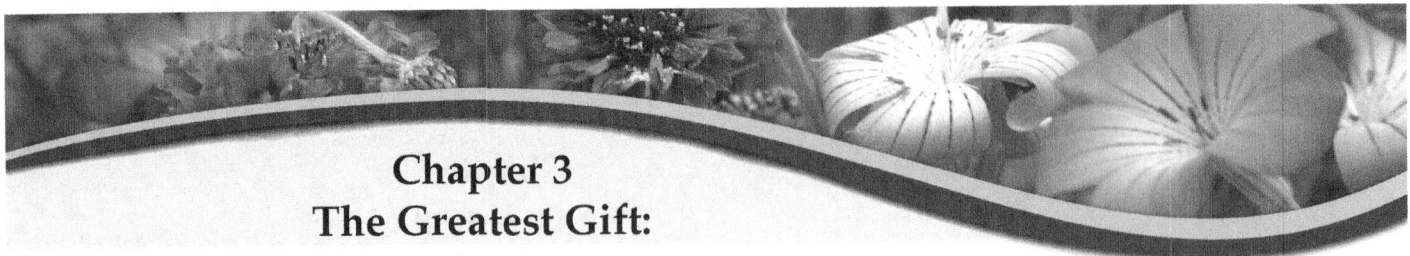

Chapter 3
The Greatest Gift:

It is so easy to use simple cliche's as a substitute for genuine communication. Here are a few more unhelpful platitudes that it would be best to avoid:

- That happened a long time ago.
- You should forget about it.
- I'm sure they have forgiven you.
- Don't worry about it.
- You did the best you could.
- It wasn't your fault.
- You were just a child. What could you have known then?
- She is in a better place now.
- It was her time to go. God took her when He was ready.
- At least he lived a good long life. You should be thankful that he's out of pain.
- You still have your children.
- It doesn't matter. Who cares?

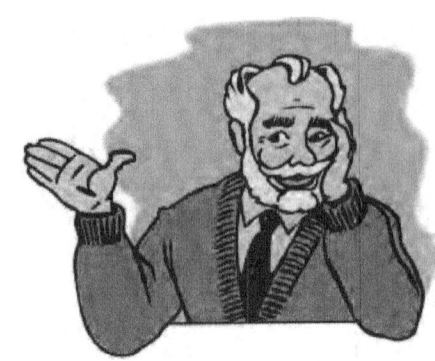

Can you think of other statements commonly made that minimize pain and shut down the person's flow of emotion? List them below:

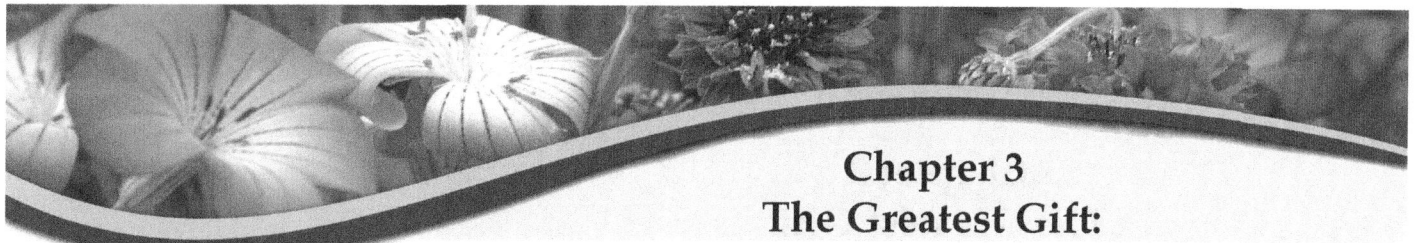

Chapter 3
The Greatest Gift:

Here are some responses that are more sensitive to the person's needs:

- I know about grief, but I don't know about your grief.
- I can see that you have a lot of love in your heart for…
- I wish I had something profound to tell you, but I don't.
- It seems like things are getting stressful for you.
- I can imagine that would feel frustrating.
- I am not sure how I can be of help, but I am willing to listen.
- Is there anything that I can do to make things easier for you?
- May I make a suggestion?
- How can I help?
- Tell me about it.

Can you think of other responses that would be supportive and helpful? List them below:

A Closer Look

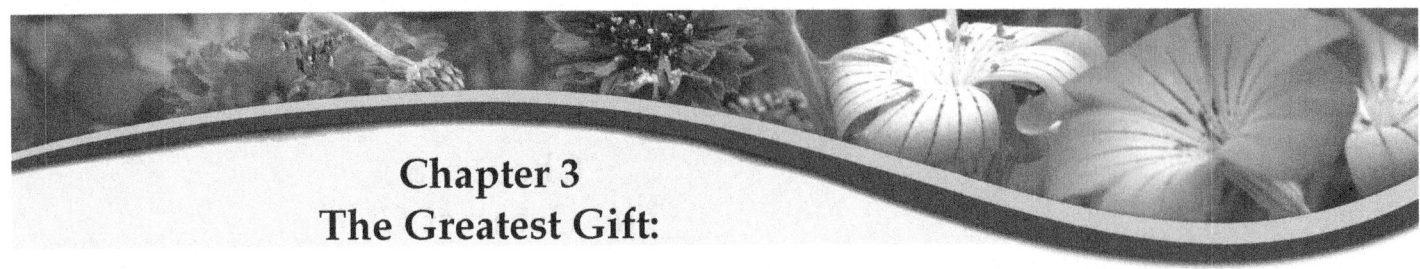

Chapter 3
The Greatest Gift:

Look over the pyramid of Maslow's Heirarchy of Needs on page 86 again. How do you see hospice providing for each level of need that the patient has?

Physiological Needs:

Safety and Security:

Love and Belonging:

Esteem:

Self-Actualization:

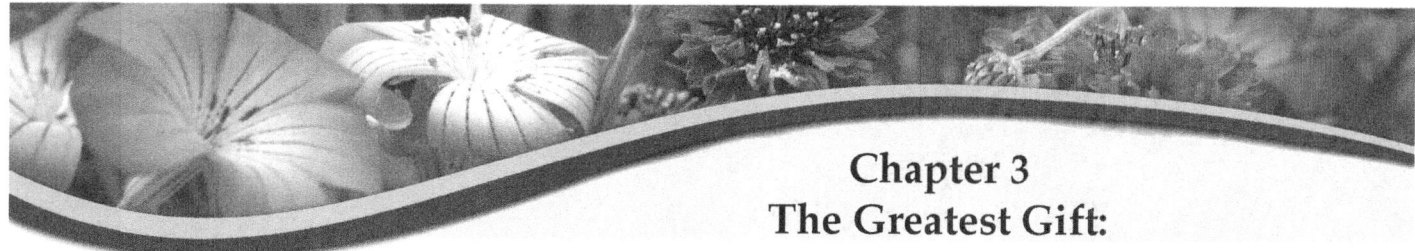

Chapter 3
The Greatest Gift:

Life Review

One way to help a patient with tasks of self-actualization is to ask them questions that will assist them in doing a life review. This is an important task at end of life and may be a key component of the patient's ability to find peace in the dying process.

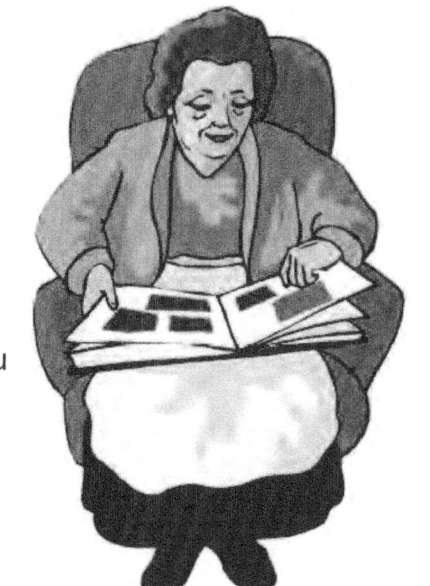

In life review, the patient talks about her life, the good and the bad, the bitter and the sweet. She may bring out photo albums to show you as she shares stories from years gone by. She also may confide in you and tell you things about her life that she has never told anyone, even those closest to her.

This is a precious time for the patient. Don't be afraid to ask questions and address real feelings. "How did you feel when your father left? That must have been really hard on your family." A well timed question will let her know that she is being heard and keep the memories flowing.

It's amazing how people tend to be protective and tip-toe around any real conversation with someone who is dying. It's sometimes difficult to tell who is protecting whom. I talked to a hospice nurse recently who told me the story of one of her patients who was dying of liver cancer. The family pulled her aside and said, "Don't tell mom she's dying. She won't be able to handle it. We're afraid she'll just give up."

When the nurse got into the patient's room, the woman asked her to close the door behind her. "I know I'm dying," the patient whispered to her. "But don't tell my kids. They wouldn't be able to handle it."

Just because someone is dying doesn't mean they are suddenly fragile or less than human. Be genuine and open. If your patient is experiencing this isolation that can happen when no one feels comfortable talking about real issues with him, he will likely be delighted at the opportunity for meaningful conversation and deep sharing of his heart.

A Closer Look

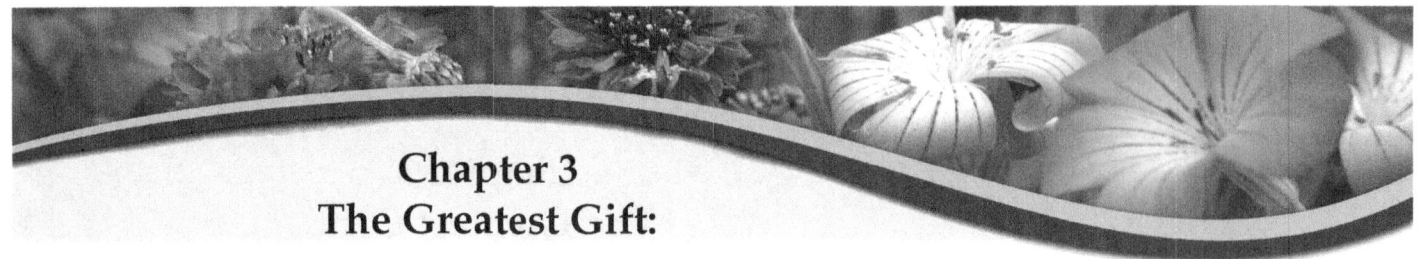

Chapter 3
The Greatest Gift:

 ## *Skill Check*

Complete the following:

1. The five emotional stages of dying are:

2. One common thread that persists throughout all the stages, whatever their order, is:

3. Five characteristics of an open family system are:

4. Five characteristics of a closed family system are:

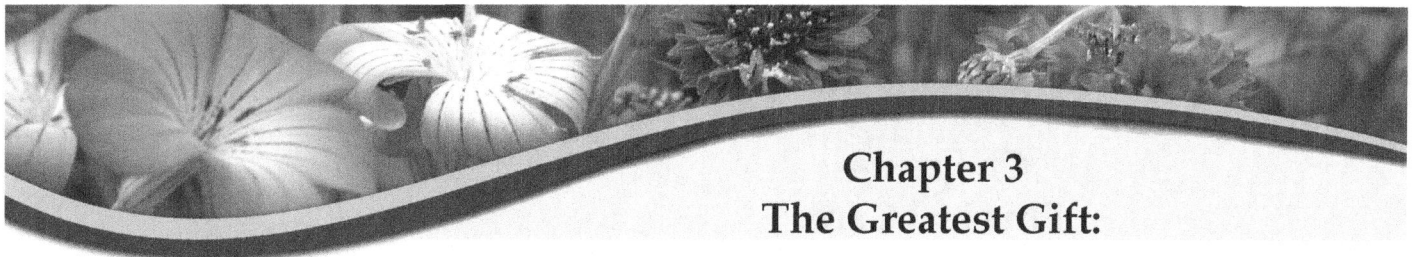

Chapter 3
The Greatest Gift:

5. List five ways to shut down communication.

6. Define and describe how you would use the following in a listening situation:

Clarifying statement

Leading statement

Prompter

Silence

Restatement

7. Describe the social worker's role in hospice.

"We do not see things as they are, We see things as we are."
The Talmud

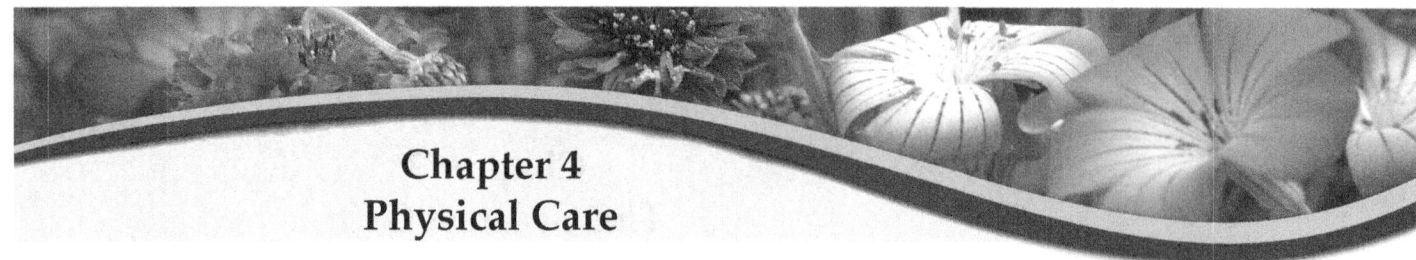

**Chapter 4
Physical Care**

4. Physical Care

When a Patient is Dying

"Just the facts, please..."

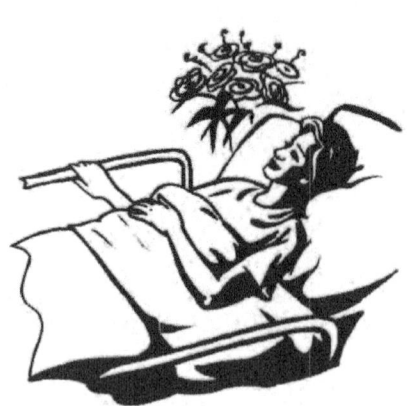

The vast majority of the patients who are admitted to hospice are suffering from end stage cancer of some kind. AIDS patients in end stage disease access hospice care, too. More and more, however, physicians are recognizing the value of involving hospice in the care of patients with end-stage renal disease, cardiac disease, respiratory disease, Alzheimer's Disease, and others. Although the symptoms of each disease process may vary, there are certain physical symptoms that are common to the dying process.

For instance, constipation can be a recurrent problem as the patient's appetite wanes and activity decreases, regardless of the actual underlying disease. Nausea, loss of appetite, weakness and fatigue, incontinence, anxiety, depression, and insomnia are other symptoms that can plague the dying patient.

The hospice focus, to help the patient free up energy to deal with issues higher on Maslow's hierarchy of needs, is on alleviating the annoying, distracting, and sometimes debilitating symptoms that accompany the dying process.

Care team members stay abreast of the latest techniques in symptom control, knowing that a patient distracted by pain or nausea may not be able to move ahead in the process of grieving and finding meaning and purpose in what he or she is experiencing.

Uncontrolled physical symptoms can also produce an inordinate amount of fear in the patient. This fear often creates a state of increased tension that exacerbates pain, restlessness, nausea, and other symptoms, which in turn causes more fear. It can be a vicious cycle with no end in sight without intervention from health care workers.

Hospice workers around the globe who have witnessed the impact that this cycle of fear can have on the dying person have expressed the conviction that it is this fear that causes the dying to want to end their lives prematurely through physician assisted suicide.

Chapter 4
Physical Care

Some questions you may be asking...

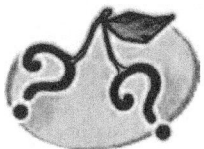 **What are some of the symptoms I may see with certain kinds of cancer?**

As was mentioned previously, some symptoms such as nausea, pain, bowel problems, anorexia, and anxiety can occur with almost any terminal illness whether or not it's cancer. A list of more specific symptoms follows.

- Lung — shortness of breath, cough, blood tinged sputum
- Breast — swelling in affected arm, tumors breaking out through the skin
- Skin — bleeding from a mole, change in color, waxy plaques
- Esophagus — decreased ability to swallow (may have a feeding tube, also called a PEG tube, to bypass the esophagus)
- Pancreas — pain, loss of appetite, jaundice, foul smelling stools
- Liver — profound weakness, loss of appetite, abdominal fullness (fluid in abdomen called "ascites", confusion
- Colon—nausea, vomiting, decreased appetite, diarrhea, constipation, fluid in abdomen (ascites), may have a colostomy (surgical procedure that brings bowel to the outside of the body via an opening in the abdomen called a stoma)
- Brain — confusion, headache, lethargy, weakness or paralysis of arm or leg, nausea and vomiting, seizures, decreased level of alertness (may go into a coma)
- Kidney — pain in lower back, blood in urine
- Bladder — blood in urine, pain on urination
- Prostate—inability to urinate, blood in urine
- Testes — enlarged testicle, late symptoms from places where the cancer has spread (pelvis, abdomen, lung, liver, brain)
- Cervix/Uterus — abnormal discharge, bleeding
- Ovary — nausea, vomiting, constipation, ascites
- Lymphoma/Leukemia — night chills and sweats, low grade fever, increased tendency to bleed, increased susceptibility to infection, weakness, pain
- Bone — pain, increased tendency to fracture

"Just the facts, please..."

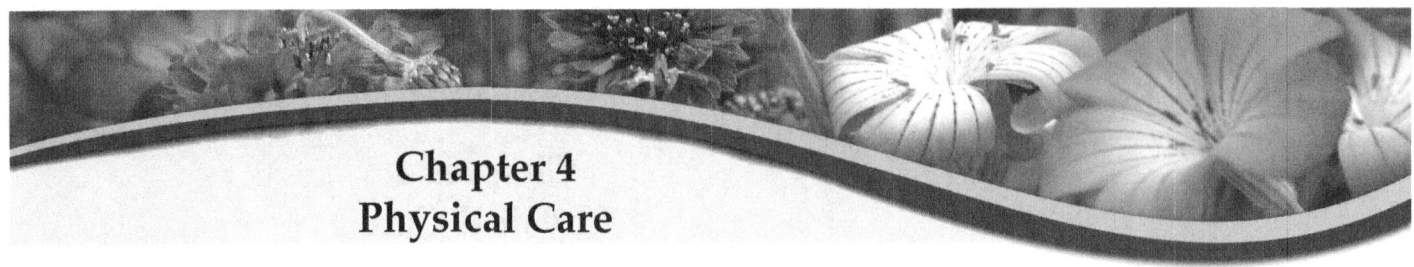

Chapter 4
Physical Care

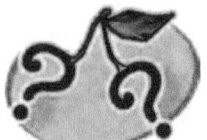 **What does the term "metastasis" mean?**

Cancer cells start in a primary site and can usually be identified even when they migrate to a different site and are found there. Metastasis (or "metastatic disease") is the term used to describe cancer that has migrated to a new area. Each cancer has a path its metastasis usually follows and often it can be predicted that, as the disease progresses, the cancer will show up in certain other places. Symptoms will then include those caused by the cancer affecting those new areas.

Here are some of the common metastatic pathways:

- **Lung to brain, liver, bone, other lung**
- **Breast to lymph nodes under arms, lung, bone, liver, brain**
- **Skin to brain**
- **Esophagus to local extension into chest, heart, lungs**
- **Pancreas to local extension into abdomen**
- **Liver is usually metastasized from somewhere else**
- **Colon to local extension within the abdomen**
- **Brain is usually metastasized from somewhere else (doesn't spread anywhere else if it is a primary brain tumor such as glioblastoma or astrocytoma)**
- **Kidney to bone, brain, lung**
- **Bladder to local extension within pelvis and into abdomen, lung, bone**
- **Prostate to bone, local extension within the pelvis**
- **Testes to local extension to pelvis, abdomen, lung, liver, brain**
- **Cervix, uterus to local extension in pelvis and abdomen**
- **Ovary to abdomen**
- **Bone is usually metastasized from somewhere else**

Chapter 4
Physical Care

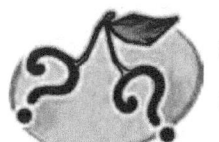 **What can I expect to see in my patients that don't have a cancer diagnosis?**

When a patient with a diagnosis other than cancer is admitted to hospice, their care is closely tailored to the actual symptoms that present. When a patient with end-stage respiratory disease, for example, is admitted he or she may or may not have pain, anxiety, bowel problems, etc. The course of the disease is much less predictable than a cancer diagnosis. The same goes with end-stage Alzheimer's, cardiac disease, and others. The following is a general outline of what you may expect to see with some of the non-cancer diagnoses:

- **AIDS** - neuropathy, dementia, confusion, depression, weight loss, weakness, infections (opportunistic, because of compromised immune system)

- **Alzheimer's** - confusion, forgetfulness, dementia, depression, insomnia, incontinence, hallucinations, inability to do self-care, seizures, pacing and wandering, sometimes violence and hostility, fatigue and anxiety

- **Congestive heart failure (CHF)** - shortness of breath, swelling in feet and ankles, rapid heart rate, fatigue, anxiety, fluid in lungs, insomnia

- **Amyotrophic Lateral Sclerosis (ALS)** - progressive loss of muscle function starting with limbs and eventually affecting swallowing and respiratory function, weakness, fatigue, depression, incontinence

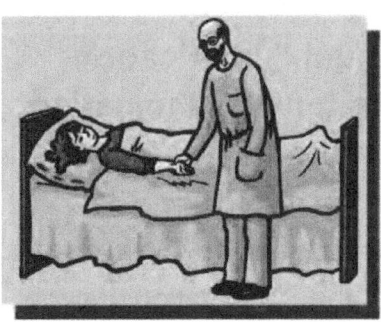

- **Liver failure** - similar to liver cancer with yellow skin and sclera of the eyes (jaundice), nausea and vomiting, buildup of fluid in the abdomen (ascites), profound fatigue and weakness, confusion, somnolence

- **Renal failure** - decreased urine output, confusion, pain in lower back, weakness and fatigue, sometimes blood in the urine

"Just the facts, please..."

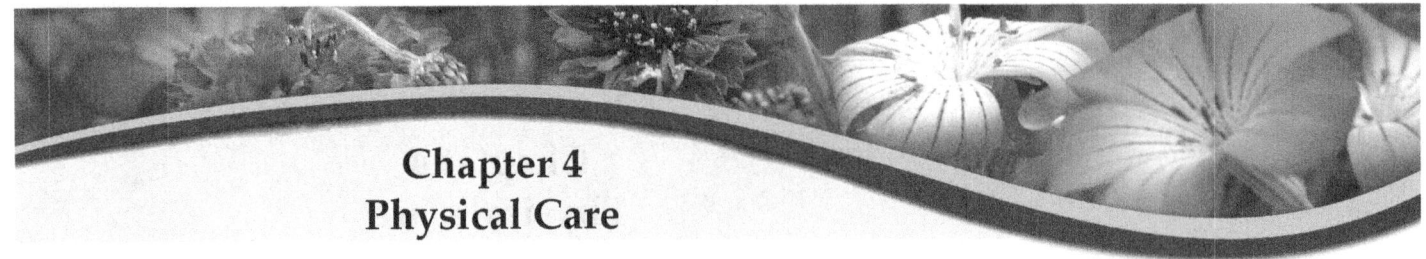

Chapter 4
Physical Care

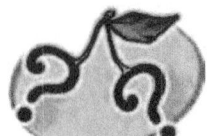 **"I've heard that cancer is a very painful way to die. What does hospice do to control the pain?"**

Cancer *is* often very painful, some kinds of cancer more so than others. Much research has been done, however, into the science of pain control in the terminal patient and, except for rare cases, there is no reason why a cancer patient has to die in pain. There are several basic principles of pain management that are essential for all care givers to understand in order to keep the patient's pain controlled.

- **Pain is a major robber of quality of life.**
  It distracts, demoralizes, drains energy, and exacerbates other symptoms. There is no logical reason to leave a cancer patient in pain.

- **Chronic pain (as in cancer) is different from acute pain (as in surgery or a short term illness).**
  It is irreversible, progressive, intractable, and meaningless. It takes special attention from the hospice team to keep it under control. Team members will address pain issues on virtually every visit or phone call they make to the patient.

- **Pain is what the patient says it is.**
  No one can judge another's level of pain. Some people are able to control outward signs of pain so that it appears to others that their pain is much less than it actually is "inside". Others have difficulty tolerating even slight amounts of pain. Hospice uses a variety of tools to "scale" the patient's perception of their pain. These tools help team members adjust pain medications so that pain is controlled to a level that the patient considers adequate.

- **There is no such thing as "too much" medication when it comes to pain control as long as the patient is experiencing relief with minimal side effects.**
  Some cancer patients may take dosages of morphine in the hundreds of milligrams. It is important for patients to know that as long as their pain continues to increase, their medication dosage can increase to control it.

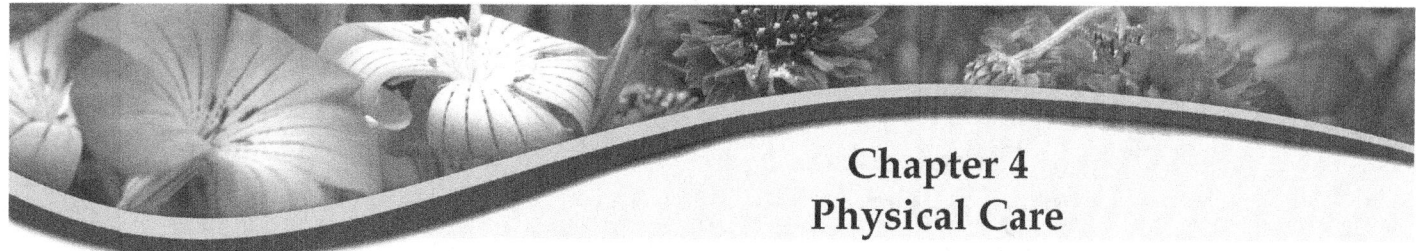

Chapter 4
Physical Care

- **Addiction is not an issue with cancer pain control.**
  Pain is a natural narcotic antagonist, which means that a certain amount of pain "burns up" a certain amount of medication. Or, stated another way, a certain number of pain receptors "bind off" a certain amount of medication. If the amount of medication given to the patient matches the number of pain receptors in the patient's body, pain control is achieved. Hospice nurses observe carefully for signs that increases in pain medication may be needed.

- **Some nonverbal signs of pain to watch for are:**

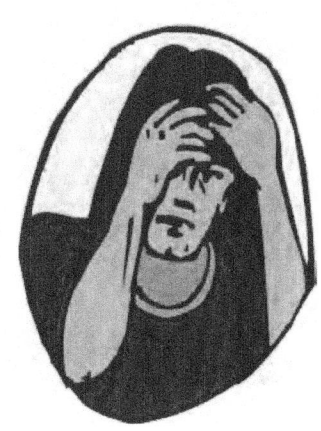

Grimacing

Wincing

Restlessness

Insomnia

Rapid heart rate

Increased or abnormally decreased blood pressure

Guarding of the body area that you know to be affected by the cancer

*Note: Sleeping is not a sign that the patient is comfortable and out of pain as patients often sleep to escape from the pain!

"How do you know which pain medication will be the most effective for a patient?"

There are several factors the hospice team considers before recommending a certain medication to the patient's primary physician. In the pain assessment, the hospice nurse will try to ascertain the location, character, strength, recurrence, and frequency of the pain by asking the patient questions about his or her sleep patterns, activity levels, and perception of the pain.

"Just the facts, please..."

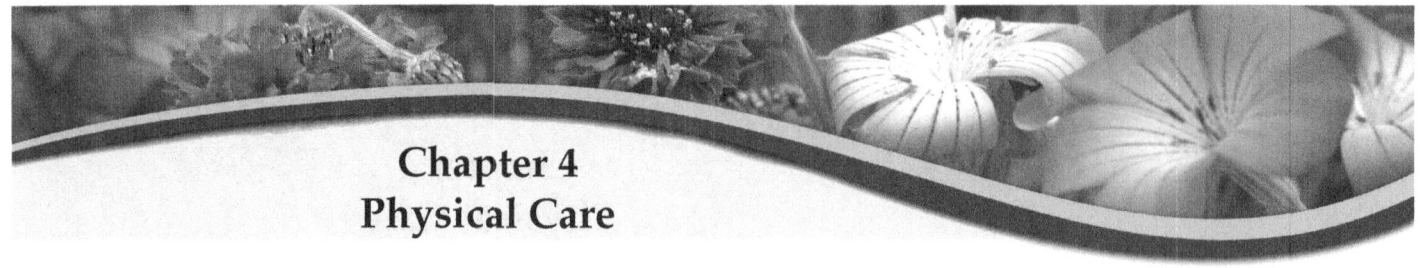

Chapter 4
Physical Care

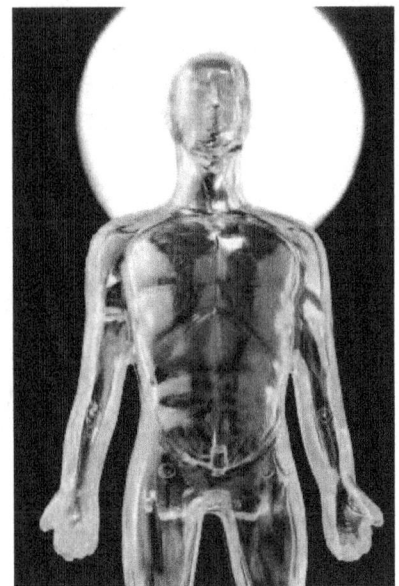

Visceral pain is a deep pain that is caused by a tumor crowding surrounding tissue. This type of pain responds very well to opiates. Morphine is the drug of choice in this category because of its effectiveness with relatively few side effects when given properly. The dosage is determined by the level of pain and the amount of medication it takes to achieve a level of comfort that is acceptable to the patient.

Morphine can be given orally, in an updraft nebulizer machine, or under the tongue (sublingually) in a fast-acting 20 mg./cc solution. This route of administration is especially useful in patients who cannot swallow because it is absorbed well through the membranes under the tongue or in the buccal pouches along the gum lines in the sides of the mouth. Disadvantages of this form of administration include a bitter taste, the need to give the medication frequently because it is only effective for a few hours, and the possibility of spilling it.

Morphine can also be given in a long-acting tablet. In this form, the medication stays in the patient's system for 8-12 hours, allowing family members to get more rest in between dosages. The pills are small and easy to swallow, but the patient must be conscious and able to swallow to take them. Because of the longer half-life of this form of morphine, hallucinations are more of a problem with long-acting morphine than with short-acting morphine. Many hospices give medications rectally when the patient isn't able to swallow anymore. You may observe the hospice nurse teaching the family to "score" or crack the shell of the tablet before inserting it to allow adequate release of the medication in the rectal vault.

Other pain medications your patient may use for visceral pain are oxycodone, hydromorphone HCL, acetaminophen with codeine phosphate, or various combinations of acetaminophen and hydrocodone bititrate. These are all short acting and usually used when the patient only needs occasional dosages of pain medication. By the time the patient needs one or two tablets every 3-4 hours of any of these meds, it is usually an indication that something stronger and more long acting is needed. The most common combination of pain medications for moderate to severe pain is long acting morphine every 12 hours with a shorter acting pain medication as needed in between for "break through" pain. The amount of long-acting morphine used increases as the patient's pain increases.

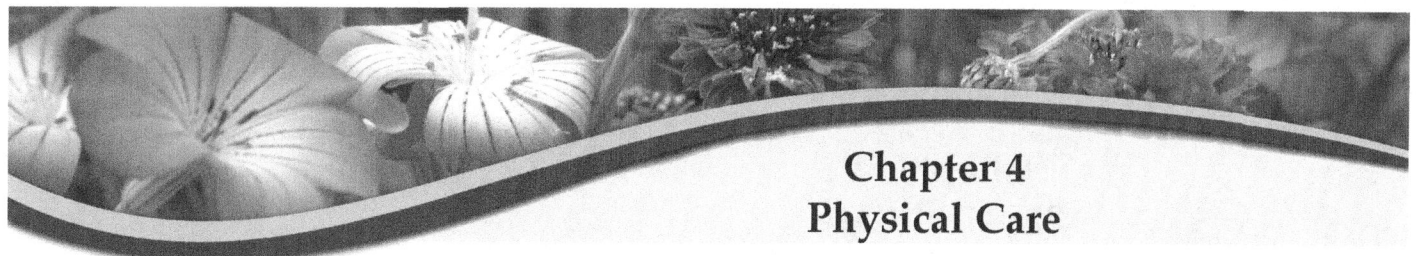

Chapter 4
Physical Care

Bone pain is caused by invasion of the bone by tumor, whether it be a primary site or metastasis from somewhere else. Bone pain is often described as a deep "toothache" type pain. It can be very severe, especially when it accompanies breast, lung, or prostate cancer.

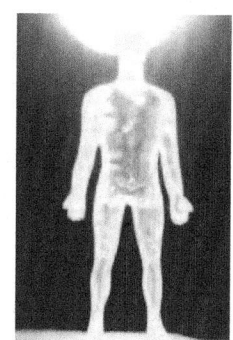

Bone pain will not respond to opiates alone. This fact is responsible for much of cancer's horrendous reputation where uncontrolled pain is concerned. If the primary physician is unaware of the need to combine different medications to control the different kinds of pain a terminally ill person may have, the patient may suffer terribly.

To achieve pain control when visceral and bone pain are both present (as in a case of prostate cancer spreading to the bone) the hospice team recommends a combination of an opiate and a non-steroidal anti-inflammatory (some type of ibuprofen or one of its cousins - also called NSAIDs).

Many physicians try to avoid using these NSAIDs because they cause stomach upset, but they are essential in controlling bone pain. If stomach upset occurs, some kind of stomach protection needs to be used and perhaps another type of NSAID tried.

Nerve pain is caused by cut or damaged nerve endings, a very common occurrence in patients who have undergone surgery, radiation, and/or chemotherapy. Neuropathy is also a very common occurrence with AIDS patients. Nerve pain is a sharp, penetrating pain that patients have described as feeling like "someone is jabbing me with a red hot poker". The pain is intermittent and intense. Sometimes, as in neuropathy in the limbs, it is burning and radiating.

Opiates won't relieve nerve pain and neither will NSAIDs. Patients whose physicians have ordered opiates to relieve their nerve pain have reported that the medication only "snowed" them so they could tolerate the pain, but it had little effect on the pain itself. Hospice physicians have discovered that one of the side effects of tricyclic antidepressants is a blocking of nerve pain impulses. Patients that have taken from 50-150 mg of certain tricyclic antidepressants have reported significant relief of their nerve pain.

Abdominal pain, when it is not caused by tumor activity (in which case it would be treated as visceral pain), is most often a result of gastrointestinal upset of some kind. A rigorous bowel management program, antacids, massage, digestive enzymes, and other interventions aimed at improving gastric function are all used to relieve this kind of pain.

"Just the facts, please..."

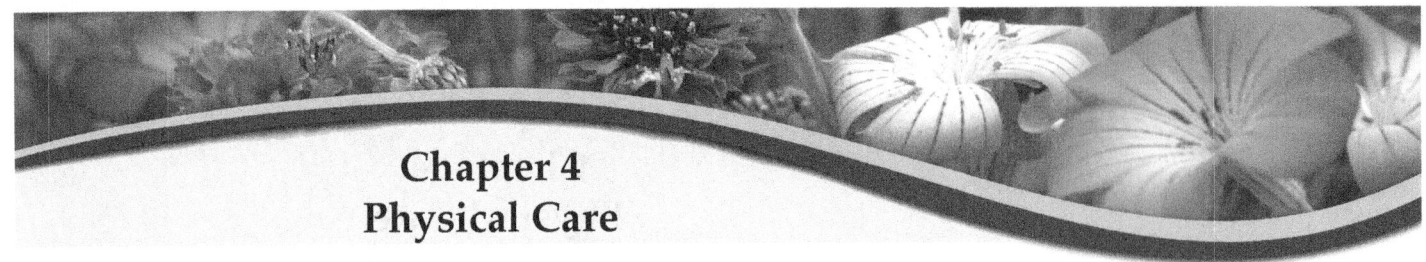

Chapter 4
Physical Care

More about pain management

Although you, as a volunteer, will not be responsible for physical assessment of the patient's pain and symptoms, it is important that you understand what is happening physically with the patient for your own comfort level and so that will develop that "gut" sense when something isn't right. You are the person who will be in the patient's presence without any external distractions. That stillness and presence will allow you to see changes that a team member coming in for a scheduled visit might not catch. The team will rely on you to report anything you notice that you feel needs attention.

Not all dying people will experience physical pain. Some will have intense pain that takes massive doses of medication to alleviate. Remember that pain is always what the patient says it is. This is their experience. No one else can say what is going on in someone else's body. We can't "compare" pain experiences and it isn't the volunteer's job to assess pain levels or decide what medications might or might not work.

If you notice that a patient seems to be in pain, however, ask them about their pain. It is also important to get permission from the patient (if they are alert and oriented) to report unresolved pain to the nurse. It seems like a small thing, but dealing with pain is an intensely personal thing. This

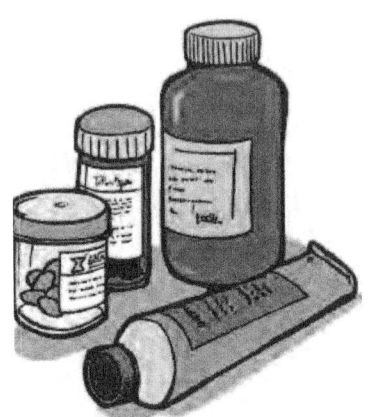

small courtesy speaks volumes to the patient about respect for their right to handle their pain in their own way. They may want the pain completely medicated and be willing to deal with possible side effects like drowsiness. Or they may want to be more alert for interactions with family and tolerate a little more pain to be able to do that.

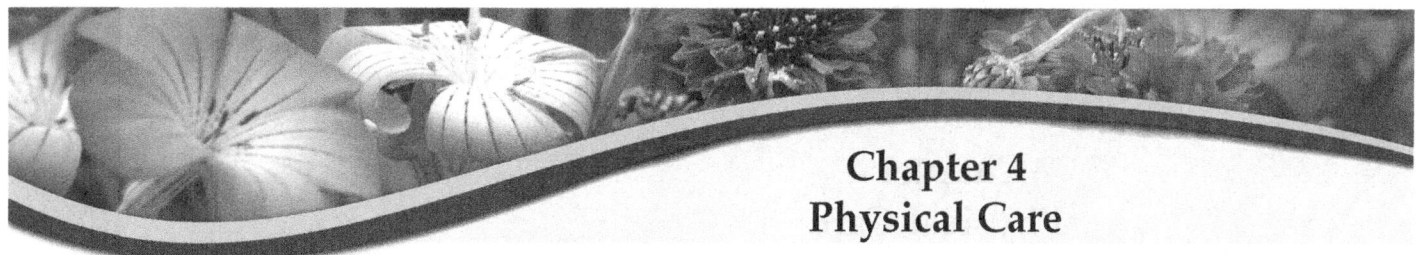

Chapter 4
Physical Care

The choices a patient (or their family if the patient is unconscious or confused) makes for a pain management regimen may be influenced by culture, family "rules", or some kind of atonement for their past "sins". In some cultures, enduring the pain is a sign of strength, endurance, and good character. If the person lived a lifestyle that they feel contributed to their current condition, they may find meaning in doing "penance" by experiencing pain now. If the patient chooses to "white knuckle it" through the pain, that is their choice and it must be honored as such. (Although a chaplain or social worker visit might help them work through the emotional and spiritual issues.)

If, however, the patient is tolerating pain because of fear of addiction to the pain medications, or misunderstanding the principles of pain management, intervention is needed to give them the information that will help them make educated choices about pain medication. The patient and family need to know that there is a difference between addiction to narcotics and tolerance to the drugs that requires increases in amount of medication to achieve the same level of relief.

Another block to effective pain management could be misunderstanding of the need for regular, scheduled doses of pain medication to "stay ahead of the pain." Once the pain builds up, the patient could go into a pain crisis in which it takes much more medication to get the pain controlled again. It is much more effective to keep an adequate, steady level of medication going and use "prn" (as needed) doses when pain spikes.

I describe this to families like this:

Our bodies, from the time we are born, have pain receptors to register the normal, everyday kinds of pain that happens (I stub my toe, I get a stomach ache, or I whack my shin on something.) Pain receptors are our friends. And our bodies produce natural opiates to bind off these pain receptors and relieve the pain.

The problem with cancer pain and pain that results from surgeries, chemo, and radiation, is that it is far more pain than our bodies can naturally handle. The opiates we use in pain management for hospice patients are very close to the body's natural opiates in structure and ability to "bind off" these extra pain receptors. The more pain receptors that need binding, the more medication is needed to bind them off. If we hit the "right " ratio, the patient experiences relief from the pain.

There are many things that can happen to increase the patient's need for medication. Progression of the disease, getting over-tired, having emotional, spiritual, or mental pain that exacerbates the physical pain, etc. Some times of day are more likely to be painful than others and some days are more difficult.

"Just the facts, please..."

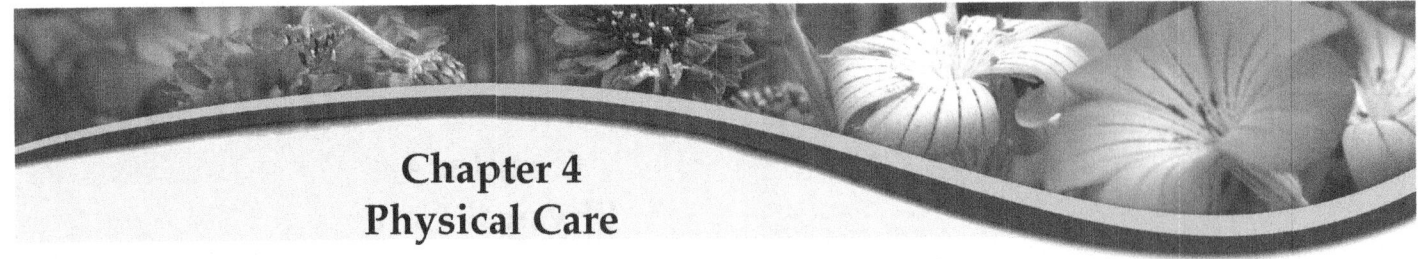

Chapter 4
Physical Care

So, I describe the patient's pain to be like a mountain range. There are low peaks and high peaks. Picture a blanket of clouds covering those mountain peaks. We try to keep the "blanket" of pain control at a steady state so it covers most of the peaks. This is done with a long acting pain medication. When the patient gets tired or something is happening in their body to increase their pain, a higher peak may poke up through the "blanket". This is when we use the short acting pain med to get the pain back under the "blanket."

Hospice nurses and physicians specialize in honing pain management to a science, with the help of the entire team. You, as the volunteer, can give valuable information as to how the patient is doing with their pain while you are there.

Occasionally, a patient will hoard medicine, acting like they are taking them, but really stashing them away, for fear that their pain will get worse later and they might not have enough medication to deal with it then. This is a situation that needs to be reported to the nurse right away. Of course the patient's pain regimen won't be effective if they aren't taking the medication as scheduled. And the patient's fear needs to be addressed by the appropriate team members to help the patient feel more safe with the process as his or her disease progresses.

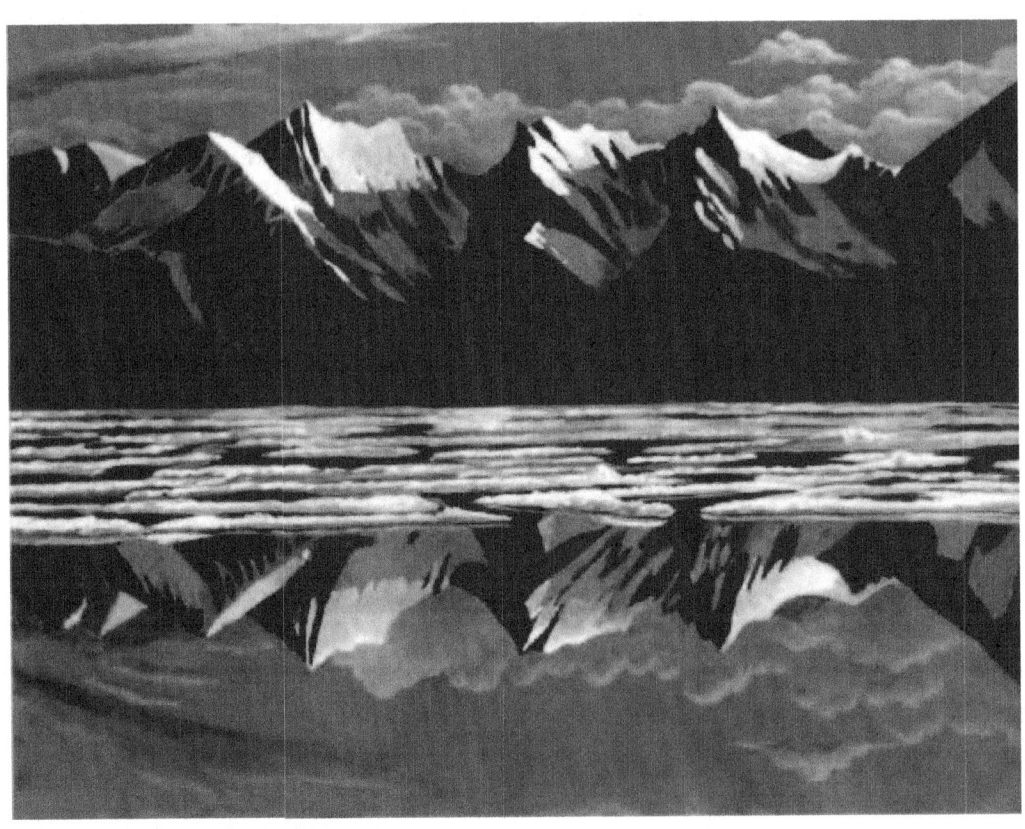

"Just the facts, please..."

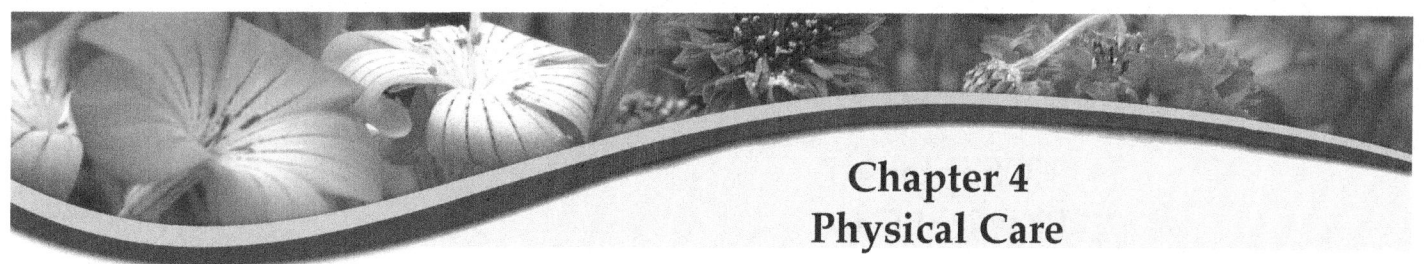

Chapter 4
Physical Care

In his wonderful little book on end of life care, written from a physician's perspective for his dying patients and their families, Dr. W. Brad Townsend says,

*"Fear is a natural and common reaction to the changes that will occur in your body as you die. As I have worked with patients, I have noticed that most of them fear not only death, but also the suffering and pain caused by their disease... Fear of death is one way in which we and our bodies express the will to live."**

Discuss: How can I help my patient deal with the fear of pain?

---

*Talk With Me About the End of Life, A Physician's Guiding Words, W. Brad Townsend, M.D., Roseburg, OR, 2009. Patients and families love this little 23 page book. Packed with beautiful illustrations and sensitively written in easy to understand language. I love it.

I've made it available at www.bordermountain.com in bulk quantities to give out to your hospice families. Or you can order them directly from Dr. Townsend at 1813 West Harvard, Suite 423, Roseburg, Oregon 97470.

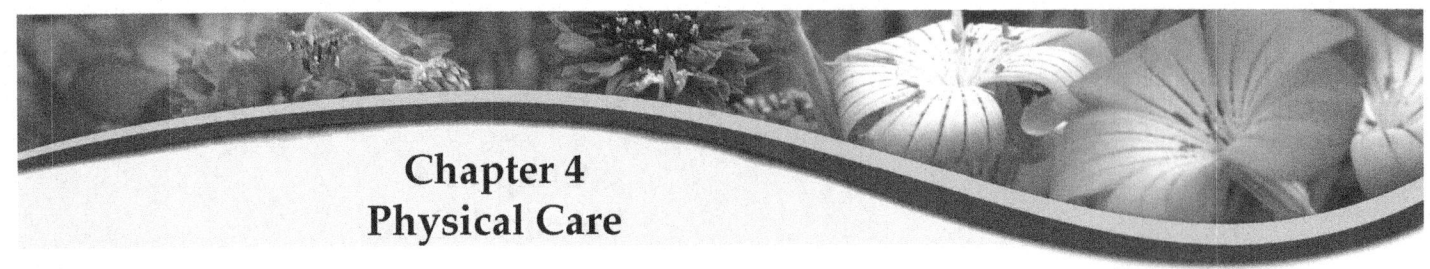

Chapter 4
Physical Care

 *At the Heart of the Matter*

Ask yourself the following questions. Think them through carefully then discuss them as a group or, if you are working on your own, write your answers in the spaces provided.

1. Do you think there is ever a time that pain could be beneficial to a person? Why or why not?

2. Have you ever experienced severe intractable pain for longer than a few days? What were the circumstances?

How did you cope?

Chapter 4
Physical Care

How did you view the pain?

How did you view those around you who were not in pain?

What impact did the pain have on your day-to-day life?

3. As used in the DVD animation sequence, "The Robber", what does the phrase "pain is a terrible landlord" mean to you?

4. Describe your feelings about taking care of someone who is in pain.

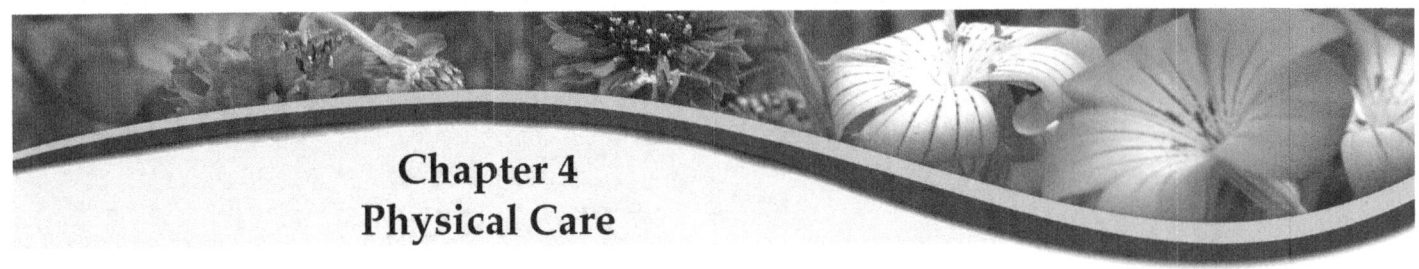

Chapter 4
Physical Care

 # Putting it Into Practice

How can you, as a caregiver, help relieve the physical suffering of a patient as their symptoms progress toward the end of their life? Here are some ideas:

- **Weakness and fatigue:**

Encourage the patient to plan activities carefully. Even a simple effort such as eating a meal can be exhausting when energy resources are limited. Work with the patient and family to ensure that the patient is getting adequate rest. Sometimes a sign on the door limiting visitors can be helpful, especially if it is signed by a member of the hospice team so family doesn't feel they are being ungracious to guests.

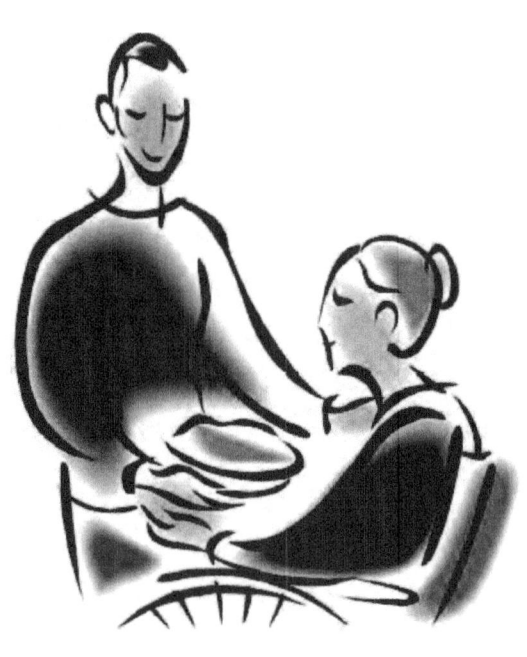

- **Loss of appetite (anorexia):**

Small, frequent meals are more easily tolerated by a patient with a poor appetite. It helps to use a small plate and limit portions, presenting them in an attractive way with garnishes and bright colors. Eat with the patient. It's amazing what a difference it can make to turn the meal into a social interaction rather than just another task to be performed.

Milkshakes made from powdered instant breakfast, with a scoop of ice cream and some frozen fruit added for richness and flavor, can sometimes tempt even the most flat appetite. They're also very nourishing. (Check first to be sure the patient doesn't have a sensitivity to milk products. Milk allergy is common and can cause uncomfortable symptoms that can be avoided with a little awareness and creativity. There are many great substitutes for dairy now available for those sensitive to milk.)

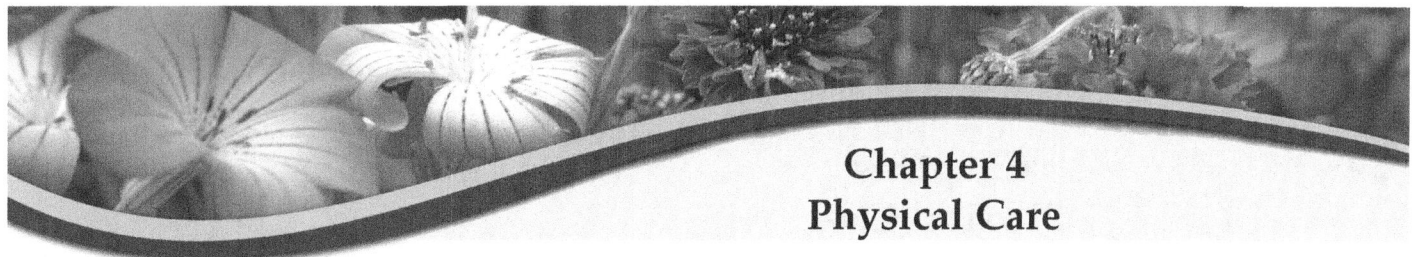

Chapter 4
Physical Care

- ## Nausea and vomiting:

Small, frequent meals help here, too. It is best not to leave the stomach empty. Cold beverages and soda crackers are sometimes soothing. Liquids are best taken between meals when they will not dilute the digestive juices needed to process food in the stomach efficiently. Encourage the patient to eat more foods when she feels better and avoid favorite foods during times of nausea. Generally, mornings are the best time of day. This may be the best time for her to eat her main meal. Encourage her to try resting or lying down after eating.

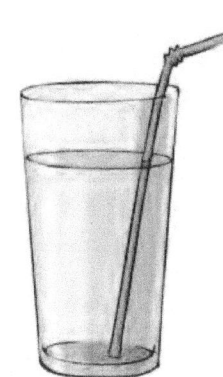

Limit the patient's exposure to foods with strong odors. Encourage the use of prescribed medications as needed (the doctor will probably prescribe Compazine or Phenergan suppositories. Ativan and Haldol sometimes help, too.)

- ## Constipation:

Increasing fluid intake helps. The hospice nurse will probably start the patient on a bowel management program that includes a natural vegetable laxative with a stool softener. If the patient hasn't had a bowel movement by the third day on this regimen, a laxative suppository will likely be given to him with one repeat dose if needed. If that doesn't work, the nurse will give an enema or do a manual removal of the stool in the rectal vault.

Narcotics affect bowel motility. With this slowing of bowel function, constipation is almost a sure thing without intervention. You can help by encouraging the patient to take medications as directed by the hospice nurse and encouraging fluid intake (as long as the patient is able to tolerate it).

- ## Diarrhea:

Encourage the patient to avoid foods high in roughage and fiber during the episode of diarrhea. She may also need to avoid milk products. Bananas help restore lost potassium, so it may be helpful to encourage her to eat them. Loose stools are not necessarily considered diarrhea unless they occur more than five or six times in a day's time. True diarrhea is treated with an anti-diarrheal such as Lomotil.

Putting it Into Practice

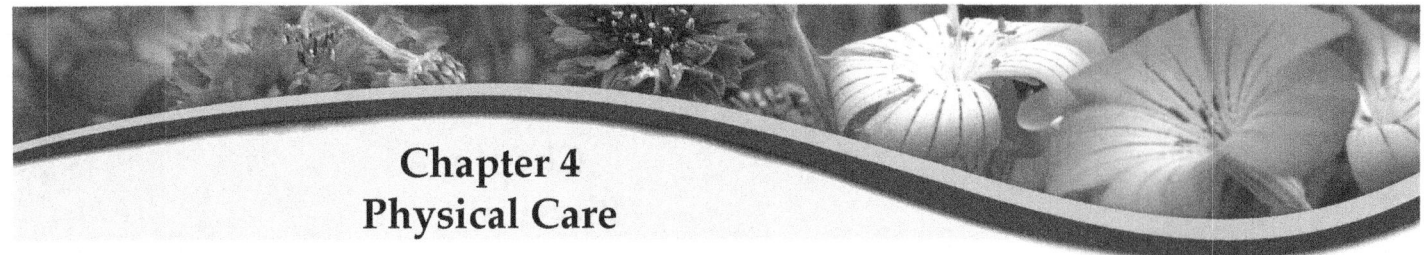

Chapter 4
Physical Care

- ## Incontinence:

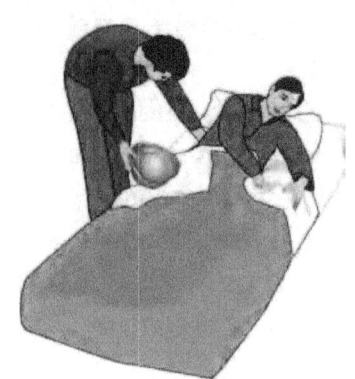

Cleanliness is important to help prevent skin breakdown when a patient is incontinent of bowel and/or bladder. Excellent perineal cleansing agents are available to keep this area clean and odor free. Bedding should be protected with disposable pads and these should be changed as soon as they are soiled.

If skin breakdown is a problem in spite of prompt changing of soiled linens, the nurse will probably ask the physician about inserting a catheter to protect the skin. Catheters increase the chance of a urinary tract infection, but in some cases the risks are outweighed by the benefits.

- ## Insomnia, anxiety, and depression:

It's important when dealing with insomnia and anxiety to find out what may be causing it. Is the patient experiencing increased pain at night? Are there unresolved issues that are running through his or her mind and preventing sleep? Are there lurking fears of death or abandonment? Is it harder for the patient to sleep lying down than sitting up in a chair because of breathing problems?

If you are aware of sleeping problems your patient may be having, bring it up to the care team. Medications may help, but rather than just masking the symptoms, it is important to find out what the root cause could be. Maybe a chaplain visit or a session with the social worker is in order. Relaxation techniques such as deep breathing, therapeutic touch, and massage can also be very helpful.

- ## Dry mouth:

Many medications cause dry mouth. This feeling of "chewing cotton" is very uncomfortable for the patient. Mouth swabs dipped in cool water and swirled around in the mouth can help. Sometimes sucking on ice chips or hard candy helps. Of course, it's important to keep fresh water available to the patient at all times.

Putting it Into Practice

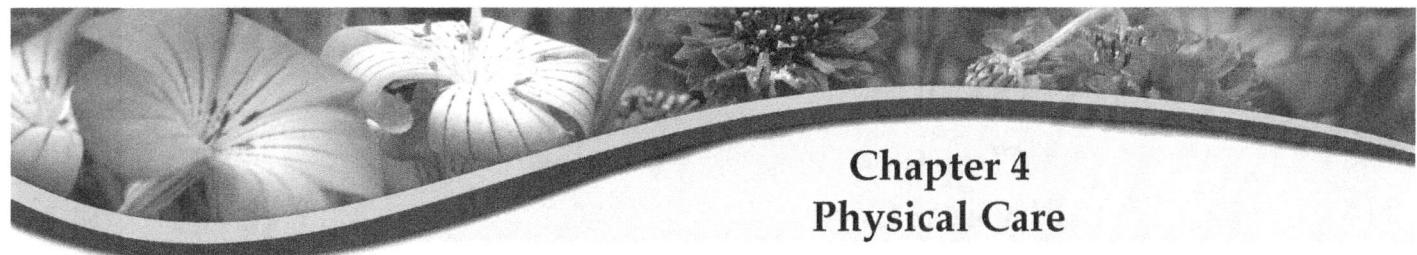

Chapter 4
Physical Care

- **Edema in the ankles, fluid in the abdomen:**

Ascites or fluid buildup in the abdomen is often caused by liver involvement or a protein deficiency because of advancing cancer. Congestive heart failure causes swelling (edema) in the ankles and lower legs. Decreasing salt intake helps, as does keeping the legs elevated above the level of the heart. For the patient with ascites, the semi-sitting position is usually the most comfortable.

Diuretics can sometimes help reduce swelling in the lower extremities, but very little will help reduce the fluid in the abdomen. The physician may tap off a quart or two of fluid from the peritoneal cavity, but the fluid usually returns quickly, making the actual value of the procedure very questionable.

Fluid can also build up progressively in the ankles, then legs, then sacral area, hips, abdomen and finally lungs when the body is in "**fluid overload**". This happens if the patient's body is shutting down in the final stages of life.

The natural progression of the body's functions at this time is to begin to shut down the less necessary functions and focus on the core body organs, such as the heart and lungs and liver. **Loss of appetite** is often one of the signs that the body is shutting down and "asking" for less nutrition. There is, in fact, plenty of nutrition available in the body's own cells for this last phase of life and the patient can quite comfortably go without much food or fluid at all for days and even weeks.

The tragedy occurs when this phase of life is misunderstood by medical personnel and the family is led to believe that a **feeding tube** and **IVs** will help keep the patient more comfortable. The fact is, pushing food and fluids through these invasive means can force the patient's body into fluid overload, characterized by progressively increasing **edema, lung congestion, nausea, vomiting** and **pain**.

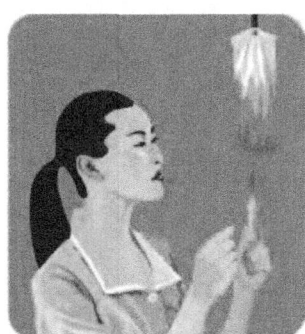

The patient's body can't use the excess food and fluid, so it isn't helping at all. Instead it is causing harm and greatly reducing the patient's quality of life at a time when he or she needs to focus energy on important tasks of closure. Family members need to be supported in their decision to respect the patient's wishes not to be **force-fed** when the patient is no longer able to eat or drink. Sometimes they may need extra reassurance that they are doing the loving thing, not the cruel thing.

Putting it Into Practice

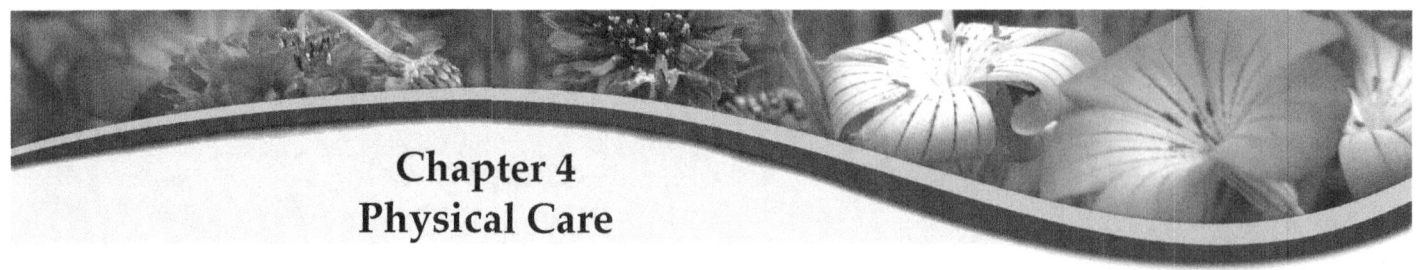

Chapter 4
Physical Care

- **Skin breakdown:**

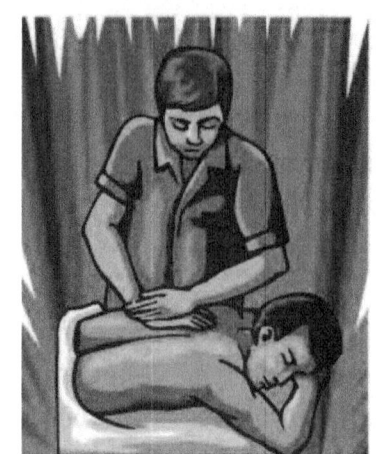

Besides keeping the patient's skin scrupulously clean, the best thing that can be done to prevent skin breakdown is to make sure the patient's position is changed at least every two hours. Try an experiment. Touch a fingertip of one hand to the skin on the back of the other hand. Apply very light pressure for a few seconds, then release the pressure. Do you see the white spot left for an instant on the back of your hand even from very light pressure?

The tiny **capillaries** that feed the skin are very fragile and easily collapsed. Tissue can tolerate having its blood supply cut off for an hour

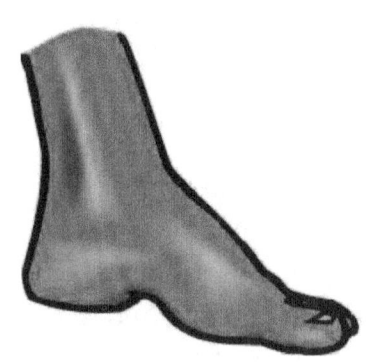

or so without damage, but if the time is extended past two hours, the tissue starts to die from the inside out. Bony prominences such as knees, elbows, shoulder blades, ankles, heels, and hips are especially susceptible because they lack the padding that can protect other skin areas.

If the patient is in bed a lot, make sure you pick the feet all the way up and look up under the heels to find the beginnings of skin breakdown. This is a notorious place for **decubitus** ulcers to form and deepen without being discovered until they are advanced enough to bleed on the bedding. Special booties that protect heels from pressure can help prevent this from happening. An ounce of prevention, in this case, is worth ten pounds of cure.

Another place to watch for breakdown is the backs of the ears. Breakdown will start as a discolored spot and the patient may complain of soreness in the area. Special dressings can help. Staying aware of positioning and keeping pressure from the area with frequent turning is the best way to prevent this type of breakdown.

It is important when positioning a patient in bed to avoid **"shearing" pressure**, where skin is pulled in one direction and the patient in another. This action is a major contributor to skin breakdown. Another contributor is the presence of crumbs or wrinkles in the sheets under the patient. Wet skin is more fragile than dry skin, so allowing the patient to lie on wet bedding will increase the chances of breakdown.

Putting it Into Practice

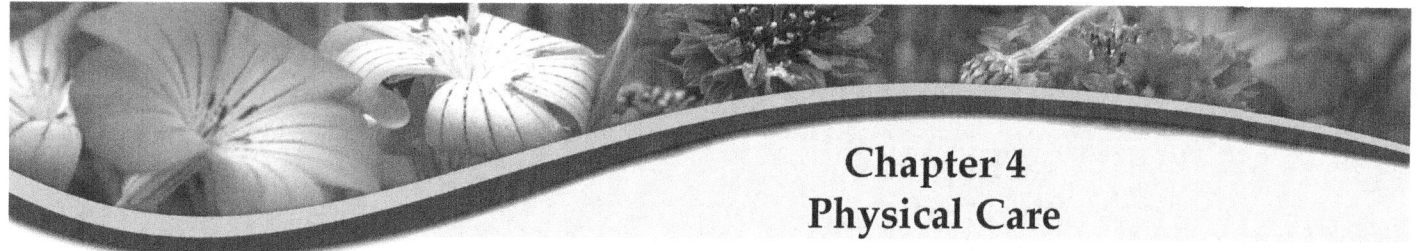

Chapter 4
Physical Care

- **Shortness of breath:**

Respiratory problems are the most common causes of shortness of breath, although cardiac episodes and general debilitation can also cause it.

It is helpful when dealing with a patient who experiences shortness of breath to keep needed objects close by, to plan activities in such a way as to conserve energy, to help the patient maintain a semi-sitting position even when resting, and to administer oxygen as needed.

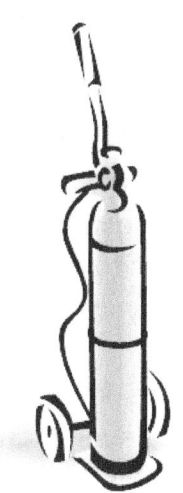

Sometimes, with a patient with **COPD (chronic obstructive pulmonary disease)** a fan blowing directly into the patient's face helps him feel that he is getting more "air." The respiratory distress that accompanies end stage respiratory disease often requires an anti-anxiety in addition to other medications for breathing.

- **Seizures:**

Seizure activity is fairly common with brain tumors, so it is important when caring for patients with brain involvement that you are comfortable with what to do when a seizure occurs. If the patient is in bed all the time and seizures are a common occurrence, chances are the hospice nurse has already shown the family how to pad the bed rails to protect the patient from injury during the seizure. If the patient is ambulatory and slumps to the floor, just be sure objects that might cause injury are moved out of the way. Loosen any tight clothing that might restrict movement. **DO NOT PUT ANYTHING IN THE PATIENT'S MOUTH, ESPECIALLY YOUR FINGERS.** If the patient chokes on emesis (vomit), turn him over on his side to let the fluids drain out.

It is important to check the time and call the nurse as soon as a seizure starts. Sometimes seizure activity can continue into a condition called "status epilepticus" which is actually a series of seizures that won't stop. The nurse, with doctor's orders, will know what medicines to give the patient to stop the seizures (usually an injection of Valium).

Putting it Into Practice

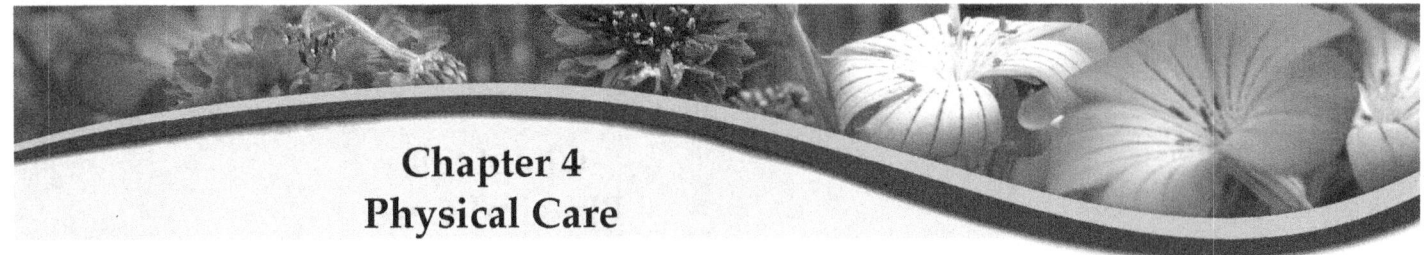

Chapter 4
Physical Care

- **Difficulty swallowing:**

Patients who have difficulty swallowing should avoid milk as it tends to be mucous producing. For some reason, liquids that have color are more easily swallowed. Warm liquids are easier to swallow than cold. Slippery foods such as Jell-O and custards should be avoided.

The speech therapist or occupational therapist, who deals with swallowing issues, may recommend thickeners to add to liquids to make them easier to swallow. He or she will also teach the patient and family ways to position the head and neck to facilitate swallowing.

At some point in the progression of the disease process, usually very close to death, most hospice patients develop an inability to swallow. This is the body's signal that it cannot tolerate any more nutritional intake. (Refer back to section on edema.)

Notes:

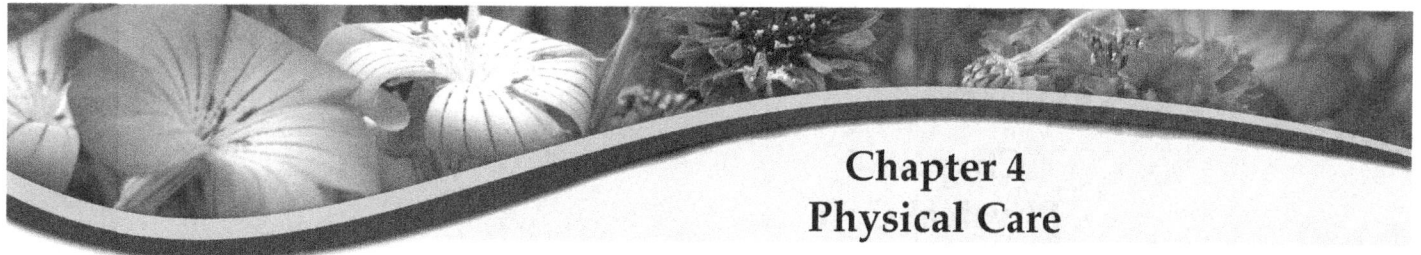

Chapter 4
Physical Care

The dietician acts as a resource in the area of nutrition. Here are some dietician's tips concerning nutrition in the terminal patient:

Foods that may help reduce nausea:

Salty foods
Popsicles
Soda crackers
Carbonated beverages
Mints
Ice cubes made of apple juice
Clear soup
Dry toast
Pretzels
Fruit-flavored gelatin

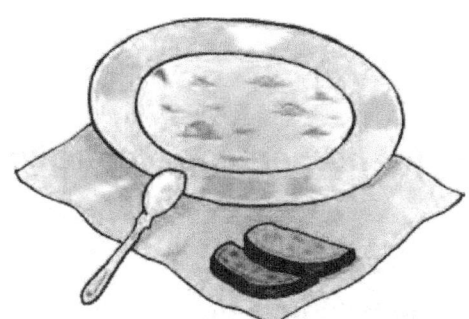

Foods that may contribute to nausea:

Very sweet foods
Spicy foods
Hot foods
Greasy foods
Smelly foods
Fried foods
Acidic foods
Ice cold foods

Putting it Into Practice

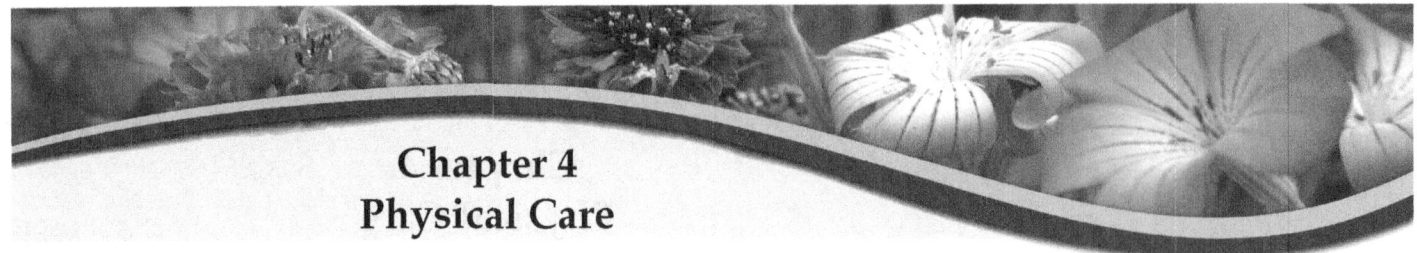

Chapter 4
Physical Care

To increase fluid intake:

- Disguise fluids in food form such as gelatin, ice milk, ice cream, and watermelon.
- Drink fluids in small amounts throughout the day. Dilute juices with water or ice. Try drinks with carbonation such as ginger ale.
- Avoid caffeinated beverages because the caffeine causes the body to lose fluid faster.

Recipe for homemade electrolyte replacement:

1 teaspoon salt
1 teaspoon baking soda
4 teaspoons corn syrup
1 six ounce can orange juice concentrate

Mix all ingredients together. Add water until you have one quart of liquid. Refrigerate in a closed container. Shake well before using. (Keeps up to two weeks if kept cold).

Tips to treat a sore mouth and throat:

Add extra fluids to stews, casseroles, and simmered foods
Blend ice into milk and milk shakes
Chop or blenderize food to change the consistency, not the flavor.
Drink blenderized foods from a cup
Moisten dry foods in liquids (crackers in soup, toast in cocoa)
Use sauces and gravies on meats and vegetables

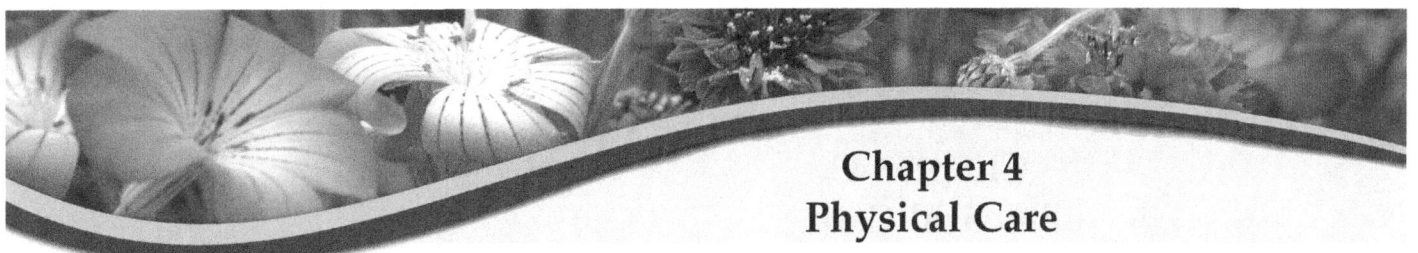

Chapter 4
Physical Care

Foods that may be less irritating to a sore mouth or throat:

- Applesauce
- Sherbet
- Cold fluids
- Cream soups
- Cooked cereal
- Yogurt
- Custard or pudding
- Eggs
- Low acid fruits such as pears and bananas
- Gelatin

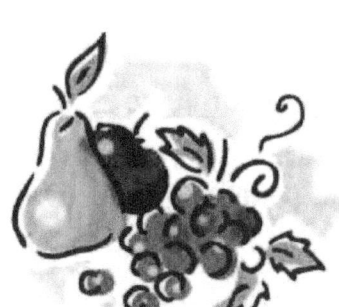

A Great Bowel Care Recipe:

1 cup applesauce
3/4 cup prune juice
1 cup unprocessed wheat bran
Mix together and store in a small container. Have patient eat one tablespoonful daily, drinking plenty of water afterwards and spaced through out the day. (Not recommended for patient's on limited fluid intake.)

Laxative Tea:

4 tablespoons of Senna leaves
1 1/2 tablespoons of Elder flowers
1 tablespoon of Fennel seeds
1 teaspoon of Anise
Pour 1 cup of boiling water over 1 teaspoon of mixture. Steep and strain. Have the patient drink 1 cup in the morning and one at night (with doctor's approval.)

Putting it Into Practice

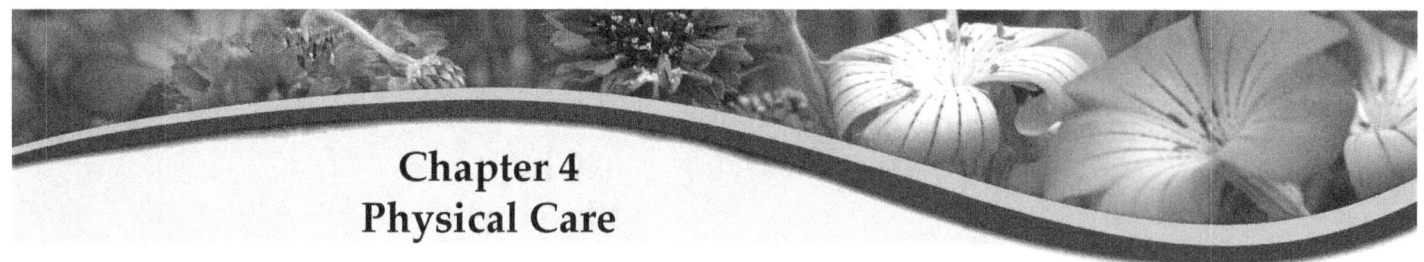

Chapter 4
Physical Care

Morning Laxative:

3/4 teaspoon salt
1 cup of hot water
Three tablespoonfuls of lemon juice

Mix together and drink. (Only with approval of a physician.)

Morning Orange Juice - Flax Laxative:

Boil two tablespoons of flax seed in three quarts of water and let cool. Store in the refrigerator. Each morning add two ounces to orange juice and mix with flax. Drink a glass every morning. (Only with the approval of a physician.)

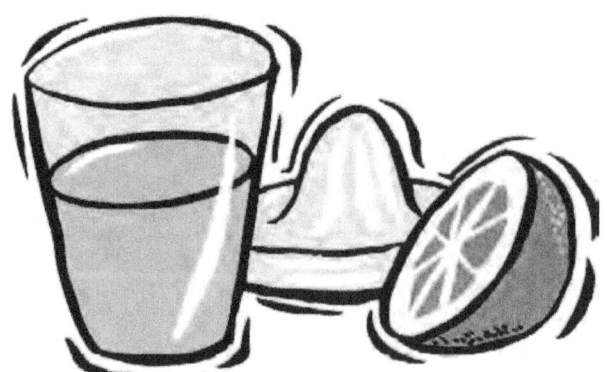

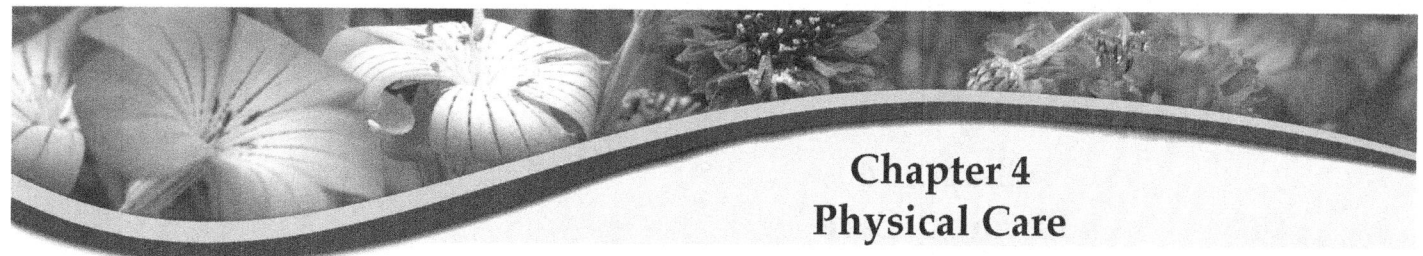

Chapter 4
Physical Care

Caring for the AIDS Patient

Caring for AIDS patients who are dying can require special sensitivity because there is still a lot of social stigma attached to the disease. Many people fear even being in the same room with someone who has AIDS. It's important to examine your own fears and beliefs about this disease and to learn everything you can about it so you will be able to provide care to the AIDS patient with genuine comfort and compassion.

Here are some basic principles to remember when caring for an AIDS patient:

1. There is no evidence to date that AIDS is transmitted in any way other than through sexual contact, through blood, or from mother to unborn child.

2. Universal Precautions (which apply when caring for any patient including those with AIDS) call for: gloves when handling any bodily fluids, mask when the patient is coughing or any secretions may become airborne, gown and eye protection when there is any danger of splashing bodily fluids, and meticulous hand washing before and after touching the patient, even if you were wearing gloves.

3. If you have an open skin lesion or a draining sore, refrain from direct contact with the patient.

4. Be very careful not to bring infections to your patient. If you have any kind of infection, respiratory or any other, stay away until you are completely well. AIDS patients are susceptible to fungal, viral, and bacterial infections because of their depressed immune systems.

5. Don't be afraid to touch. AIDS patients are just people who have a terrible disease that is killing them. They need caring touch as much as any other human being does.

Putting it Into Practice

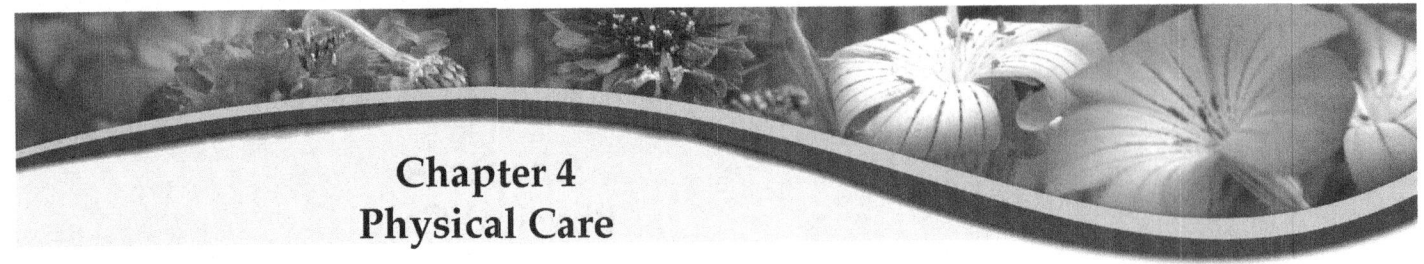

Chapter 4
Physical Care

Medical Marijuana

The use of medical marijuana in the treatment of pain, nausea, anorexia and cachexia has been controversial at best because of a long history of fear and misinformation about it. Because of a growing body of research, however, that demonstrates its effectiveness in treating symptoms, many states have now legalized it.

The states that have legalized marijuana for medical use regulate who may use it and how it can be distributed. Designated dispensaries in many states distribute different forms of medical marijuana and provide education in using it for their condition.

It is still illegal at the federal level, though and because there is a discrepancy between state and federal law, people could still be arrested and charged with possession in a state where medical marijuana is legal. At the time of printing of this manual, the US Attorney General Sessions just revoked the Cole Memorandum, which had provided protection from federal prosecution in states voting to allow medical or recreational marijuana use. Considering the many potential benefits of using medical marijuana to alleviate hospice patient symptoms, it would be well worth the time to investigate the current status of legal use of marijuana in your state.

Some states have approved growing industrial hemp (a genetic strain of the marijuana cannabis sativa plant that yields very low amounts of the psychactive ingredient THC) under controlled circumstances. This hemp can be processed in several ways to produce CBD oil and other CBD products. The industrial hemp CBD provides many of the beneficial marijuana health benefits without any psychoactive effects. Depending upon the processing methods, many of the beneficial turpenes and antioxidants in industrial hemp can be retained in the hemp CBD oils and other products. Properly prepared, hemp CBD products may have significant pain control and anti-seizure properties. Note that product labeling is confusing as many hemp products are marketed as "hemp oil", which is made from hemp seeds, which have no CBD content at all. Unless purchasing "hemp CBD oil" with a declared amount of mg of CBD, patients may not be receiving any benefit of CBD from their hemp product.

At this time hemp CBD is not legally considered marijuana, and can legally be transported between and used in all states. However, the laws concerning hemp and marijuana are certainly volatile and may change at any time.

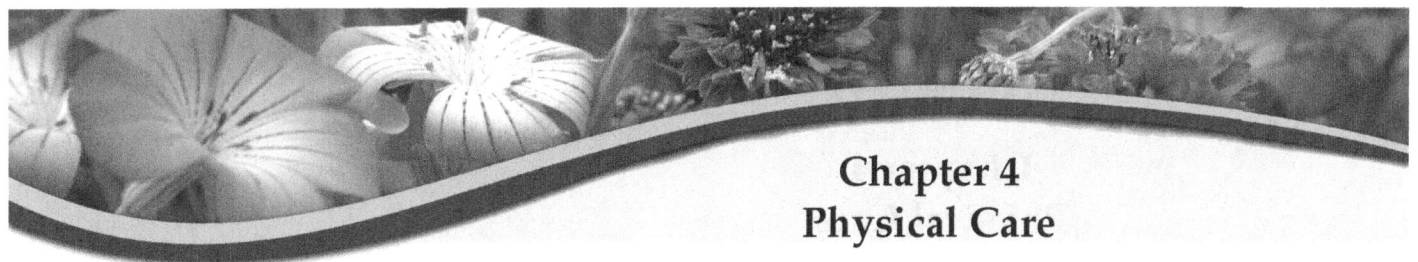

Chapter 4
Physical Care

Marijuana is made from the dried buds and leaves of various strains of the Cannabis sativa plant that are bred specifically for high content of psychoactive THC. There are a variety of ways it can be taken, including inhaling it as a vapor, adding it to food or tea, or smoking it. Cannabis oil can be rubbed on externally or taken internally.

Dronabinol (Marinol, Syndros) and nabilone (Cesamet) are drugs made from synthetic forms of the ingredients in marijuana. Some people find relief from them and others say that the synthetics are not as effective as the real plant.

Some of the conditions or diagnoses that medical marijuana has been demonstrated to help relieve are:

- Chronic Pain
- Nausea
- Vomiting
- Severe wasting associated with cancer treatments
- Anorexia due to cancer or HIV/AIDS
- Muscle spasms
- Crohn's disease
- Epilepsy or seizures
- Multiple Sclerosis
- Amyotrophic lateral sclerosis (ALS)

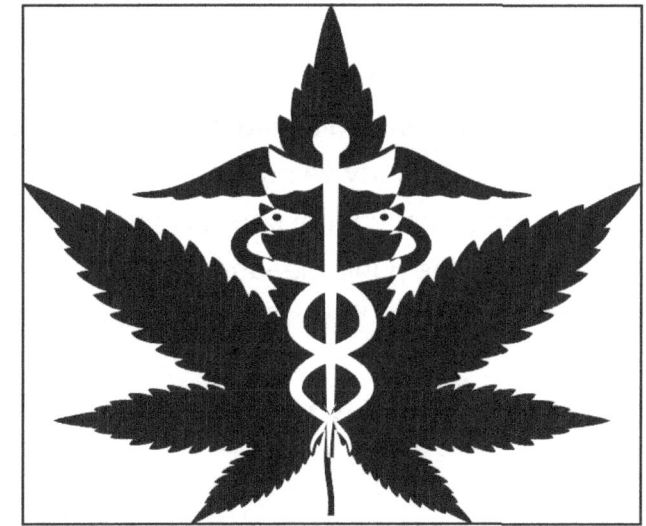

While it is unlikely that your patient will have medical marijuana prescribed by hospice, it is very likely that they will have obtained it from another source and be using it to treat their symptoms. Becoming educated about it and maintaining a non-judgmental stance toward your patient's use of it is an important part of creating a safe, supportive atmosphere for providing care.

*More information can be found about the use of medical marijuana on the Mayo Clinic, the Arizona Department of Health Services, and the Minnesota Department of Health websites.

Putting it Into Practice

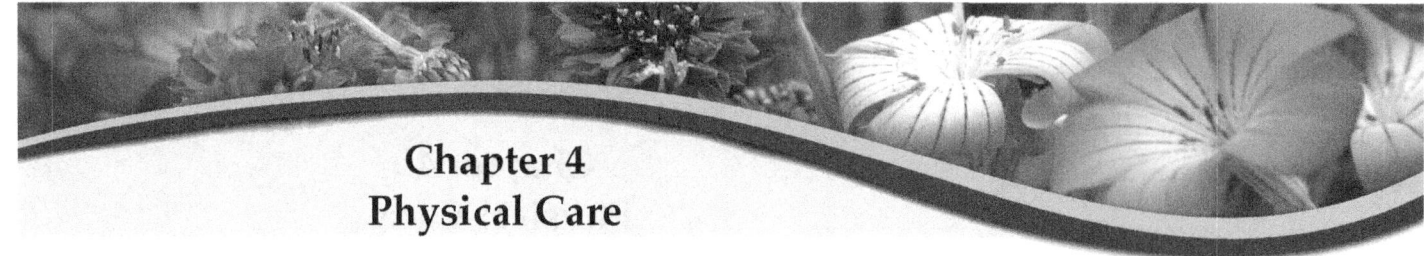

Chapter 4
Physical Care

Infection Control

It's hard to believe that infection control in health care is only about sixty years old. In the early 1950's a severe outbreak of Staph infections prompted health care workers in England to approach infection control in a whole new way. Guidelines to prevent the spread of infection were recommended and carried out in health care settings.

To implement infection control everyone needed to be on the same page as far as understanding how infection was spread. In 1969, V.W. Greene published Microbiological Contamination Control in Hospitals, a series of articles that identified six links necessary to spread infection.

With all the attention that has been placed in recent years on the spread of infectious illnesses such as avian flu, swine flu, and an upswing in tuberculosis cases, these six links are as applicable today as they were forty years ago. Almost every office waiting area, grocery store, and restaurant today provide a container of sanitizing hand gel or lotion for patrons to use. Every care team member interacting with the public needs to know these links and the techniques they can use to prevent the spread of infection, to themselves or to others they come in contact with.

The six links necessary to spread infection are:

1. An *infectious agent* such as bacteria or a virus that can cause an infection.

2. A *place* for the bacteria or virus to lurk. These places can include equipment used to care for patients, the health care provider's or family member's hands, items in a room that an infectious person has had contact with, etc.

3. An *exit point* from the place where the germs are harbored.

4. A *method of transmitting* the germs from their lurking place through the exit point and to the person being infected. (Human hands serve as the most effective method for transferring germs!)

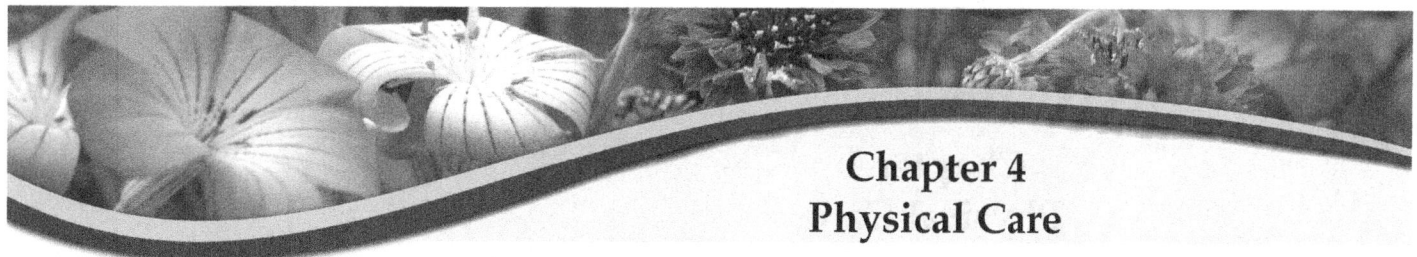

Chapter 4
Physical Care

5. An *entry point* into the person being infected. This could be through the lungs, through the eyes (rubbing eyes with contaminated hands is a great way to help germs enter the body), through a break in the skin, through nose tissue, or through the mouth or other body orifice.

6. A *susceptible person*. The very old and the very young are the most susceptible to infection, as are those on corticosteroids or antibiotics. Patients who've had surgery, foley catheterizations, or respiratory infections are highly susceptible to infection and of course, anyone with a terminal illness is especially at risk.

The removal of just one of these links is all that is necessary to stop the spread of infection. The easiest to link to break is the "method of transmitting " **link**.

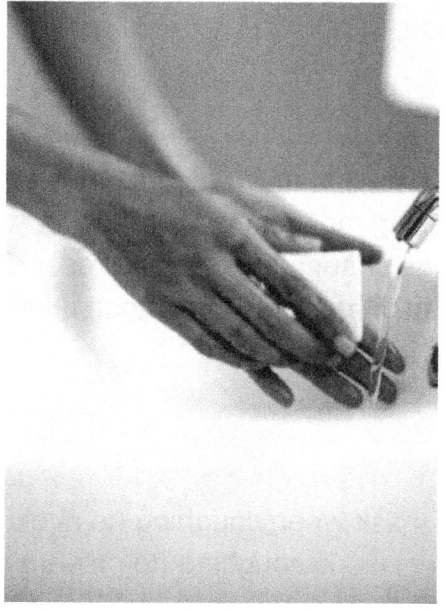

> **Good hand washing
> is the single most important action
> you can take to
> break the chain of germ
> transmission in all care settings,
> including the home.**

Putting it Into Practice

Chapter 4
Physical Care

Techniques That Limit the Spread of Infection

1. Hand washing

It is very important to always wash your hands before and after every contact with a patient or family member, whether it is in a healthcare setting or in the home. No other action is as effective in preventing the spread of germs as this simple principle. Scrub for a full 20 seconds. Make sure you dry your hands with a paper towel or a hand towel that has not previously been used. Use the paper towel to turn off the faucet to avoid picking up the germs left there when the water was first turned on (or from others who have used the same sink.)

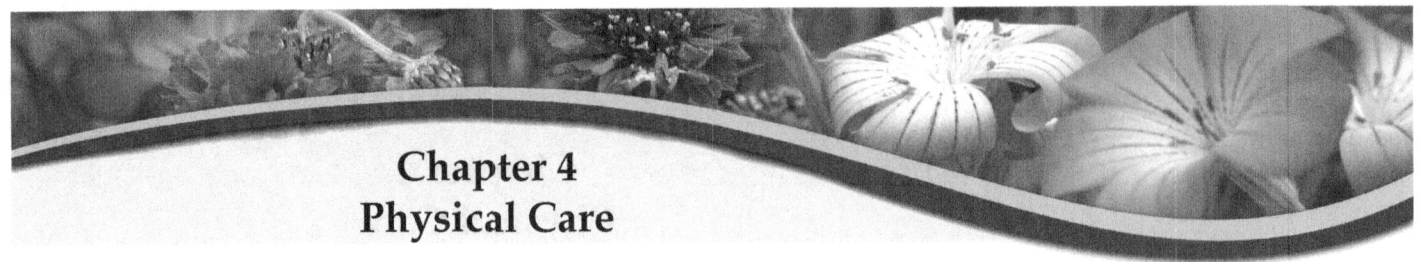

2. Gloves

Always wear gloves when touching items that may be contaminated with any kind of body fluids, when touching mucous membranes, or when emptying fluid drainage containers such as urinary catheter bags or suctions machine reservoirs. Wear gloves when cleaning surfaces of any kind of contamination such as incontinent stool, urine, or emesis. And always wash your hands immediately after removing your gloves.

3. Masks/gowns/goggles

All care team members must wear a mask when coughing (to avoid spreading airborne germs to others) and when working with a patient who is coughing (to prevent inhaling the patient's germs). Wear goggles, gowns, and gloves when there's a chance that blood or other body fluids could be splashed or sprayed into the air.

4. Good sanitation practices

If you are a care team member working in a health care setting, do not place bed linens, clean or dirty, on the floor. Bag dirty linens immediately where they are removed. Don't sort them in the patient care area. Keep urinals and bed pans away from the surfaces where food and mouth care items are placed (a bedside table.)

Putting it Into Practice

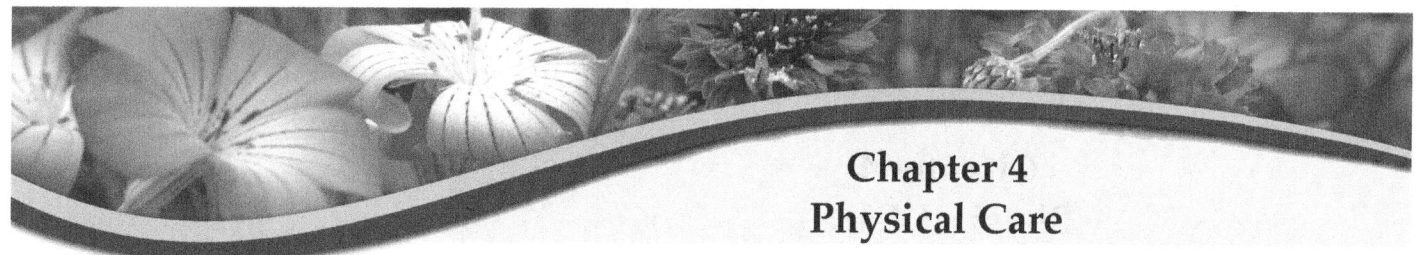

Chapter 4
Physical Care

5. Disposing of hazardous waste safely and using caution with hazardous materials

If you will be exposed to any kind of sharps or other hazardous materials, be sure you know how to dispose of them properly. Needles should NOT be recapped, bent, or broken, but placed immediately into a puncture-proof container. Do not try to jam a needle into an already full container. Cleaning supplies can cause damage to respiratory tissue or to skin. Make sure the area in which you are working is well-ventilated. Always use gloves when handling toxic chemicals. Make sure all containers that contain these chemicals are clearly labeled and stored out of reach of children or adults with vision problems, or those who may not be able to read the label.

6. Safety with food

Make sure that hot food is served hot and cold food is served cold. Harmful bacteria can grow in food if it is not kept at the appropriate temperature . All cooked food has the potential for transmitting harmful bacteria if it is not cooked at a high enough temperature. Don't keep leftovers in the office refrigerator for longer than three days. Mark all food with the purchase or preparation date so all will know how long it has been stored in the refrigerator, to avoid the danger of food poisoning.

7. Maintaining a strong immune system

The best thing you can do to prevent the spread of infection is to maintain a healthy immune system. Important ways to do this are with a balanced diet (80% of your nutrition from alkaline foods such as fresh fruits and vegetables and 20% from acid foods such as nuts, grains, and lean meats to maintain a healthy acid/alkaline balance in your body), adequate rest, eight to twelve glasses of water a day (not soda or sugary fruit juices which create a highly acidic state in the body and suppress the immune system), and limited stress. These allow your body to fight off potential infections and prevent you from becoming a carrier of germs to your clients and coworkers.

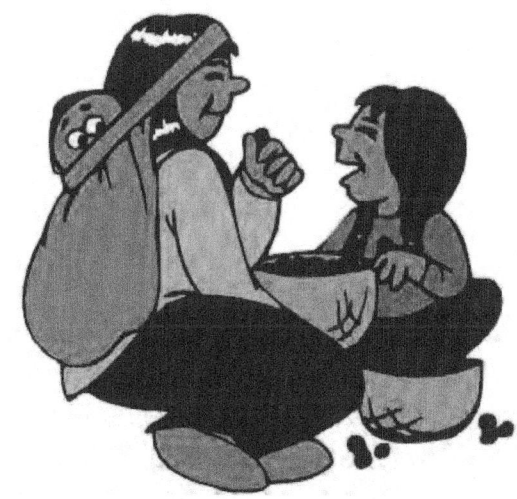

Putting it Into Practice

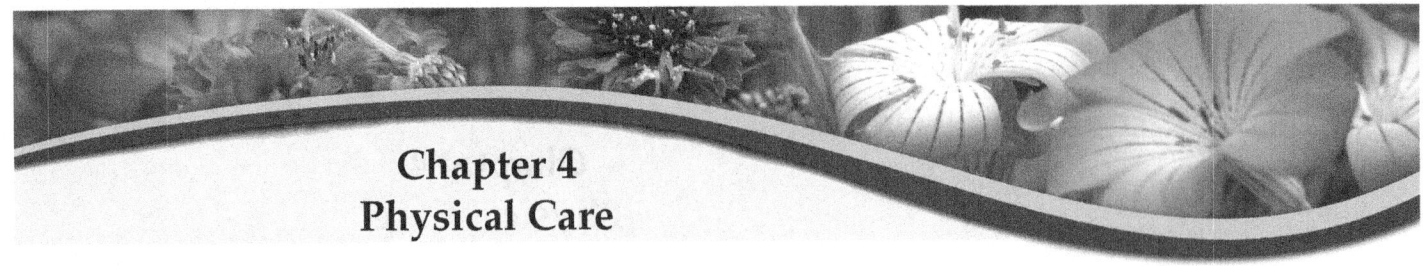

**Chapter 4
Physical Care**

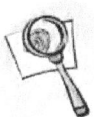 A Closer Look

The medical director, the team member ultimately responsible for the patient's physical care, attends team meetings to receive updates on the condition of each patient and offer direction to the team in providing physical care. He or she is also available between meetings to make recommendations concerning medications and treatments as the patient's condition changes.

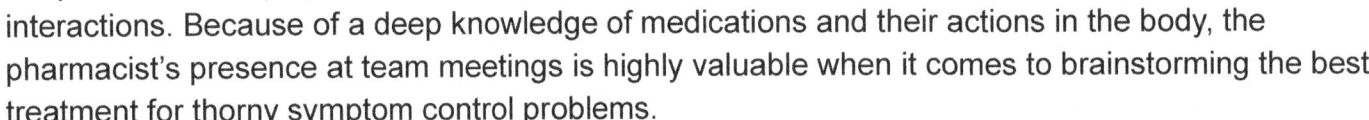

The pharmacist acts as a resource to care team members, recommending medications that may be most effective for the patient and staying alert for signs of untoward medication interactions. Because of a deep knowledge of medications and their actions in the body, the pharmacist's presence at team meetings is highly valuable when it comes to brainstorming the best treatment for thorny symptom control problems.

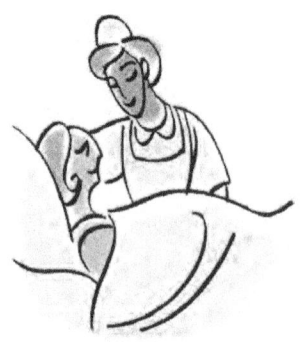

The nurse is in many ways the backbone of the care team. It is usually the nurse that does the initial assessment and provides direction to the rest of the team as to how to proceed with the patient's care. Whenever the nurse visits your patient and his or her family, you will notice that he or she is continually scanning the environment, watching for clues that will help provide the best possible symptom control for the patient.

The nurse's responsibilities include supervising the nursing assistants, assessing the patient for pain and other untoward symptoms, and developing and continually updating a care plan that addresses any problems the patient might be having.

The nursing assistant provides personal care based on the care plan developed by the nurse. Duties may include bathing, range-of-motion exercises to maintain flexibility, shaving, shampooing and combing hair, changing linens, light housekeeping chores, and simple food preparation. Often, the nursing assistant is the first to notice uncontrolled pain, skin breakdown, or other symptoms because he or she is so close to the patient.

Chapter 4
Physical Care

There are lots of practical ways that you can help relieve the physical symptoms caused by the progression of your patient's disease process.

To be forewarned is to be forearmed is an old saying that applies here perfectly. What do you need to know about your patient to be able to provide support to them and to the family in a knowledgeable way? This information will be provided to you by your volunteer coordinator before your first visit.

- Patients name, gender, age, diagnosis, and history

- Do they speak a language other than English? Is he or she a veteran? Is there any abuse in their history?

- Does the patient have any communicable diseases that require special precautions, such as AIDS or MRSA (drug resistant bacterial infection)?

- Are they in a facility or at home? (Address, directions, special information about parking, etc.)

- Which hospice team members are visiting the patient?

- Level of responsiveness. Are they fully conscious? Drowsy or confused? Comatose?

- Any special needs such as walker, wheelchair, bedside commode, hearing aides

- Can they see? How well can they hear?

- Do they have any special equipment in place? IV pump, medication pump (CADD), oxygen concentrator or tanks?

- What is their nutritional status? Eating? Drinking? Feeding tube? Able to swallow? Dietary restrictions?

- What family members are present in the home (or, if the patient is in a facility, regularly visit)?

- Are there young children in the picture?

A Closer Look

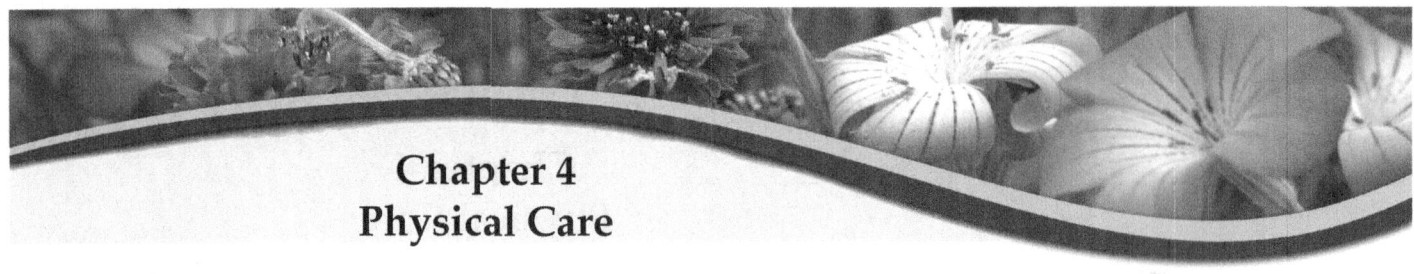

Chapter 4
Physical Care

A Volunteer Survival Kit

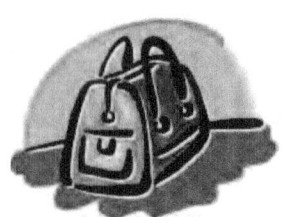

A small travel bag that contains:

- *A toothbrush and toothpaste*
- *Hand sanitizer*
- *A comb*
- *Chap stick or lip gloss*
- *Mini deodorant*
- *Baby wipes*
- *Fingernail clippers and an Emory board*
- *Lotion (for you, not the patient. Only use their lotion on them.)*
- *A change of underwear*
- *A whistle (for safety in parking lots, etc.)*
- *CDs for playing music for your patient if appropriate*
- *Coloring book and crayons for children present*
- *A book to read at the bedside when sitting for long periods– this gives the patient the privacy to sleep or do what they need to*
- *Note pad and pen for taking notes on your visit as things happen (don't rely on memory. Things could get hectic and you may forget important details to report back to the team.)*
- *A watch to keep track of and note the times of significant occurrences*
- *A small stuffed animal, if your patient is restless - this gives the patient something to do with their hands*

> Remember to dress comfortably with shoes that are not only supportive, but easy to slip off in a "no shoe" household. Dressing in layers works best as many homes or facilities can be very cool or very warm. Layers allow you to adjust your own comfort level regardless of the temperature.

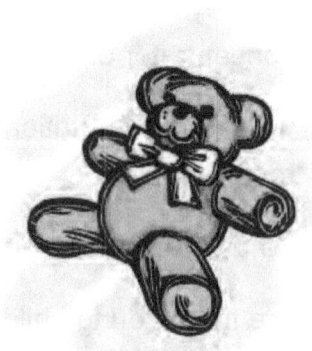

A Closer Look

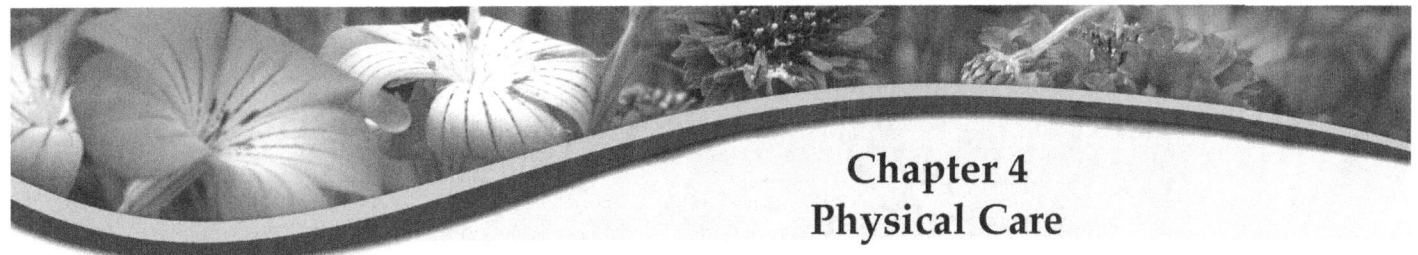

Chapter 4
Physical Care

Because you, as the volunteer, will be one of the closest team members to the patient and family, having built a foundation of trust with them, it is very possible that the patient will choose to die while you are there. Familiarize yourself with the changes you will see in the patient as he or she approaches death.

As in any of the previous stages, what the patient and family need most from you at this time is your mindful presence. Keep in touch with the hospice team as things change. It is likely that several of them will be there with you now, especially the nurse and the chaplain (if the patient has a relationship with the chaplain already).

Signs That Your Patient May Be Beginning the Active Dying Process

- **The patient will have a tendency to sleep more**

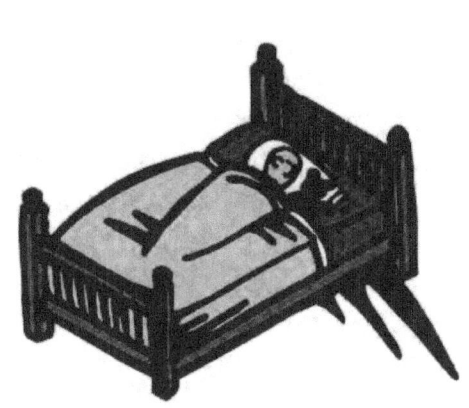

As the patient gets closer to the end of life, they may start sleeping more and more and be harder to arouse when they have been asleep. It takes a lot of energy for the body to fight the disease. Changes are also occurring in the patient's metabolism that cause drowsiness. This is normal.

- **You may see periods of confusion and withdrawal**

It can be very difficult for family and friends to see the patient lose interest in things that he or she was once passionate about and begin to withdraw. The patient may completely withdraw from loved ones, too. It's easy for family members to take this personally and be hurt by what seems to be a rejection of them on the part of the patient. Reassure them that it is not. This is a natural part of the process as the patient "lets go" of this life and prepares to transition to the next.

If they are restless and fidgeting, place something in their hands to feel. Stuffed animals work well for this. It can be very comforting to touch something soft.

A Closer Look

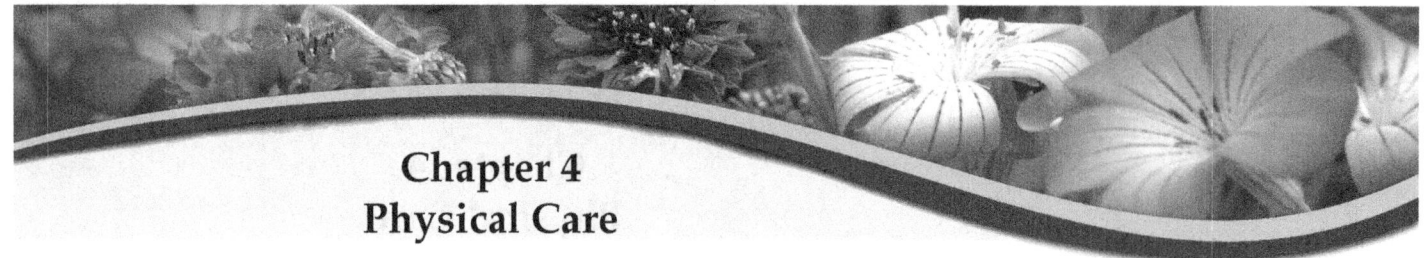

Chapter 4
Physical Care

- **Decreased appetite/thirst**

As the body begins to shut down and concentrate its energy on the internal organs, the urge for food and fluids will decrease and the patient will start refusing to eat or drink more than a few sips or bites at a time (and these usually to please an anxious family member urging them to eat.)

The patient isn't suffering from hunger at this point. In fact, as the body shuts down its systems one by one, it is no longer able to process food and fluids. Forcing them, via IVs or feeding tubes, just causes nausea, vomiting, edema in the body, and fluid to build up in the lungs. This increases discomfort and creates a great distraction for the patient as they are trying to tend to the emotional and spiritual tasks of letting go.

Encourage and reassure family members that, even though those drastic measures may be available in our highly advanced world of medical technology, they are not in the best interest of the patient and will causes more suffering. Focus on what they can do, such as ice chips in the mouth to combat the feeling of dryness or moistening the mouth with a swab. Popsicles are a good alternative to ice chips if the patient is still able to swallow without difficulty.

- **Swallowing difficulties**

Patients almost universally lose their ability to swallow toward the very end of life. This is part of the body's natural shutting down process (the body saying, "I can't handle this. Don't feed me.") Do not give a patient having difficulty swallowing any foods or fluids by mouth. The risk of aspiration (fluid going down the wrong way and ending up in the lungs) is very high.

You may see the nurse giving fluids at times, under special circumstances, but do not give them yourself, even if the patient requests it. Tell the nurse if the patient asks for a drink or ice chips.

Sometimes, when a patient has lost their ability to swallow before coming onto hospice, you may see a feeding tube has been placed to bypass the swallowing difficulties. This feeding tube also greatly increases the risk of aspiration and of swelling, vomiting, and general misery if food or fluids are given to this type of patient by mouth.

- **Losing weight**

Most patients lose weight as they get closer to death. The weight loss can be dramatic and is because of their loss of appetite and other health considerations.

A Closer Look

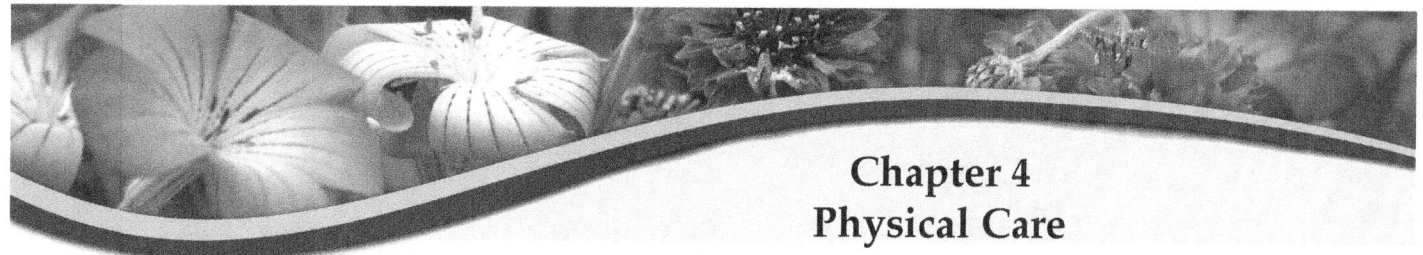

Chapter 4
Physical Care

- **Changes in vision**

The patient's eyes may become dry (artificial tears help) or vision may become blurry at times. The most common vision change is actually in the eyelids themselves, which tend to relax, giving them a "zoned out" look. They may fixate on one area in the room, staring in that direction while awake. Some patients keep their eyes open even while asleep at this stage.

- **Relaxation of the jaw**

The jaw tends to relax toward the end of the dying process and cause the mouth to fall open. This can be disconcerting to family members, who try to close the patient's mouth, only to have it fall open again. Explaining to the family that this is caused by relaxing muscles may help them accept it. Giving them a task to do, like keeping the patient's mouth moistened with swabs and their lips lubricated with lip balm, can help them feel more in control.

- **Decrease in urine output**

As the body shuts down, so do the kidneys, and the urine output will decrease dramatically. The urine will become more concentrated and darker in color. This is partly because the patient is taking in less fluids. If the patient has a catheter, the urine is visible to all, so the family may question you about what they are seeing. Reassure them that scanty, dark urine is normal at this stage.

- **Incontinence**

Although there is a significant decrease in the amount of urine the body produces and the patient may not be eating at all, they may still have some waste materials produced. It is very common for the patient to lose control over bowels and bladder and have "accidents". This can be embarrassing for the patient and the family, so be sensitive in your responses when it occurs. Letting family know that it is not unusual and is part of the process will help alleviate the sense of shame that can accompany losing control of bodily functions.

A Closer Look

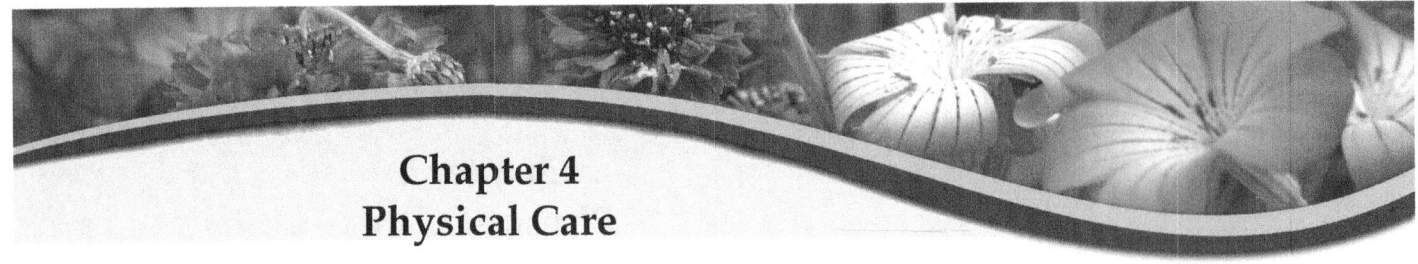

Chapter 4
Physical Care

- **Edema and swelling**

The kidneys begin to do less filtering of fluids as the body shuts down, so the excess fluid can build up in the lower body. It usually starts with the feet and ankles, moving up to the legs and sacral area, then the abdomen, then the lungs will start to fill up. Diuretics can help a little but usually aren't very effective as they cause more problems than they solve. The best approach is to limit fluids to what the patient's body is saying it can tolerate.

- **Spiking temperatures**

Because of the body's natural dehydration process, the patient may have spikes in temperature, sometimes as high as 104 degrees. Antibiotics don't help because this is a natural body process and not caused by infection (although the patient may develop concurrent infections as the circulation decreases and the immune system weakens.)

Cool washcloths and ice in a cloth can help (never put ice directly on the skin.) The patient may have a high temperature and cool skin on their extremities at the same time. This is because of a shutdown of circulation to the arms and legs as the body reserves blood supplies for the internal organs.

- **Blood pressure changes**

Blood pressure may go up and down during the dying process, but it usually plummets very low just before death.

- **Heart rate**

Heart rate will fluctuate as well, but it usually goes up as the blood pressure goes down. If the heart rate stays at 120 beats per minute for long periods of time, this is a late sign. It's okay, unless the family just really wants to know what vital signs are, to just let it be and don't spend a lot of time focusing on vital signs. They will be what they are.

- **Mottling of the skin**

This is caused by decreased circulation to the lower extremities. The feet (especially the big toes), then the legs, may appear purple and splotchy.

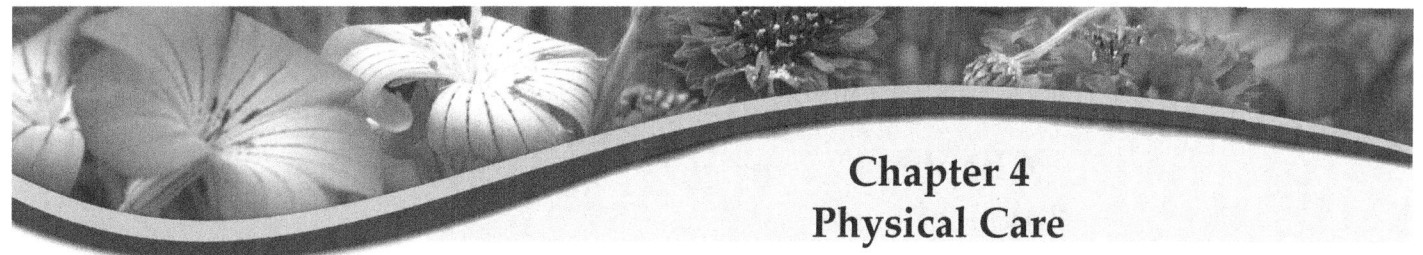

Chapter 4
Physical Care

- **Seizure activity**

This can be caused by fevers or in a patient who has a brain tumor or metastasis from some other primary cancer site to the brain. Keep the patient safe by clearing away anything that they could hit with their hands or legs while seizing. Record the time and length of the seizure to the nurse.

What to do when your patient is actively dying

At some point in the care of your hospice patient, you will come to the point at which you realize your patient is actively dying. Not knowing what to expect as death approaches can lead to anxiety and a feeling of helplessness, especially for the family. It is important for you to understand what to expect so you can offer support and information with confidence to your hospice family.

The following list will give you an idea of what you may see as your patient approaches death and what you can do to help make him more comfortable.

- **Changes in facial appearance, sight, speech, and hearing**

The patient's facial muscles may relax, causing the cheekbones and chin to become more prominent and the eyes to appear sunken. The skin may take on a pale, ashen color. Sight gradually fails and the eyes may remain half open and glazed. Hearing is the last sense to go.

Remove the dentures if it seems more comfortable for the patient. Give good mouth care using moistened swabs. Keep the lips well lubricated with lip balm (not petrolatum based, as it is flammable and your patient may need oxygen.) Keep the room comfortably lighted and sit near the head of the bed where you can be seen more easily. Insert artificial tears into the eyes if the patient isn't blinking. Talk to the patient, offering comfort and explanations of what you are doing. Always assume he can hear and understand you even if you see no outward sign of acknowledgment.

A Closer Look

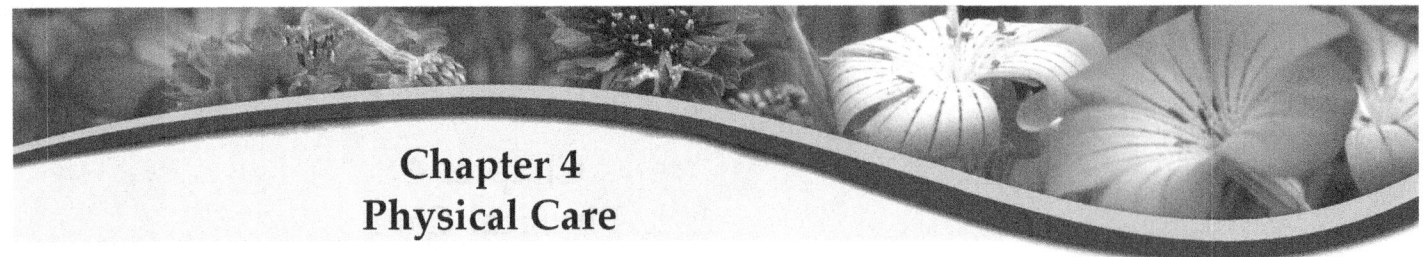

Chapter 4
Physical Care

- **Changes in skin, muscles, and bone**

The muscles begin to relax as they lose their function, limiting the patient's ability to move. As the body shuts down, circulation diminishes to the arms and legs and they may feel very cool to the touch. The skin may appear pale and mottled and may be covered with perspiration.

Even though the skin is cool to the touch, most dying persons aren't aware of feeling cold. It is best to keep clothing and bedding light and make sure there is fresh, circulating air in the room. Carefully inspect the patient's skin, especially over the bony prominences, for any sign of breakdown. Turn and position the patient comfortably at least every two hours.

- **Changes in the respiratory system**

Breathing may become rapid and shallow or very slow with a snoring type of sound. Sometimes periods of rapid, heavy breathing may alternate with short periods of no breathing at all. Wet, gurgling, or "rattling" breathing is caused by secretions building up in the lungs.

Elevating the head of the bed to a 45 degree angle helps the patient to be able to cough more effectively and may be more comfortable than lying flat. Turning him on his side to let secretions drain out can help prevent choking. If the patient is alert and restless due to difficulty breathing, oxygen often helps.

Offer comfort and support to the patient through your touch and presence. Speak to him even though he may not be able to talk back.

- **Changes in mental status**

The patient may be confused about time, place, or who is present in the room. Some of this may be due to changes in metabolism, changes in vision, or increased sleeping. She may become restless and may hallucinate or engage in repetitive motions. Or she may slip into complete unresponsiveness.

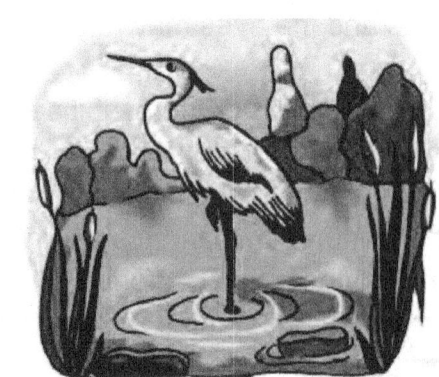

140   **A Closer Look**

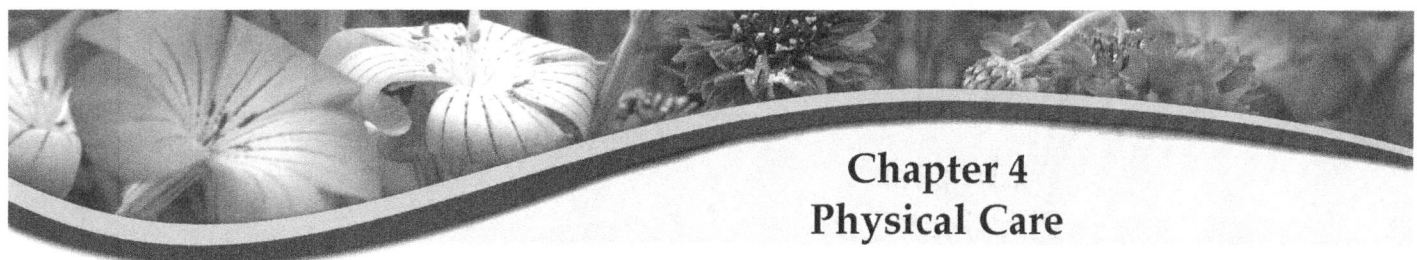

Chapter 4
Physical Care

Someone needs to stay with the patient to provide comfort and support. Don't try to restrain repetitive motions, but speak quietly and naturally to the patient.

Don't try to give food or fluids to an unconscious patient or to one who has difficulty swallowing. Assist a conscious patient in orientation by surrounding them with familiar objects such as pictures of loved ones, clocks, and calendars.

- **High temperature**

It is not unusual for a patient to spike a temperature of 104 degrees or higher as they draw closer to death. This is the body's "last ditch" attempt to fight the disease.

Use light clothing to cover the patient and use cool, moist cloths on the his forehead or on the back of his neck. Tylenol suppositories can be helpful in bringing the fever down, too.

- **The Final Moments**

In the last minutes of the patient's life, breathing often changes to a very shallow, gulping pattern, as if they were trying to swallow. They may vomit or become incontinent of bowel and/or bladder. After providing any personal care that might be needed for comfort, honor this time by staying close and offering loving presence and reassurance without distracting the patient from his or her task.

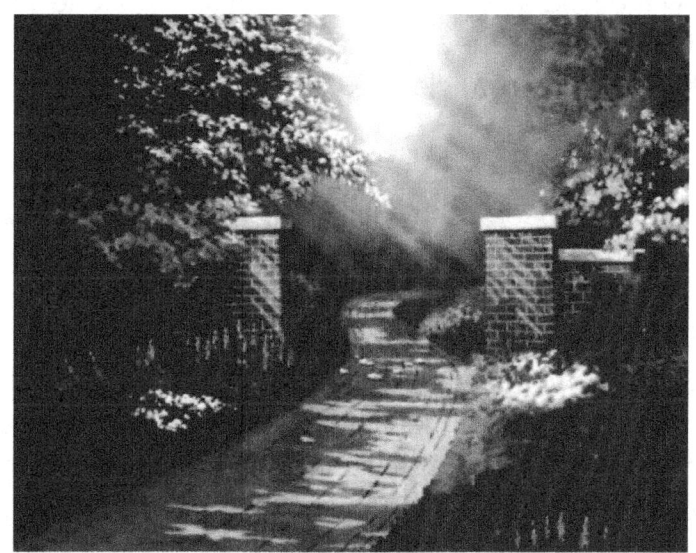

Encourage the family to stay close but not to interfere with the process. Soothing music can help create an atmosphere of peace and tranquility during this transition. When the patient's heart stops and they take their last breath, note the time for the record. Offer support to the family. And be sure to find support for yourself. This is an intense experience and you need to process it with someone you trust.

A Closer Look

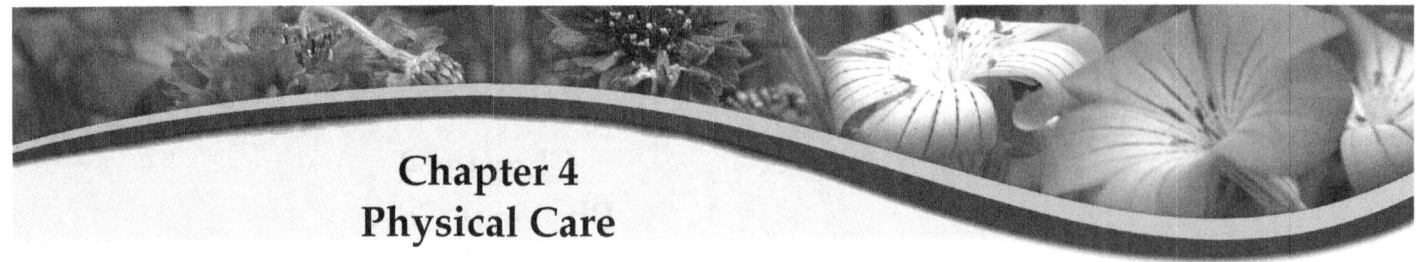

Chapter 4
Physical Care

What to do when your patient dies:

If you think your patient has died (you don't see any rise and fall of the chest with breath and you don't feel a pulse), call hospice so the nurse can come out and pronounce the patient. If your patient is in a facility, notify the nurse in charge of the patient and also call hospice.

Don't tell the family that the patient has died, because it isn't within your scope of practice to pronounce the death. (Sometimes the patient can look very dead and then start breathing again for a few minutes.) Do, however, make note of the time you discovered the patient was no longer breathing and give it to the nurse when he or she arrives.

The nurse will do an examination of the patient and notify the doctor of the death. The nurse will also notify the medical examiner, depending on state laws. Then the mortuary will be notified. The family can take as long as they want to take with the patient. It is their call as to when the mortuary is notified to come and pick up the body. They may not know this, so you can reassure them that it is up to them to say how long they need to say their good-byes and be with their loved one's body.

Offer comfort and support to the family while waiting for the hospice nurse to arrive. Take this time to tell the family thank you for allowing you to be part of this important time in their lives. Let them know they did a wonderful job with their loved one's care. Offer to give family members time alone with the patient. They may have unfinished business and have something they need to say to the patient for their own closure.

Don't judge any of the family's responses. Some people cry at the time of death and some don't. Often, it has been such a long difficult journey that many of the tears have already been shed. It's up to you to just accept them where they are and with whatever response they need to have to their loved one's passing.

Gently help the family decide whether to stay in the room when the mortuary comes or not. It can be difficult for family members to see their loved one placed into a body bag. Sensitive mortuary staff accomplish this task with dignity and sensitivity and leave the patient's face uncovered until outside and out of sight of the family.

A Closer Look

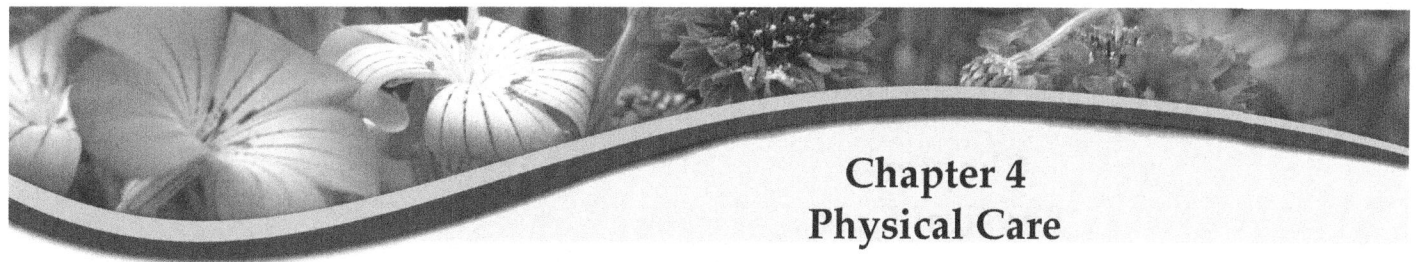

Chapter 4
Physical Care

While waiting for the mortuary to arrive, family members may feel tense or lost. This is an odd transition time, with the body still in the room, but the person they loved "gone." It sometimes takes the mortuary an hour or more to arrive. This is a good time to tell heartwarming and funny stories about the patient. You may even want to suggest a circle in which each person tells of a favorite memory or something special about the patient. Some families may want to have a prayer.

After the mortuary arrives and takes the body, offer support and comfort to each family member and remind them that bereavement services are available for the next year. Give them contact information and any brochures you might have with you. Let them know they can call hospice at any time, day or night, and someone will be available to talk to them if needed.

If your patient is in a facility, take the time to connect with the staff before you leave the building, thanking them for caring for the patient so well and offering hospice bereavement support (via the bereavement group) for them as well.

A Closer Look

Chapter 4
Physical Care

Skill Check

1. List four diagnoses (besides cancer) that might be seen in hospice.

2. Explain why fear increases pain.

3. List ten common symptoms that you might see in a dying patient and what you could do to help relieve the discomfort of each.

4. Define the term "metastasis".

5. How could you determine whether or not your patient was in pain if he couldn't speak to you?

Chapter 4
Physical Care

6. Describe the hospice nurse's role on the team.

7. What are some of the foods to encourage a patient to avoid if she is nauseated?

8. Describe five major changes that may occur as a patient is actively dying and what you can do to make him more comfortable.

9. Define the universal precautions to be used in patient care.

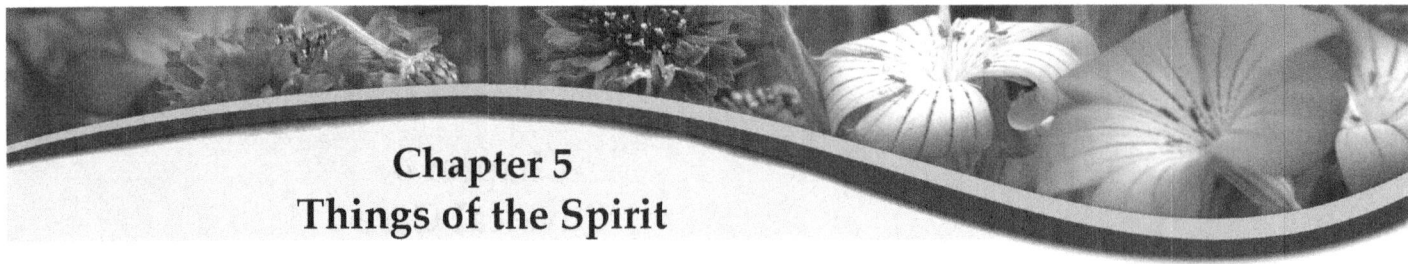

Chapter 5
Things of the Spirit

5. Things of the Spirit
Providing Spiritual Care

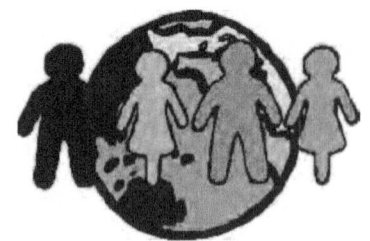

"Just the facts, please..."

Spiritual care is a major component of the holistic approach to providing for the needs of the terminally ill. This concept has never been disputed since the very beginnings of hospice. Exactly how to go about providing spiritual care for individuals from widely differing backgrounds and ideologies has presented more of a challenge.

It's important for end of life care providers to have a basic understanding of what spirituality is and what spiritual needs are likely to arise as the person faces death.

Spirituality, by its very nature, is difficult to quantify. It's easier, initially, to approach it from the angle of what it is *not*.

- Spirituality is *not* morality. Morality is an instilled set of social mores, an inner yardstick for measuring what is good for the society in which the individual functions. Sometimes what is immoral in one society may be perfectly accepted in another. A person may experience *spiritual pain* if his behavioral choices are in conflict with his moral code, but *morality* and *spirituality* are not synonymous.

- Spirituality is *not* psychology. Psychology deals with the emotions, with human relationships and how they function. Psychological problems can *cause* spiritual pain, but psychology is not spirituality. Spirituality deals with the *why* of life, not the *how*.

- Spirituality is *not* religion. It is here that some hospice care givers become confused about exactly what they are expected to provide to the dying person. Religious systems have attempted to address spiritual needs while providing moral structure. Sometimes these religious systems have succeeded in enhancing spiritual growth, sometimes they have inhibited it.

Chapter 5
Things of the Spirit

Some questions you may be asking . . .

If spirituality isn't morality, psychology, or religion, what is it?

Spirituality could be described as transcendent values versus human limitations. Human limitations are those things that "chain us to the earth", the practical, everyday tasks such as paying bills, changing the flat tire, folding the laundry, etc. Spirituality encompasses those things that are above human limitations, such as faith, hope, loyalty, and love. The world of the physical is not an enemy of the soul, rather, the choices we make in the real world (such as how we dress, what we spend our money on, etc.) reveal something about our spiritual values.

Spirituality is characterized by questions rather than answers. The physical world can be quantified, measured, and judged. It relies on scientific proof for validation. There are no such parameters for the spiritual. It has been said, "The things that mean the most in life can't be proven."

One job of the human spirit is to seek purpose and meaning on an individual level. No one can accomplish this task for another. Each individual's story will be different, fashioned and shaped by his or her unique experiences in life. Questions arise based on this need to clarify the meaning of one's existence. Who am I with all the distractions of life stripped away? What have I contributed to the lives of others? What do I fear? What do I value?

What if I have a different religious belief system than my patient? Can I still provide spiritual care to them?

Absolutely. It is not necessary that you personally subscribe to the patient's particular belief system in order to offer spiritual support. What is necessary is that you treat the patient's beliefs with the utmost respect and honor. Each hospice patient will need to find meaning within their concept of the "big picture" of life. Inner peace comes from seeing oneself as part of a "big picture" that makes sense and that one has faith in. It is important that you, as a hospice spiritual care provider, develop a basic understanding of the patient's "big picture" so you can support him in it, especially if performance of certain rituals or practices are necessary for the patient to be in harmony with his or her belief system.

"Just the facts, please..."

Chapter 5
Things of the Spirit

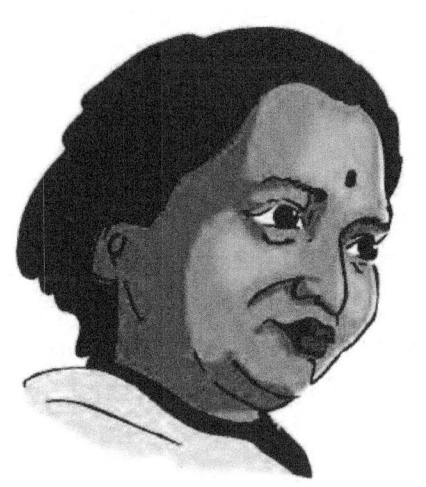

Life review is an important part of the patient's finding a place in the "big picture". One patient spent the months preceding her death painstakingly writing out her memoirs, chronicling each contribution she felt she had made to her family, to her church, and to society. She shared on paper what she considered to be the most valuable in life and who she was personally. Her daughter typed the manuscript, had it bound, and presented it to her before her death.

Others do verbal life review with trusted companions or care givers. The social worker often has opportunity to encourage life review with gentle questioning that gives "permission" for the dying person to begin this task. One occupational therapist in hospice assists his patients with organizing old photos to be videotaped. He then audiotapes the patients as they tell the story behind each picture. Each patient that participates in this process experiences a satisfying life review and the family gains a priceless memorial of their loved one.

The key to providing spiritual support to a person engaged in life review is active listening. It is important not to judge, analyze, or trivialize the content of the speaker's words. Reflecting the patient's thoughts back, slightly rephrased so he or she can hear their ideas out loud and evaluate them, is a great gift to them. In a nutshell, end of life spiritual care is helping the dying put a voice to their inner beliefs. It is conversation, not conversion; and support, not control. It is allowing the patient to ask questions, not providing answers for them.

End of life spiritual care is **soul care** in the very deepest sense of the word. It practices the principles of spiritual growth by providing an atmosphere that places the free choice and dignity of the patient as paramount. Care is based on values that transcend philosophical or religious differences, the most important of which are faith, hope, and unconditional love.

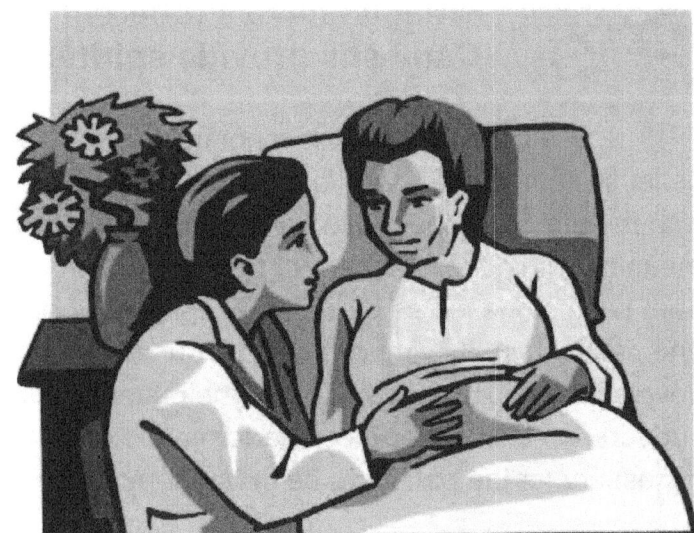

Chapter 5
Things of the Spirit

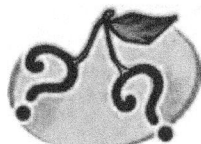 **How will the care team know how to address the specific spiritual needs of a patient and/or family that have very different beliefs from those of hospice team members?**

It is an excellent idea, if it is at all possible, to consult or involve spiritual care providers whose belief systems are similar to the patient's who will be able to better identify, understand, and meet the spiritual needs of the patient. Your local chamber of commerce should have an up-to-date listing of local religious groups that you could access. The ministerial association in your area is another good resource.

Learn the special needs inherent in each major faith tradition so you will know when to suggest or seek guidance from a spiritual care provider from that tradition. Here are a few of the major faith traditions and special spiritual care needs that you might encounter. Keep in mind that, although your patient and family may subscribe to a certain faith tradition, participation in the rituals of that tradition varies widely according to the individual. For example, don't assume that just because someone is Jewish that he or she will be Orthodox. Find out what is important to your patient and family within their own personal spiritual experience.

How Some Different Cultures May View the Dying Process

While it is important to remember that every family situation is unique, sometimes it is helpful to know some of the general features of a particular culture's view of death. This information is not intended to advance stereotypes but to increase understanding. The best way to learn about a family's belief system and their culture's special spiritual needs is to ask them.

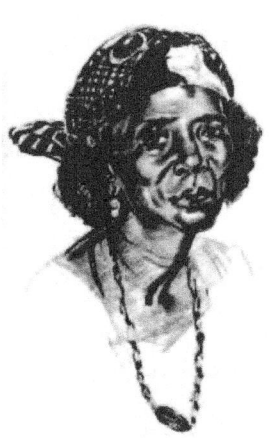

African American

- **Often strong Christian heritage**
- **May be Muslim**
- **Most African Americans die in a hospital, so "going to the hospital" can signify being ready to die - thus staying home to die, as in hospice, can be seen as neglect of the patient and unloving**
- **Strong emphasis on family and community support**
- **Emotion may or may not be expressed openly**

"Just the facts, please..."

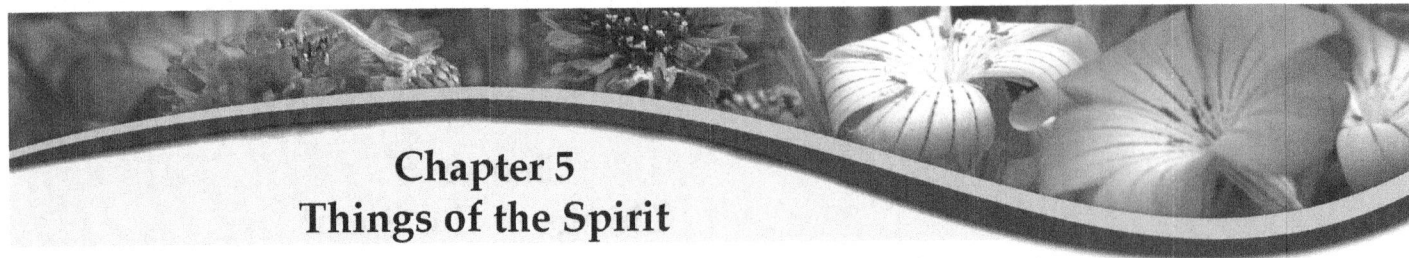

Chapter 5
Things of the Spirit

- Music is often a powerfully important part of expression of faith and grief and hope in seeing the loved one again in the afterlife
- Support and value the dying/deceased person's "good fight"
- Funeral is very important- may be rituals based on African traditions

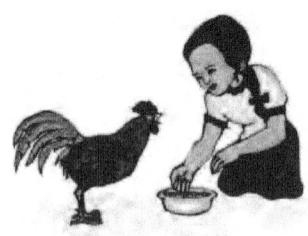

Hispanic American

- Strong Catholic influence
- May consider death nature's method of clearing the way for new life to emerge
- May associate yellow flowers with death, using them to decorate the home or grave of the recently departed
- Last rites by the priest are very important, so be sure and have the priest's contact information handy as the patient declines and notify the clergy with any changes in the patient's condition to ensure opportunity for this ritual to take place before the patient's death
- Children are socialized to accept death at a young age
- Close family ties and great emphasis on support of family and friends
- Body may lie in state in the home on top of a table or stand, with herbs and candles burning underneath
- The funeral service, held in the church with a priest officiating, is very important; and the response from young and old alike is open and demonstrative
- Novenas are said for nine days after the funeral

Buddhist

- Believe all aspects of life are temporary
- Goal is Nirvana, a state of being beyond pain and suffering, which is reached after many rebirths in which the person learns to develop true compassion and wisdom
- Great emphasis on the importance of maintaining a clear, calm, unruffled response to life to keep from bringing bad karma, or results, in a future life

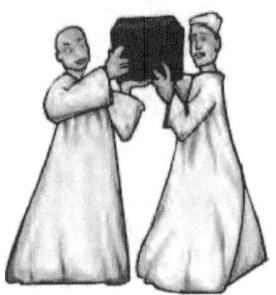

Chapter 5
Things of the Spirit

- May chant certain sutras, or teachings of Buddha, to calm the dying person's mind and prevent any evil from influencing his rebirth process negatively
- May follow a 49 day ceremony to guide the person through the transitional state between lives
- Family may wear traditional white cloth and openly show emotion following the death
- Both cremation and actual burial may be practiced

Jewish

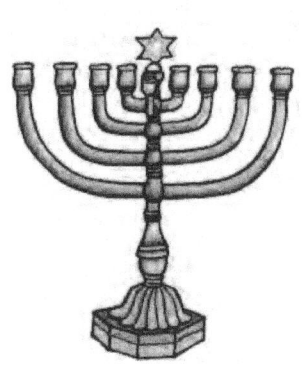

- Emphasize balance of embracing life with passion and accepting death with equanimity
- "Rite of confession" as death approaches allows the dying person to ask forgiveness, say final prayers of comfort and hope together, and say goodbye.
- Value honoring the dead and comforting the mourners
- Immediately following death, the body is moved to a place where it can be prepared for burial (washing and shrouding it, done by specially trained volunteers)
- Autopsies are considered disrespectful to the body unless there is good for mankind to be gained from doing it
- Coffin is usually very simple and basic, so as not to interfere with natural decomposition
- Body is guarded constantly during the time between death and burial
- Funeral begins with the cutting of a black ribbon which symbolizes the "cutting away of life"
- A special meal to console the family follows the service
- Official mourning, shiva, lasts for seven days, then is followed by sheloshim, lasting for thirty days, then the period of mourning extends for a full year
- Each period has special customs

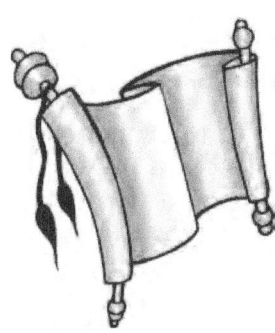

"Just the facts, please..."

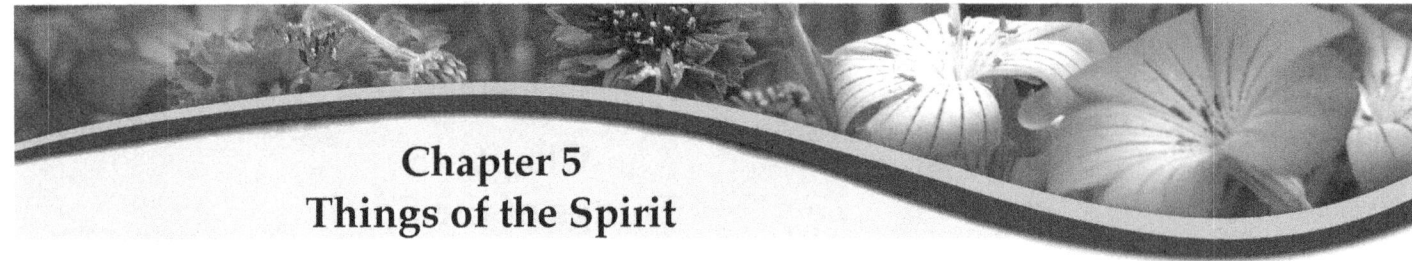

Chapter 5
Things of the Spirit

Native American

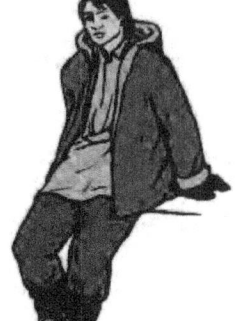

- Beliefs and traditions surrounding death may be a mixture of Christian and tribal elements
- Death is not feared, but considered a natural part of the cycle of life
- Strong belief in the afterlife
- Deep respect for the body
- Mourning is considered natural and normal, with strong expressions of grief by both men and women. Women may wail and men often sing mournful, emotional songs
- Strong family support
- Taboos surrounding death, especially the sight or sound of an owl, which it is believed means that someone will soon die
- Body may lie in state for three days, during which the family and loved ones grieve openly, touching the body
- Family may either burn or give away the deceased person's possessions before the burial
- A lock of the deceased's hair is often kept in the family home throughout the year-long period of mourning. This hair and its container are burned at the anniversary service, during which the deceased is honored by the giving of gifts and money by the family to those special people who have been invited to the service

Islam

- Death is considered a natural part and process of life
- Strong belief in one God, Allah, and that there is a day of judgment and a life after death, in which one's actions from earth follow him
- Believe that after they die, they can observe the lives of family members from heaven, even visiting them periodically in the form of a bird

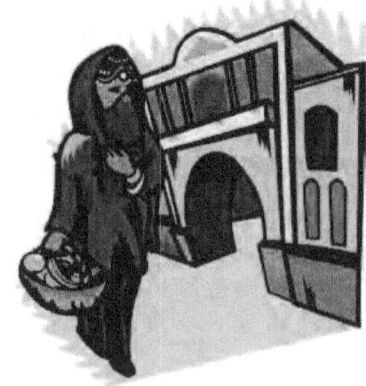

152 "Just the facts, please..."

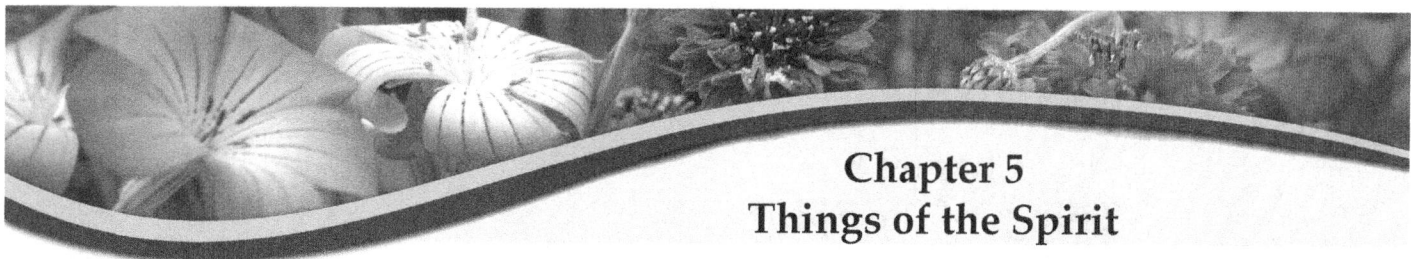

Chapter 5
Things of the Spirit

- A close relative stays beside the patient as they are dying, reading the Koran and praying for God's blessing, until the last breath is taken
- The body is not left alone
- Immediately upon death of the patient, all friends and relatives are notified by one family member, while someone continues to read the Koran, and another family member does the following:

1. Turns the body so that it faces Mecca
2. Closes the mouth and eyes, then covers the eyes and face
3. Stretches the person's hands out at their sides and straightens the legs
4. Bathes the body and covers it with white cotton

- Males wash male bodies and females wash females
- There are always two people to bathe the body
- Three kinds of water are used– water with leaves of the plum tree, camphorized water, and pure water
- At the burial, family and friends gather with a religious leader and weep and pray for forgiveness, letting their sorrow out
- Tea, sugar and sugar syrup are made available at the service for those who weep so much they faint.
- A meal is served after the funeral and then close relatives stay for a week, continuing to cry and pray together. It is believed that the more the family prays during this week, the easier the deceased's life will be in the afterworld
- After seven days, a stone is placed on the grave with fresh flowers on top
- Close relatives wear black for 40 days

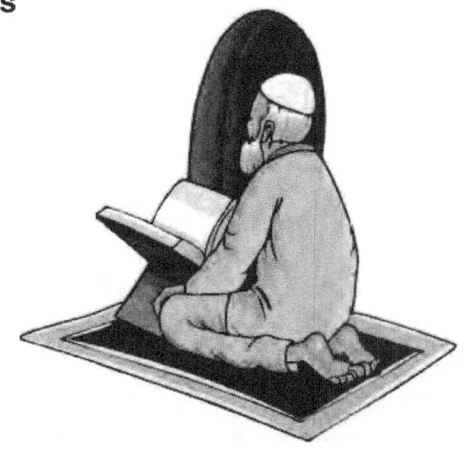

"Just the facts, please..."

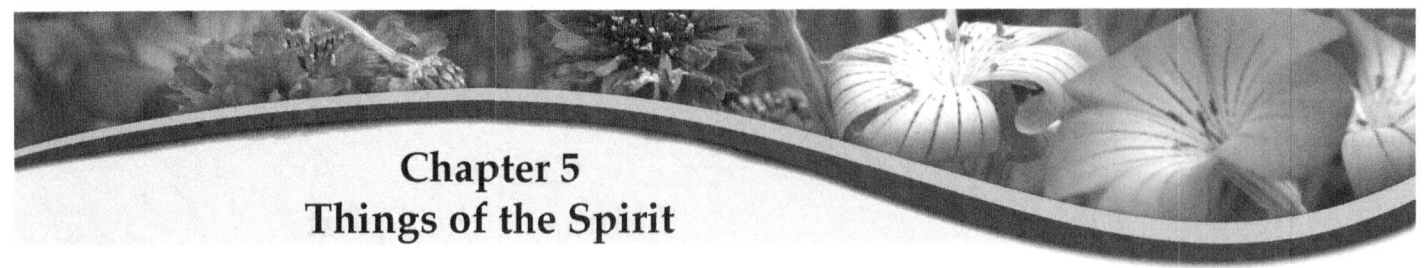

Chapter 5
Things of the Spirit

 *At the Heart of the Matter*

Why do you want to help others by being an end of life caregiver? The fact that you are still pressing forward with this caregiver training expresses your commitment to helping those who are dying. What are your reasons? Have you had the opportunity to dig down deep within yourself to find out why you need to reach out to others in such a profound way?

We have explored the spiritual needs of the dying patient and his or her family. It is equally important to explore our own spiritual needs as they relate to helping others. Let's look at some of the basic spiritual components of the helping process. Notice that, as is usually the case, delving into the spiritual realm involves more questions than answers.

- Unconditional Love

What do I believe about love? How is it best expressed? What if I offer love and acceptance to someone and they reject it? Where does love come from? What does it look like? Is it possible to give without receiving anything in return? What is my concept of God's love?

My thoughts about love:

Chapter 5
Things of the Spirit

- *Hope*

What is my definition of hope? Is it possible to live without hope? In what ways is hope nourished? Where does hope come from? What is hope's role in my day to day life?

My thoughts about hope:

- *Faith*

What is faith? Which is more important, the faith you have or the object of your faith? Is it possible to have faith in someone you don't know or something you don't understand? Where does faith come from? What makes faith grow? Is it possible to survive without faith in anything? What impact would that have on one's life? Can you impart faith to another person? How?

My thoughts on faith:

At the Heart of the Matter

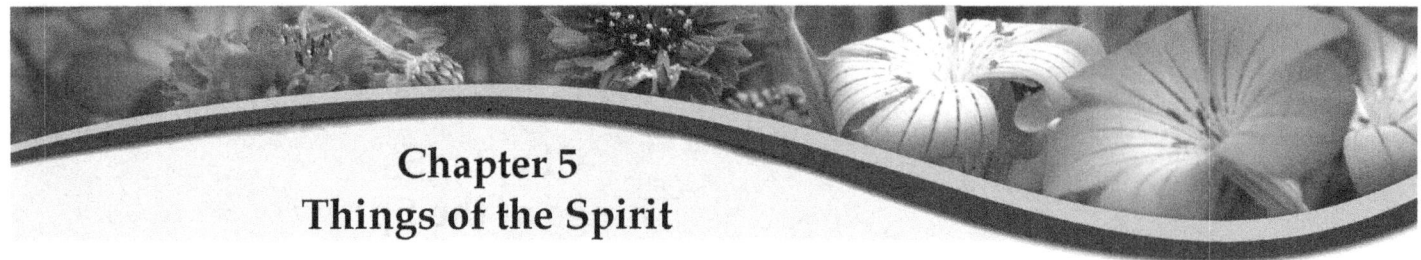

Chapter 5
Things of the Spirit

- *Humility*

What is humility? On what is humility based? If I am truly humble, how will that exhibit itself in my innermost attitudes? Is humility a weakness or a strength? Why? In what ways will my level of humility impact the care I provide to others? How is humility developed?

My thoughts on humility:

- *Commitment*

What does commitment look like? What attitudes work together to determine the level of commitment I choose to have toward others? Is it possible to be over-committed to my own spiritual detriment? How is a healthy balance achieved?

My thoughts on commitment:

Chapter 5
Things of the Spirit

Most religious systems (and many other systems of belief not based on any religion) teach that helping others is of paramount importance. The sayings "it is more blessed to give than receive" and "the good person serves mankind rather than himself" are commonly repeated in cultures all over the world.

While giving to others is crucial to our spiritual growth no matter what our world view may be, there are ways to "help" others that not only damage the giver, but also damage the receiver.

Is your giving helping or hurting others?

Take the following quiz to help you determine your true helpfulness quotient:

1. Are my own needs being neglected to the point that I have become "stroke deprived" and find myself helping others to get the "strokes" I need to feel valued as a person?   Yes   No

2. Do I usually feel that the people I am helping couldn't make it on their own and that my intervention is necessary to their well-being?   Yes   No

3. Do I sometimes find that people turn on me and make me feel like I'm the "bad guy" when I was only "trying to help"?   Yes   No

4. When things go wrong in a situation in which I am the helper, do I feel deep in my heart that somehow I must be to blame for things not turning out as they "should have"?   Yes   No

5. Do I find myself blaming the person I am helping when things do not turn out perfectly? ("She really doesn't want to have her pain controlled, she's just using pain as an excuse to get attention" or "He just isn't trying hard enough")   Yes   No

6. Do I ever begin to help someone without checking with them to see if the help is wanted or needed?   Yes   No

At the Heart of the Matter

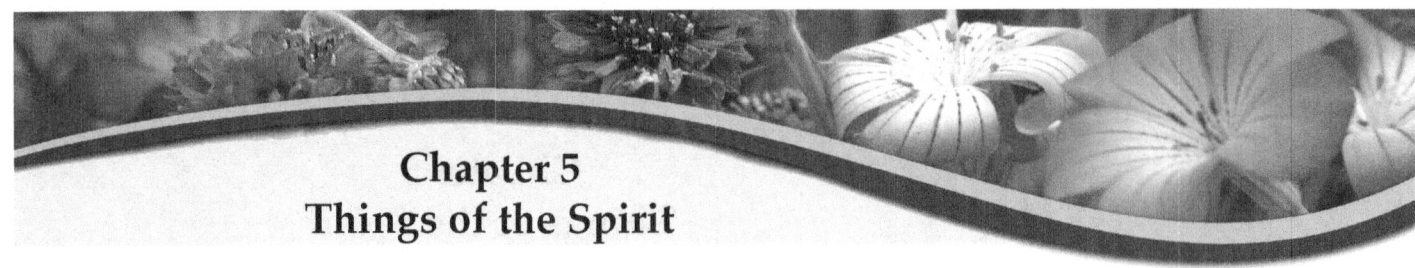

Chapter 5
Things of the Spirit

If you answered "no" to all of the questions in the quiz, your helping quotient is probably at a healthy level. Any "yes" answers deserve a very close look. You may be a rescuer instead of a true helper. Even if you do have tendencies to be a rescuer, however, bringing unhealthy behavior patterns out into the light of day is the biggest step toward transforming them into healthy ones.

None of us are perfect and our responses are seldom "cut and dried". Our behavior patterns are usually somewhere on a continuum rather than set in one place. Where would you place yourself on the following scale?

Refusal to Help   Rescuing

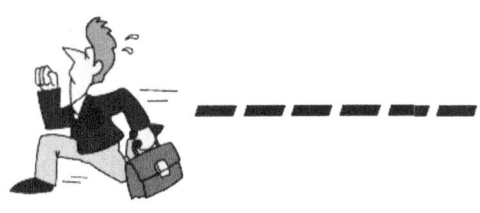 **Healthy Helping**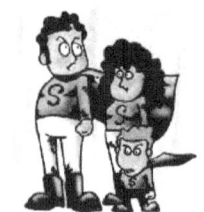

Underlying belief:　　　　　　　　　　　　　　　　　　　　　　　Underlying belief:
(because it's all his fault)　　　　　　　　　　　　　　　　　(because it's all my fault)
"He's no good"　　　　　　　　　　　　　　　　　　　　　　　　　　"I'll keep trying"
"They are all that way"　　　　　　　　　　　　　　　　　"Maybe if I give enough…"
"It's no use wasting your energy"　　　　　"Maybe if they admire me enough
Judgment and blame (of others)　　　　　　　　　　　　they'll do what I want"
　　　　　　　　　　　　　　　　　　　　　　　　　　　　　　Judgment and blame (of self)

We've all known those hard-nosed scrooges who "bah humbug" even a sniff of the milk of human kindness. They are quick to judge anyone who isn't "tough enough" to meet their harsh standards. Their behavior is so radically different from the rescuer's that it is hard to believe that it is simply the opposite end of the same scale. Their "blame the victim" mentality is almost assuredly a result of their own helplessness in the face of early childhood abuse.

Rescuers are also quick to judge, but instead of judging others, they judge themselves. (Just as harshly, I might add). Their own emptiness, also a result of unmet needs for safety, security, and love in childhood, drives them to find some kind of relief in helping others.

Chapter 5
Things of the Spirit

Rescuers were usually considered the "responsible" ones in their family of origin and they probably received the message from their parents that they were only valuable as long as they took responsibility for "fixing" everything dysfunctional in the family. The inevitable failure to fix things produced a sense of inadequacy that, unless dealt with in an emotional recovery program, they probably carry to this day.

As a result of this inner emptiness, rescuers tend to look outside themselves for meaning. They seem to be dysfunction magnets, finding someone to "fix" to recreate that familiar childhood scenario. They may exhort, urge, persuade, or bombard their victim with advice or they may act really nice, hoping the person they have targeted will change his or her behavior through their example.

Spiritually Healthy Helping

In spiritually healthy helping, however, there is no blame involved. Stereotypes are not indulged in. There is no wise/foolish, saint/sinner, judge/judged. The helper is truly equal to the one being helped, fully realizing that the tables could be turned anywhere along their journey and the one being helped could become the helper.

Feelings are expressed in a healthy helping situation without fear of blame, anger, sorrow, or loss of fact. Most people have no problem dealing with their positive feelings. It's the negative ones they may need help with.

Being able to express their fear and anger to someone who accepts them totally just as they are, without shaming them or trying to get them to "cheer up", is very healing.

Helping is a two-way process, involving two people, and both sides of the interaction must be healthy for the outcome to be positive. To give help really means to offer someone an opportunity to change. Any other kind of help is simply a bandage until the next breakdown, helping for the moment, but of no lasting significance.

Chapter 5
Things of the Spirit

A Helper:

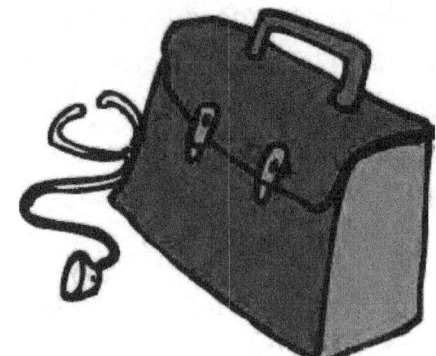

1. *Listens for a request.*
2. *Presents an offer of help.*
3. *Gives only what is needed.*
4. *Checks periodically with the person to make sure what is offered is still what is needed and wanted.*
5. *Checks results. Is the person functioning better? Are the goals being met? Is the person resolving problems independently? Are they using suggestions successfully?*

A Rescuer:

1. *Gives when not asked.*
2. *Neglects to find out if the offer is welcome.*
3. *Gives more help for a longer time than is needed.*
4. *Doesn't get feedback from the person.*
5. *Doesn't check results. Feels good if help is accepted and bad when help is turned down.*

Here are some basic principles to remember in setting healthy spiritual boundaries for yourself and respecting the spiritual boundaries of others:

- **Freedom of choice**

This principle is at the very heart of true spiritual health. As care providers, we must have total respect for the other person's freedom to choose. This is the basis of treating another with dignity, one of the pillars of the hospice philosophy.

True helping is offering something (tangible or intangible) in such a way that the person can choose to use it to effect change in his life. This choice to change is one of the most difficult things a human being can do and anyone who makes the choice deserves the utmost respect and support.

Chapter 5
Things of the Spirit

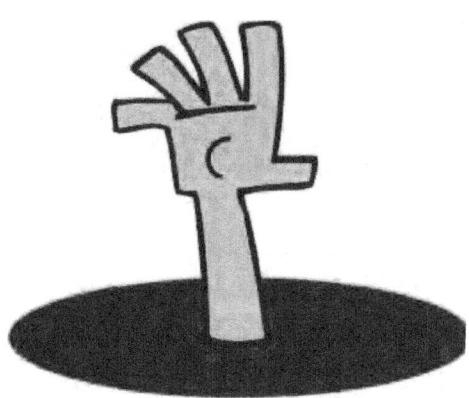

The choice to change is so difficult because it involves:

a) admitting failure
b) putting oneself for a little while in the power of another and letting him take part in your life
c) a lot of hard work, because the choice can't just be made once, it has to be made again and again in different contexts,
d) risking the unknown; giving up what is familiar and known, even if it is painful, for a "good" that can't yet be seen.

• A sense of the "real"

We can't hide behind politeness, glossing things over with pleasant but meaningless chatter, and still be genuine. Our relationships must deal with the real issues of life for us to maintain spiritual health. As we discovered in chapter three, one of the characteristics of a dysfunctional family is a refusal to talk about things as they really are. The fear of being real with each other can stifle spiritual growth.

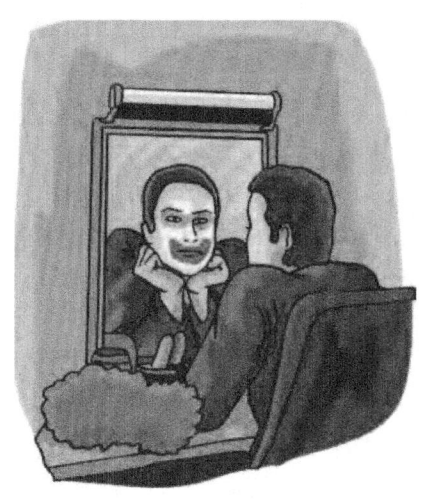

• A basis of trust, hope, faith, and acceptance

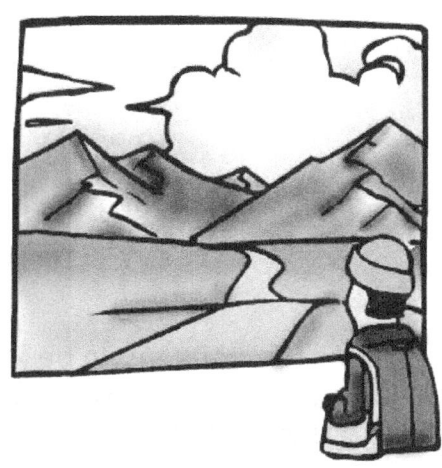

To truly help another, you must believe that he can be helped. You must believe in the power of hope and in the healing energy of love. And you must be willing to accept his decisions, even if they are not what you would have chosen for him. A "positive" choice is only really possible where the opposite is also possible and acceptable.

Keith Lucas in **"The Nature of the Helping Process"**, *says, "The person who makes the wrong choice is much closer to help than he who makes no choice at all."*

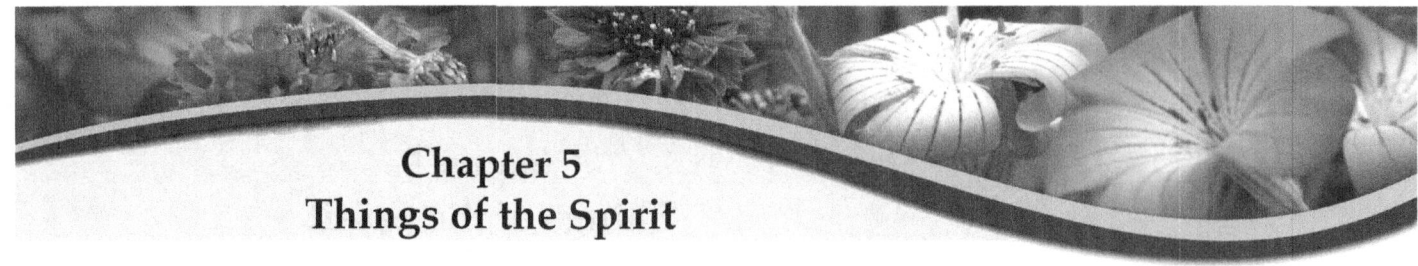

Chapter 5
Things of the Spirit

- ## An attitude of humility

There is no possible way for any of us to know what is best for another person (we're fortunate if we know what is best for ourselves!) Arrogantly spouting solutions to someone who has not asked us for information dishonors them.

The choice to be helped has to be made entirely by the person that needs the help. It cannot be made, or even too passionately wished, by the helper because even the wishing on the helper's part can take away from the will of one being helped and stand in the way of forward momentum.

- ## A willingness to commit yourself

Are you tough enough to really help? When the going gets rough (and sometimes it can get very rough) are you willing to hang in there? Are you willing to say to someone who needs your help, "I will never force you in any way, but nothing will shake my willingness to help you if you ask"?

Mother Teresa was willing to commit herself to those who need her help. So were Martin Luther King, Florence Nightingale, and the Mahatma Ghandi. We may not be as historically prominent as these people, but our work in end of life care is every bit as important as each of theirs.

The Prayer of St Francis of Assisi

(Christian Tradition)

Lord, make me an instrument of Your peace. Where there is hatred, let me sow love; where there is injury, pardon; where there is doubt, faith; where there is despair, hope; where there is darkness, light; where there is sadness, joy.

O, Divine Master, grant that I may not so much seek to be consoled as to console; to be understood as to understand; to be loved as to love; for it is in giving that we receive; it is in pardoning that we are pardoned; it is in dying that we are born again to eternal life.

Chapter 5
Things of the Spirit

A commitment to spiritually healthy helping is the hallmark of the hospice volunteer. In the space below, write or draw your own picture, prayer, poem, psalm or story that illustrates your personal passion for helping others.

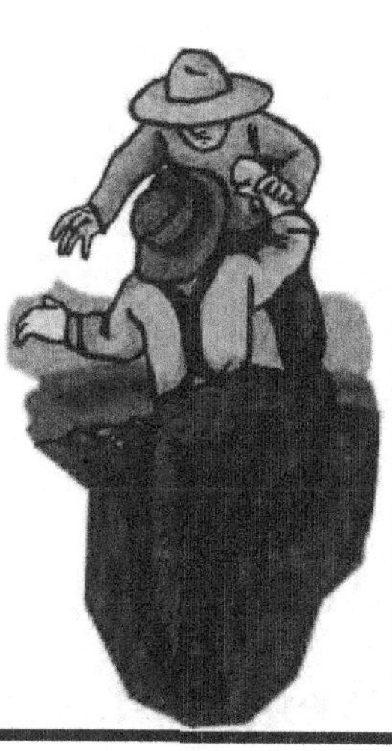

At the Heart of the Matter

Chapter 5
Things of the Spirit

 # Putting it Into Practice

How can you, as a caregiver, identify spiritual discomfort in your patients and their families? What are the clues that someone is in need of some spiritual guidance? What should your role be in providing spiritual care?

The following are some of the outward symptoms that may be signaling inner spiritual pain. Identifying just what those symptoms mean in a particular patient's experience takes a cooperative effort on the part of the patient and the care givers. What do they mean to you?

- **Fear**
- **Anger**
- **Bitterness**
- **Despair**
- **Depression**
- **Loneliness**
- **Hopelessness**
- **Confusion**
- **Rage**
- **Apathy**
- **Shame**
- **Hatred**
- **Helplessness**
- **Vengefulness**

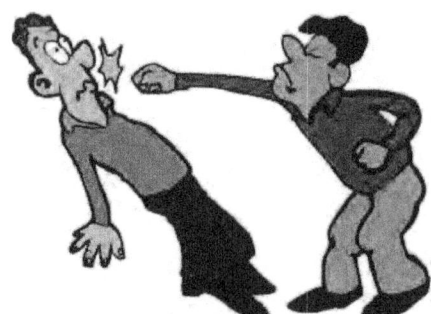

Chapter 5
Things of the Spirit

Do you think spiritual issues can be dealt with by counselors and other care team members as well as by the pastor or chaplain? Give the reasons for your answer.

Discuss the signs of spiritual pain. Do you know anyone who you believe suffers from this condition? How can you tell?

How would spiritual pain affect a person's ability to accomplish a satisfying life review as death approaches?

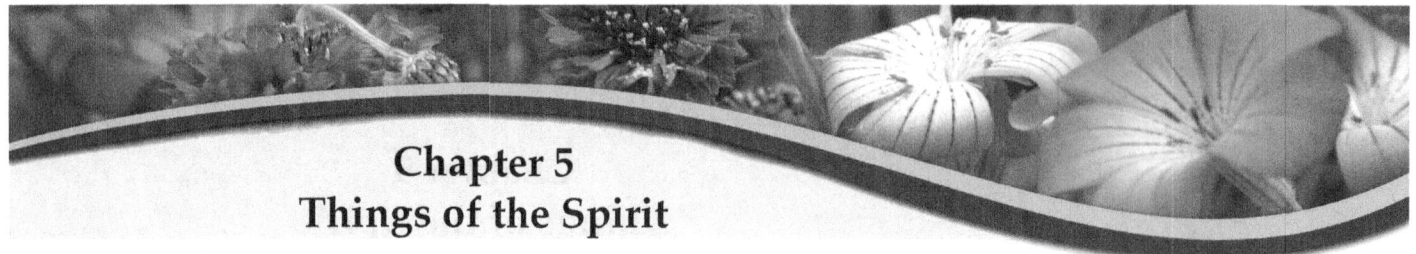

Chapter 5
Things of the Spirit

Spiritual pain can affect the patient's ability to move through the tasks of dying even more profoundly than can physical pain. This is why the chaplain is such an integral part of the care team. It is often the chaplain's role to identify and address unresolved spiritual pain.

If you have a hospice patient who suffers from unresolved spiritual pain, you may have the opportunity to observe the way the spiritual counselor works with them. It is a good idea to understand the mechanism behind this condition so you will be better able to support and help the care team in carrying out an effective care plan for this person.

Interventions for this condition are simple, but effective. They consist of:

- **Active Listening**
- **Affirmation**
- **Offering healing "tools" (if appropriate and desired by the patient). Often, and perhaps most effectively, shown through modeling**

The interaction may look something like this:

1. The spiritual counselor offers opportunity for the patient to express her pain, perhaps using encouragers like "How do you feel about..." or "I noticed you got really quiet when _____ came up. Is there something you'd like to talk about concerning that?" or "It must be hard to have _____ happen."

2. The counselor hears the patient out completely, empathizing and acknowledging her feelings.

3. The counselor will always give the patient "permission" to address or not address the problem. If the patient indicates that she doesn't want to talk about the issue, no matter what the reason, the counselor does not try to change her mind or talk her into working on it. The counselor's body language, attitude, and speech all continue to communicate complete acceptance of the patient and respect for her decisions.

Putting it Into Practice

Chapter 5
Things of the Spirit

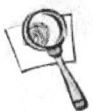 # A Closer Look

There are certain basic practices that greatly enhance spiritual health and offer comfort and a sense of safety to patients and their families. All care team members can practice these principles to create that sense of "safe haven" for all who come into their sphere of influence.

Discuss each of the following and how they can be applied to helping someone at end of life. How can each be modeled without actually directly addressing them? What is the importance of each in spiritual practice and why?

Acceptance

Appreciation

Encouragement

Chapter 5
Things of the Spirit

Forgiveness

Gratitude

Prayer

Chapter 5
Things of the Spirit

Spirituality is at the core of the hospice concept. Everything we do in end of life care is done with an eye to what is going on with the dying person's spirit. This is not about their religious tradition, for they may not have one. Things of the spirit transcend cultural and religious differences.

In the space below, describe soul care. You can use words or a song you remember or draw a picture that illustrates some aspect of soul care. Discuss your observations with the group.

A Closer Look

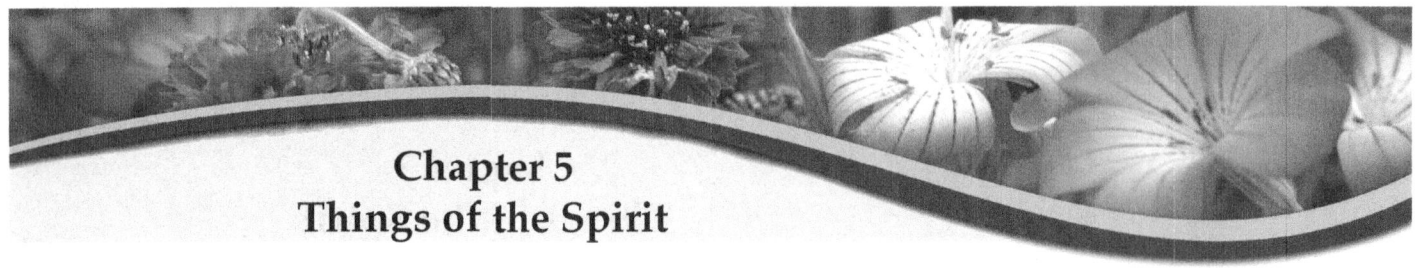

Chapter 5
Things of the Spirit

Working with people from different cultures at end of life

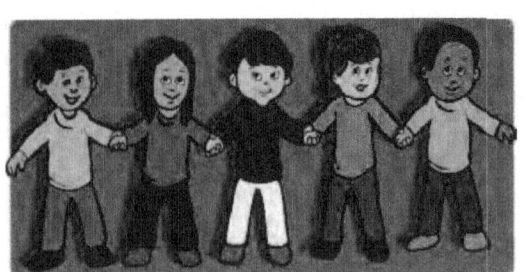

Our world is shrinking. In days past, people tended to live out their lives and die within a few miles of the place they were born. Communities and cultures had distinct boundaries and very little mixing of cultures happened. Not so much any more.

Even though we are a melting pot of cultures now, there are still cultural influences that affect how a family experiences death and dying. While it is a mistake to pigeonhole anyone into a cultural stereotype, it is helpful to understand the needs of different people groups and spiritual traditions. Always check with the individual, however, to clarify how much of his or her experience is actually based in that cultural "norm."

Because of some of the cultural differences, misunderstandings can easily come up. For example, in some cultures, eye contact between certain people is highly offensive where in another culture, not making eye contact would be just as offensive. In some cultures, emotion is expressed very openly and in others, it is more acceptable to be stoic and keep your feelings to yourself.

Here are some general guidelines to follow in working with people from a culture different than your own:

- **Don't generalize or make assumptions**

No one likes to be stereotyped and labeled. Customs in Korea are very different from those in Thailand, although both are Asian countries. Don't label someone as "Chinese" when they could actually be from any number of Asian countries, all very different in many ways. The same goes for African countries. Don't assume that just because someone looks Asian that they are from another culture. They may have grown up in Valdosta, Georgia and talk with a southern accent.

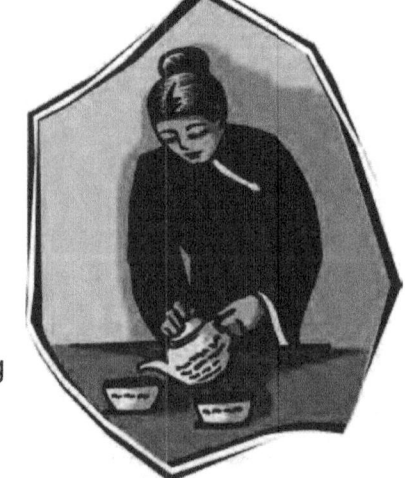

- **Don't be afraid to ask questions**

I have found that people love to talk about their homeland (if they are from another country) and culture. As long as the questions are springing from a sincere desire to understand each other, they will very likely be welcomed and answered happily.

A Closer Look

Chapter 5
Things of the Spirit

- **Learn to embrace differences**

There is much to be gained from the different perspectives that our cultural differences bring to this planet. As we welcome and honor differences, asking the deeper questions and truly listening to the answers, we are all blessed by the interchange. That's how we grow!

- **Remember that the key to understanding is *respect***

People are people - human beings who have the same basic needs for love and belonging, meaning and purpose, honor and respect. As long as we remember that, we will be a long ways down the road to understanding each other.

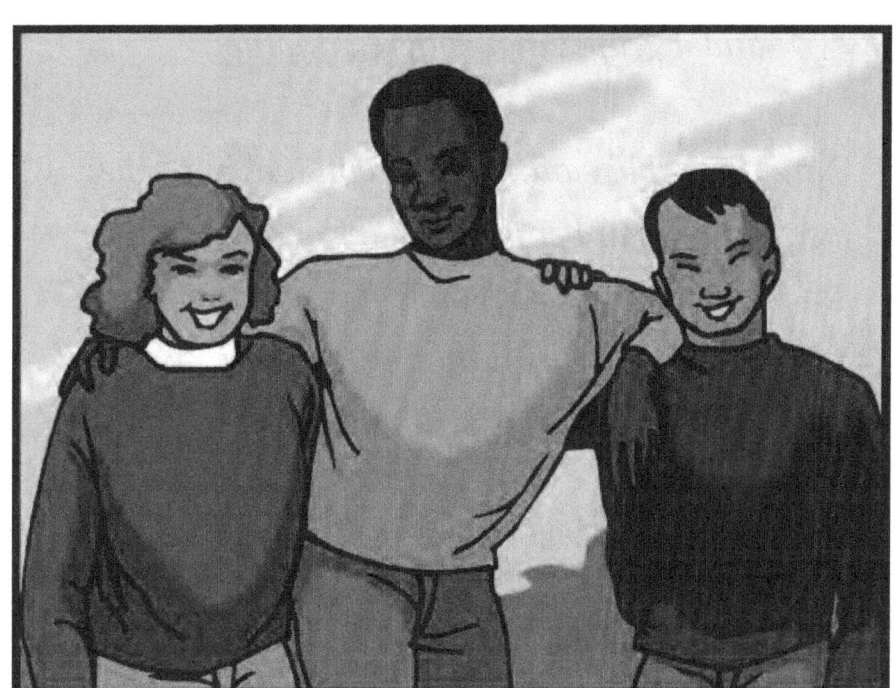

A Closer Look

**Chapter 5
Things of the Spirit**

"When is Dawn?"

*A rabbi put this question to his students:
"How can we determine the hour of dawn,
when the night ends and the day begins?*

*"When from a distance you can distinguish
between a dog and a sheep," suggested one.
"When you can distinguish between a fig tree
and a grapevine," offered another.*

*"No," the rabbi said. "When you look into the
face of a human being and have enough light
to recognize that person as your brother or
sister. Up until then it is night,
and darkness is still with you."*

Auther Unknown

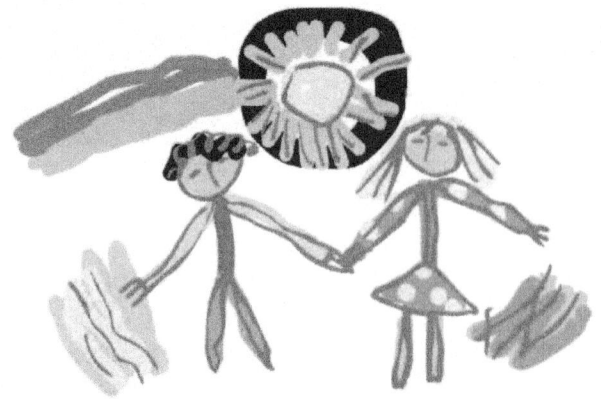

172   **A Closer Look**

Chapter 5
Things of the Spirit

Outward signs of spiritual pain can be very disconcerting to family members as well as the person who is experiencing the inner pain. While you can't change the situation for them, other than encouraging chaplain visits, there are some things you can do to support the patient and family. The following are some behavioral situations that might occur and suggestions for interventions that may help:

- **Terminal agitation**

There may be no obvious connection between what is happening currently and the patient's restlessness and agitation. You may have checked for physical discomfort in the environment and found nothing amiss. They may reach for things in the air that no one else sees and engage in seemingly meaningless movements. When this happens, there is often something inside them that is unfinished that they are working through.

This is where music can make a tremendous difference. Music reaches into the soul and brings up emotions that nothing else can. Try playing music for or singing lullabies to your patient. You will know right away if your efforts are helping or increasing the agitation. If sadness comes up for the patient, this isn't a bad thing. It is a normal part of the grief process. Be truly *with* the patient in this process, not just *near*.

- **Combativeness**

Watch your patient's facial expressions and body language for clues to the reasons for his combativeness. If it's pain, talk to a nurse about it. If not, look closer. Could it be fear? Despair? Anger?

Again, music can "soothe the savage beast." Music brings out what needs to be externalized. It's like a conduit for emotional expression.

Provide a calm, comforting atmosphere by moving any commotion and tension out of the room. Tactfully ask any family members or staff carrying on loud conversations in the room to take them out to common areas. If the television is on, turn it off. Dim the lights to a soothing level. Make sure the temperature in the room is comfortable for the patient.

A Closer Look

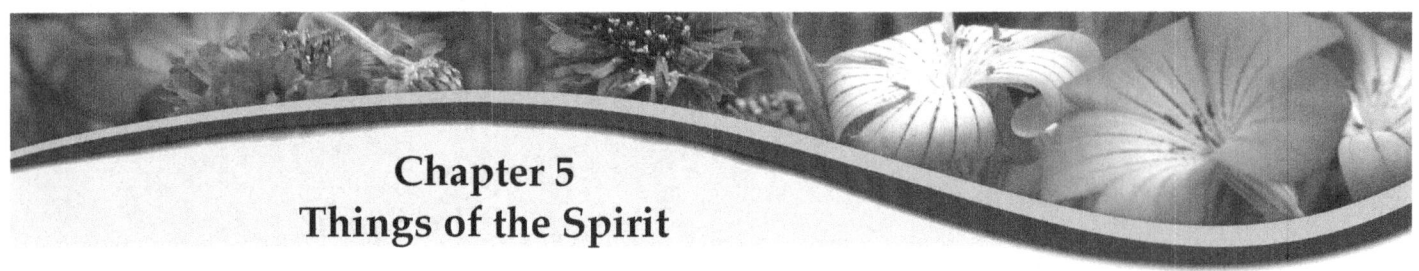

Chapter 5
Things of the Spirit

What the patient and family need from you to feel spiritually supported

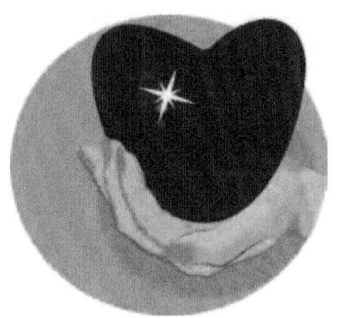

- **Acknowledge them**

As the patient and family share things with you that are difficult for them, they don't want or need you to solve the problem (unless it's a practical issue that they are specifically asking you to solve.) They simply need acknowledgment that they are in a tough situation and that it hurts. Acknowledgment says, "I see that you are struggling. You are not invisible. You have a witness to how hard this is."

- **Be present to help in tangible ways**

Supporting them with your presence means you ask them what their needs are and help them in those ways. Be specific, because a general inquiry will likely be turned down. "Is there anything I can do?" "No." Better to say, "Would you like a cup of tea? I'm making one for myself." Honoring and respecting their decisions is a way of being present.

- **Help them maintain their dignity**

You maintain a patient's dignity by always treating them as a unique human being. Any time you approach them, you identify yourself by name and call them by name and ask permission to provide the care. This says to them, "Who you are as a person is important to me. You are not just a body in a bed, but an irreplaceable special person, worthy of respect."

If the patient, in their restlessness, accidentally exposes themselves by flipping back the covers, pull them down or pull the curtain closed. If the patient is able to get up to the bathroom, pull their bedroom door closed to provide privacy. They are small gestures, but they speak volumes about the worth and dignity of the person being shielded from unnecessary exposure.

Chapter 5
Things of the Spirit

In that same vein, use the word garments or underwear when referring to the incontinent briefs a patient wears when they are incontinent. Diapers are worn by babies and the connotation for an adult is demeaning. Keep hair combed nicely and fingernails trimmed, with polish if the patient is a woman and likes nail polish. Keep men freshly shaved with hair combed.

- **Advocate for them**

For some families who are not familiar with the medical system, being at its mercy at such a vulnerable time for their loved one can be frightening. Let the patient and family know you are here to fight for them, whatever is needed.

Especially if they are in a facility, the staff changes frequently and details of a particular patient's needs can unfortunately get lost in the shuffle. You can be an advocate for the patient in the area of continuity of care. If you notice that something isn't right or that something the patient needs is being overlooked, speak up (tactfully, of course, and with a collaborative, rather than an adversarial attitude.)

It may be something as simple as advocating for getting a pitcher of water and glasses to drink it out of for the family who are gathering in the room. Or asking that the patient be repositioned if you see signs of discomfort and you know it's time for her to turn over.

- **Listen with respect**

When there is a concern, hear them out completely, allowing them to express their pain fully. Empathize, acknowledge their feelings and give them "permission" to address the problem or not. Active listening involves the whole person, with full mindful attention to what the other person is saying. Nothing you do as a volunteer could be more important than this.

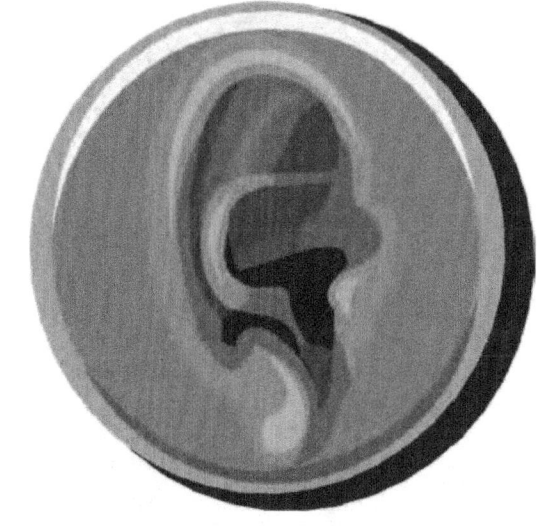

A Closer Look   175

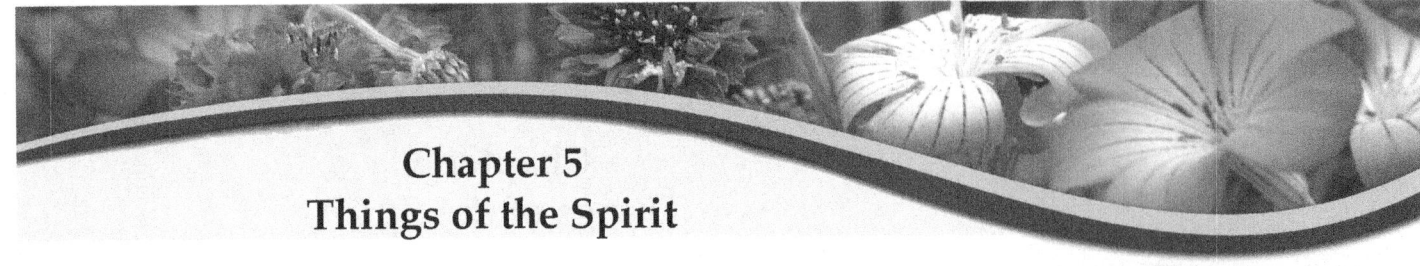

Chapter 5
Things of the Spirit

Communicating with an Unresponsive Patient

What if your patient is unresponsive? How can you communicate acceptance, appreciation, encouragement, forgiveness and gratitude?

You can! Hearing is the last sense to go and the likelihood is high that what you are communicating is getting through, if not at the level of cognizance, at least at the level of the spirit.

Talk to your unresponsive patient just as though he were awake. Introduce yourself and call him by name. Suggest to family members and friends who visit that they do the same. Use music to communicate. Sing old hymns if your patient has a history of loving them. (Don't assume that all older people love hymns. Ask the family what kind of music would be meaningful to the patient.)

Do this while applying lotion to the patient's hands or brushing her hair. Touch is a powerful communicator of worth and breaks the isolation that the unconscious state is creating. Watch carefully for the patient's response. You will be able to tell if she relaxes into the song and the physical touch or if her energy becomes more tense. If you are pulling her away from her task of letting go, she may need you to stop and give her space to do what she needs to do.

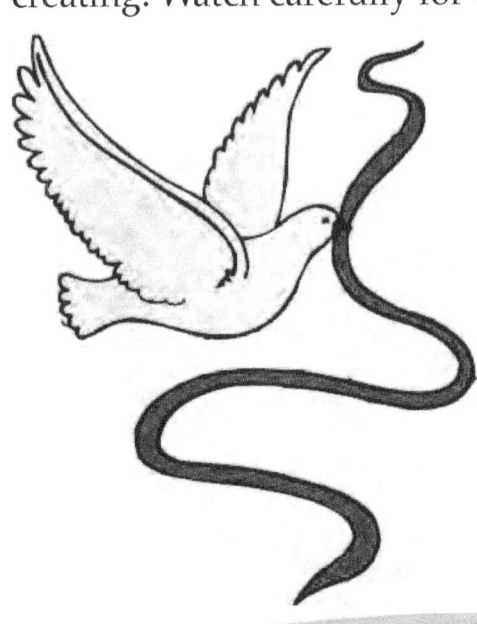

If you are in a facility and your patient is on vital sign monitors, watch her blood pressure, pulse and respiratory rate. Is her pulse going down? Is the top number of her blood pressure going down? Is her respiratory rate changing? These could be signs that your intervention is working and you are connecting with her spirit, soothing her with your verbal and non-verbal message of hope, love, and connection.

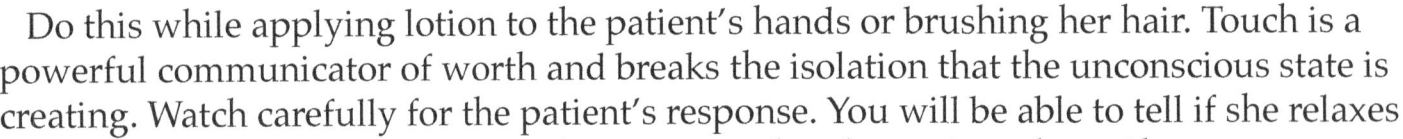

A Closer Look

Chapter 5
Things of the Spirit

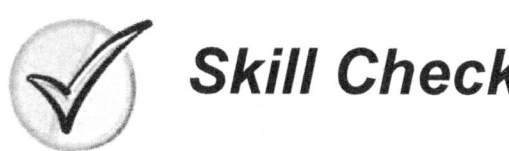 **Skill Check**

1. Define spirituality.

2. What role does life review play in a hospice patient's spiritual preparation for death?

3. List five characteristics of a rescuer.

4. List five characteristics of spiritually healthy helping.

5. What are some of the possible signs of inner pain?

"We are all one."
Louise L. Hay

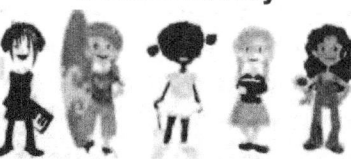

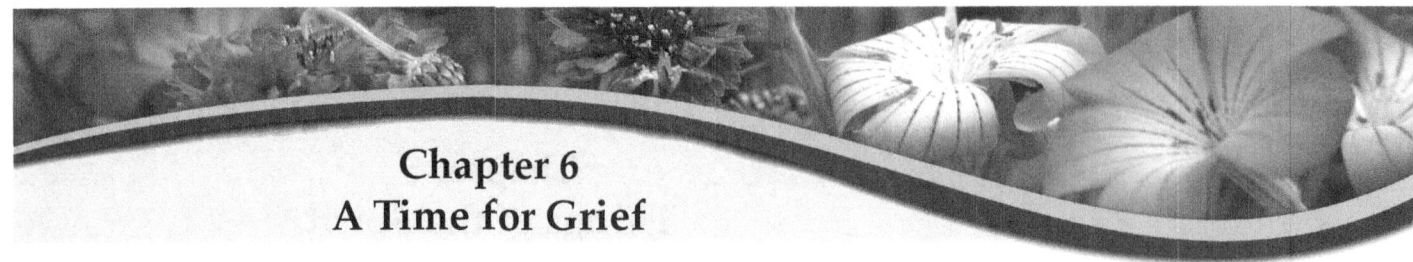

**Chapter 6
A Time for Grief**

6. A Time for Grief
Understanding Bereavement

"Just the facts, please..."

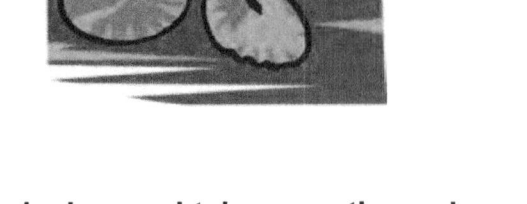

The surgeon makes a skillful cut across the man's chest, revealing layers of muscle tissue and bone. He performs an intricate cardiac operation, then carefully stitches the parts together again.

The man spends days and even weeks experiencing acute pain from the operation. Although he was an active mountain climber before the surgery, he puts off his next climb until the next year, knowing he'll need time for his body to heal and his heart to recover from the trauma of the surgery.

Even a year after the operation, when the scar has healed to a pink line and the doctors have given him a clean bill of health, the man continues to feel the reminders of his trauma. Occasionally, searing pain in the scar area lets him know that damaged nerves have not yet recovered.

A loss can affect human emotions in much the same way the surgeon's knife impacts the body. Any kind of a loss creates an emotional wound. The bigger the loss, the more severe the wound will be. And, just as a physical wound takes months and sometimes years to heal, so healing from an emotional wound takes time.

Because emotional wounds leave no visible scars, our society is less tolerant of the need for healing time. Comments like, "It's been a month since her husband died and she's still holed up in the house. She's going to have to pull herself together", are far too common. The impatience with which we treat those who are grieving only serves to increase their feeling of brokenness, isolation, and despair.

Someone once said, "Grief is not a problem to be solved, it is simply a statement that you have loved someone." The pain of separation is love's price tag and those who have had the courage to love deeply in spite of the potential pain of loss deserve our support through the difficult days of the healing process.

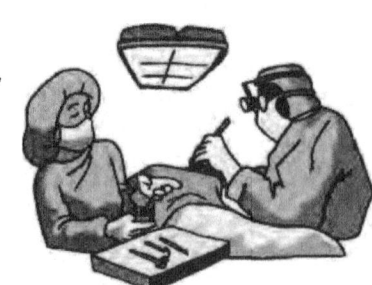

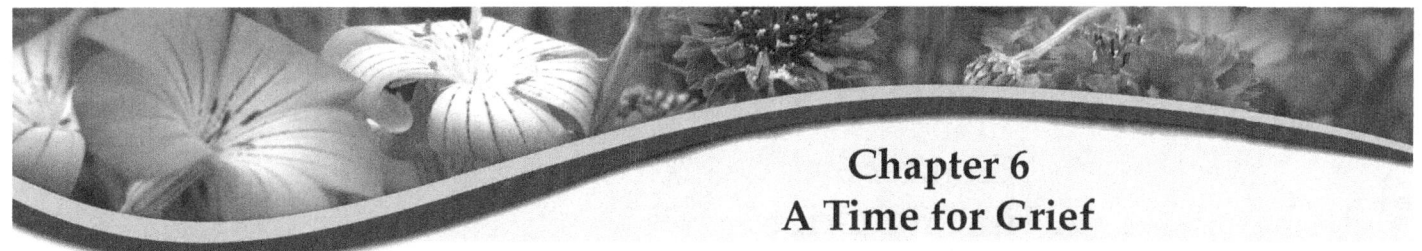

Chapter 6
A Time for Grief

Phases of the Grief Process

Loss is a wound and the more the loss affects our most important relationships, the deeper the wound. We looked the five stage model of the emotional stages of grief in Chapter Three. Let's take another look at these basic stages of grief and their primary identifiers. Remember that grief is not a neatly packaged, linear process that moves along from A to Z in a predictable manner. Grief, like life, is messy and full of surprises.

One of the most telling factors in how a person will respond in their grief process is called **resilience.** There are many things that determine a person's resilience level when the bottom drops out of their world. Among these are family system support, genetics, personality, birth order, and culture. The more underlying resilience a person possesses, the more strength they have available to them to deal with the loss in a constructive (for them) way.

- **Denial**

The surgeon steps close to the patient to begin his work. As skilled as he is, he wouldn't even consider making that first incision until the patient is properly anesthetized.

The shock and denial phase in the grief process is as necessary when an emotional wound has occurred as the anesthetic is in a surgical procedure. Major loss assaults the emotions and the impact can be overwhelming. A total nervous breakdown could very well occur as a result were it not for the softening, distracting effect of denial.

Family members and friends may be concerned during this phase that the grieving one isn't "facing reality". They may bring the "facts" of the loss to the griever's attention, trying to get them to acknowledge the "truth" and make decisions concerning the future.

The truth is: the mind will accept the loss as it is ready to. While the griever consciously denies the reality of the loss to some extent, his subconscious is busily at work preparing him for the pain of full acknowledgment.

Physical symptoms are very similar to those of a post traumatic stress disorder victim. The body is speaking of the loss, even if the person isn't ready to fully face it yet. In many ways, major loss can be as traumatic as being in a war zone.

"Just the facts, please..."

Chapter 6
A Time for Grief

Some things to watch for are:

Dark circles under eyes
Fatigue
Feeling detached from others
Not caring if you live or die
Being on "auto-pilot"
Headaches
Loss of appetite
"Nervous" eating-- no satisfaction from food
Pacing
Nightmares (especially those in which the person relives the loss)

Frequent urination
Sleeplessness
Irritability
Emotional "Numbness"
Difficulty concentrating
Uncontrollable shaking
Chest pain
Breathing too fast/shallow
Dizzy spells
Cold feet and hands
Pale skin

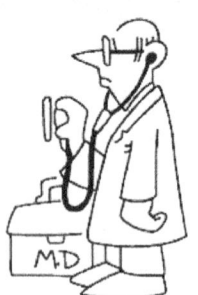

- ## Anger

The purpose of the anger stage of grief is to provide energy and motivation to deal with the added responsibilities created by the loss. Anger mobilizes the brain to begin the tasks of grieving. It helps to create enough emotional momentum to push past any "walls" of denial that may prevent emotional honesty, and provides an opportunity for processing old unresolved issues.

Some Signs of the Anger Phase of Grief:

- Fear - of the future, of the dark, of going on with life, of not being able to go on with life, of being of alone...

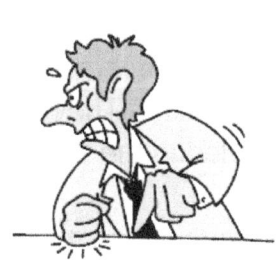

- Reliving the loss over and over and over again, trying to make sense of it

- Feeling estranged from God--anger at God for allowing the loss to happen

- Physical symptoms such as sleeplessness, tension headaches, muscle tightness, chest pain, etc.

"Just the facts, please..."

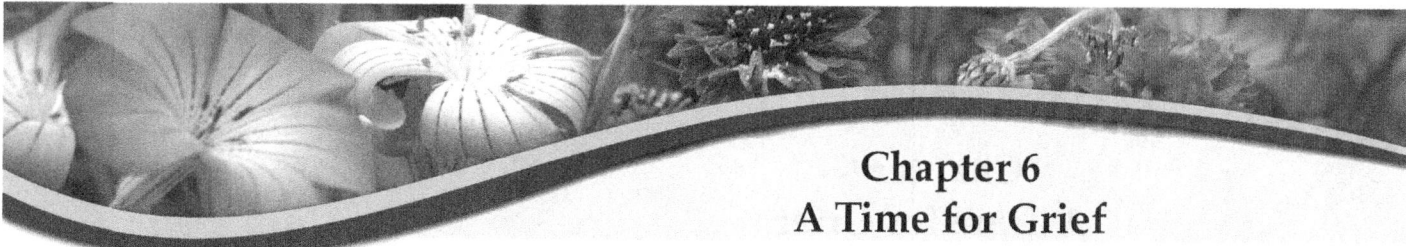

Chapter 6
A Time for Grief

- Feeling irritable with those who are moving on with their lives as if the loss didn't make any difference to them

- Feeling of wanting to "run away" from life as it is now

- Difficulty concentrating on tasks--the person's mind always going back to the loss and the implications for his life

- Seeing others with their loved ones and feeling angry that she doesn't have her loved one now

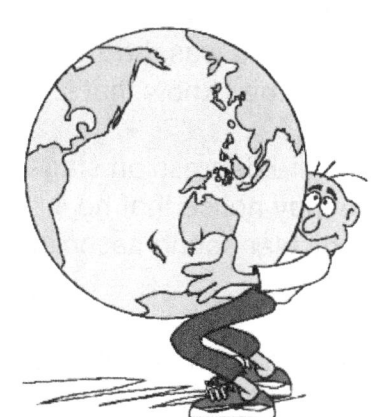

- **Bargaining**

Once the anger phase of grief has subsided, it is common for a grieving person to move into some form of bargaining. It may not be obvious. Bargaining can be totally non-verbal and the bargainer may not be aware of his behavior at all.

Making a choice to stop a bad habit, becoming compliant and easy-to-please, throwing oneself into community or church activities, increasing donations to charities... These can all be a form of bargaining if done in an effort to regain "control" over one's life and somehow help relieve the pain of loss.

- **Deep Sadness**

This stage in the grief process is characterized by a sense of deep and profound sadness. The full impact of the loss is hitting, without the numbing benefit of denial or the distractions of anger and bargaining.

Here are some reflections on how it feels to be in the depression stage of grief from those who have experienced it:

"It felt as if I were falling into a dark chasm with no bottom. I couldn't see any end to the pain."

"For a long time, I felt so angry that he had died and left me. I focused on the bad things that had happened in our relationship to try to convince myself that I am better off without him. Then the deep sadness hit and I could remember it all, good and bad, and a deep, keening sense of loss took over. I thought it was going to smother me."

"I couldn't even get out of bed in the morning. Every small task of everyday life felt impossible to me. How could I go on with my life when the best part of me, the part I gave to her, is gone?"

"Just the facts, please..."

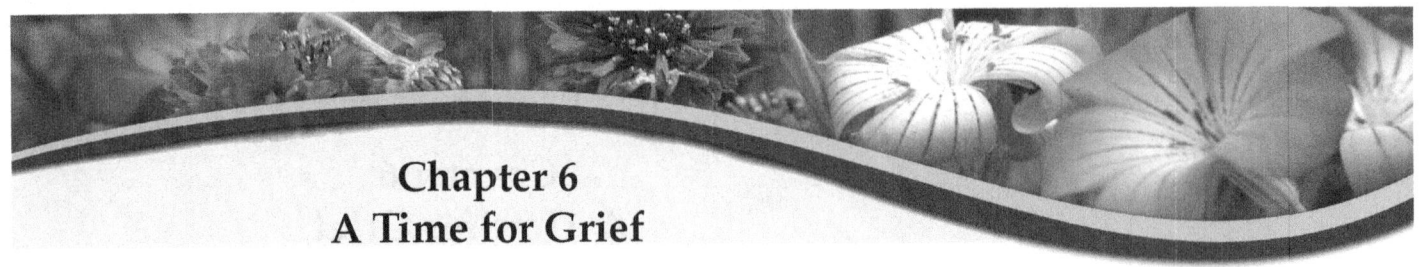

Chapter 6
A Time for Grief

"It surprised me each day when the sun came up and everyone just went on with their lives as if everything was the same as ever. I wanted to scream at them that nothing is the same and deep inside me I know that it never will be again."

In the depression stage of grief, because the person's heart is fully aware of its pain and loss, he may notice that he is "triggered" a lot. A familiar place, a certain scent, the way the air feels, a particular sound associated with the loved one, all can send him tumbling into the abyss of active grief.

It is tempting when this happens to do anything possible to relieve the pain and try to feel better again. As natural as this urge to anesthetize is, growth and healing happens when one allows themselves to fully experience the loss.

- **Acceptance**

You may have heard it said that one never recovers from grief. This is partly true, in that your life will never be the same as it was before your loss. There is, however, recovery from grief. The sunshine **does** return. A room in your heart will always be reserved for that special loved one and no one will ever take their place, but once the acceptance stage of grief is reached, life **will** begin to have meaning again.

Those who have experienced deep grief and have worked through the stages to acceptance have a different outlook on life than those who have never loved and lost. It has been said that grief is the instrument that reams out depths of compassion, understanding, and empathy in the human heart that could never be reached any other way.

In his "Growing Through Loss" workshop, grief counselor Bob Deits speaks of his experience over 25 years of working with those who have lost loved ones, many in very tragic circumstances. He calls the bereaved "adventurers" because he has found that those who have experienced and conquered grief share more about what they have **found** than what they have lost.

They are not in denial about the past, but they focus more on the future and what opportunities for growth lay ahead. They possess a deep sense of joy because they have experienced tragedy and survived. They know that there is no curve ball life could throw that will get them down. They are compassionate, patient, and sustain a deep reverence for life and the importance of relationships.

"Just the facts, please..."

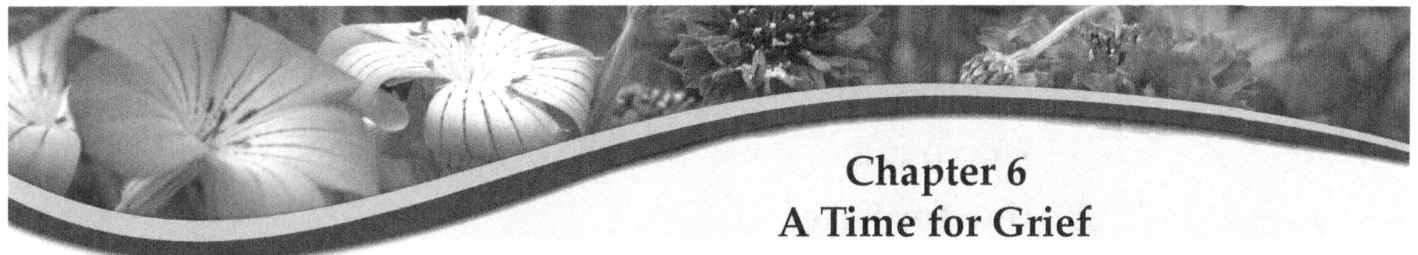

Chapter 6
A Time for Grief

Some questions you may be asking...

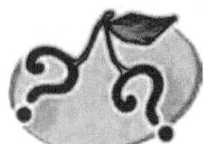

What is the difference between bereavement after the patient dies and the anticipatory grief the patient and family experienced before the death?

Not much, actually. A loss is a loss and the patient felt the pain of impending loss in many of the same ways the family and friends feel the loss after the death occurs. The reality of the actual loss often brings the grief response out more acutely with more varied reactions. Grief counselors often find that it is helpful to look at the grief process in terms of ten stages, although, as in the stages of dying, these may occur in any order at any time.

1. Shock

Even when a death is expected, family and friends usually experience a period of emotional denial of the death. Day-to-day functioning tends to be rote and may be described later as operating on "auto-pilot" or stumbling through a fog of unreality.

2. Emotional upheaval

When the shock of the death begins to wear off, the bereaved person is often distressed to find that strong emotions such as anger, fear, remorse, and extreme loneliness start to wreak havoc in his life. The person may begin to realize how much he depended upon the person who died and may feel the loss acutely. These feelings can lead to a loss of self-esteem and feelings of inadequacy.

3. Depression

As the bereaved person's feelings of anger, fear, and loneliness intensify, feelings of helplessness and hopelessness are often added. They may long for death themselves as a release from the pain. This time of deep depression can be the most acutely uncomfortable phase of the whole grief process and require the most acceptance and understanding from loved ones.

"Just the facts, please..."

Chapter 6
A Time for Grief

4. Physical Symptoms

It is very common for the bereaved to develop physical symptoms that correlate to those of the one who died. If the person died of a heart attack, the spouse may feel tightness in the chest during this stage of grief.

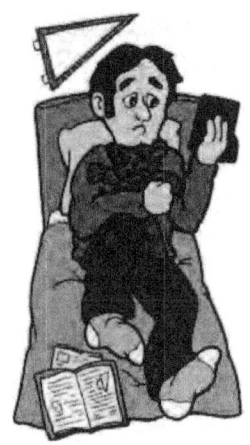

5. Anxiety

During this stage, the bereaved may fear losing the memory of the deceased. They may have vivid dreams, waking and sleeping, in which they see their loved one. This is a very disturbing time and problems with eating and sleeping are common.

6. Hostility

The bereaved may experience a period of rage about 6 weeks after the death of the loved one has occurred. It can be a very confusing and distressing to the person experiencing it, as well as those around him. He may be frightened by the intensity of his anger and see it as inappropriate, but feel unable to defuse it. He may act in very "positive" ways toward others but turn the rage he feels inward, in self-abusive ways.

7. Guilt

"Should" is the favorite word of someone experiencing this phase of the grief process. "I should have stopped in to see him that day" or "I shouldn't have yelled at her about cleaning her room before she left" are common types of statements. Death has a way of amplifying whatever issues existed between the deceased and the survivor before the death occurred and problems that seemed insignificant while the person was still alive can become major obstacles to the bereaved now.

8. Fear

The bereaved experience fear in many forms. Fear of being alone in the house where the person died, fear of going out, fear of any new relationships no matter what their nature, fear of never being happy again, fear of being happy and feeling guilty about it, fear of waking up in the morning and feeling the pain of being so alone...

Chapter 6
A Time for Grief

9. Memory Healing

During this phase of bereavement, memories both good and bad ebb and flow through the bereaved person's mind. It is usually easier to process the bad memories first, because in many ways, the good memories are the most painful to recall.

10. Acceptance

Accepting the reality of the loved one's death and forgetting them are two different things. As with the healing of any serious wound, a scar will always remain to remind the bearer of the injury. The bereaved person will never be the same, because loving and losing someone special changes them forever. Although an acceptance and "letting go" usually takes one or two years to achieve, 100% healing never happens.

Are there any guidelines as far as what to expect at certain times after the loss?

Each person's grief is unique to them and no time schedule will fit everyone's grief experience. There are, however, some general guidelines that can help in understanding where someone might be in their healing process. They have been called the "critical time intervals".

First 48 Hours

The shock from the death can be intense during this time and the emotions frightening. Denial may be very strong during the first few hours.

First Week

Many of the actions during this time are automatic: funeral planning, calling relatives, taking care of business. This time of gathering strength to do what has to be done may be followed by a time of emotional and physical exhaustion.

"Just the facts, please..."

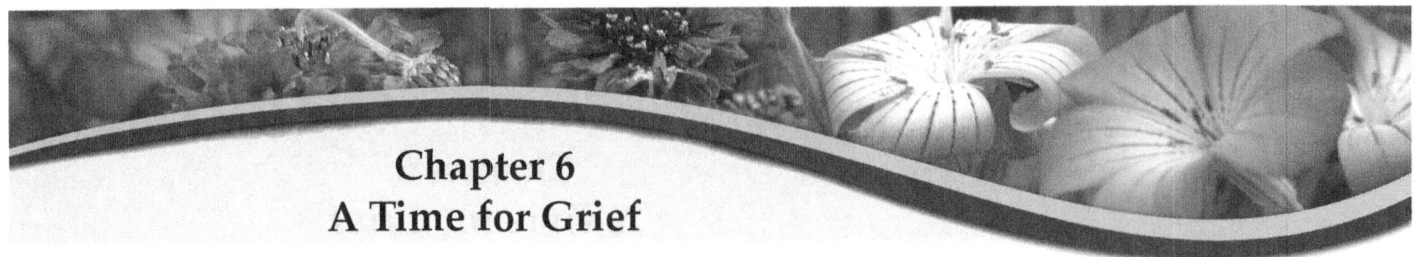

Chapter 6
A Time for Grief

Second to Fifth Weeks

This time period is often characterized by a feeling of abandonment as friends and family members return to their normal routines after the funeral. If the bereaved is trying to maintain a job, her employer may expect her to be recovered and fully functional at work. Some residual denial may still be insulating her from the full impact of the loss, so she may say things like, "Well, it's not as bad as I thought it would be. I think I can handle this".

Sixth to Twelfth Weeks

It's during this time that the anesthetic of denial may wear completely off and the reality of the loss hits full force. Some of the things the bereaved person may experience during this time are:

- **Sleep changes**
- **Unpredictable, uncontrollable bouts of crying**
- **Onset of fear, sometimes paranoia**
- **Wanting to "punish" something or someone for the pain**
- **Changes in sexual desire/activity**
- **Fatigue and generalized weakness**
- **Muscle tremors**
- **Loss of motivation**
- **Extreme mood swings**
- **Inability to concentrate**
- **Change in appetite**
- **Desire for isolation**
- **Need to talk about the deceased**
- **Physical symptoms of distress**

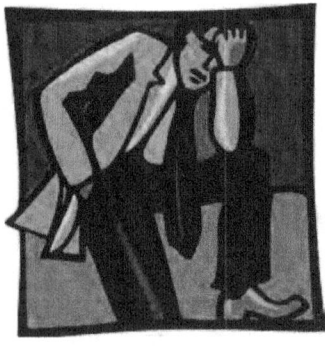

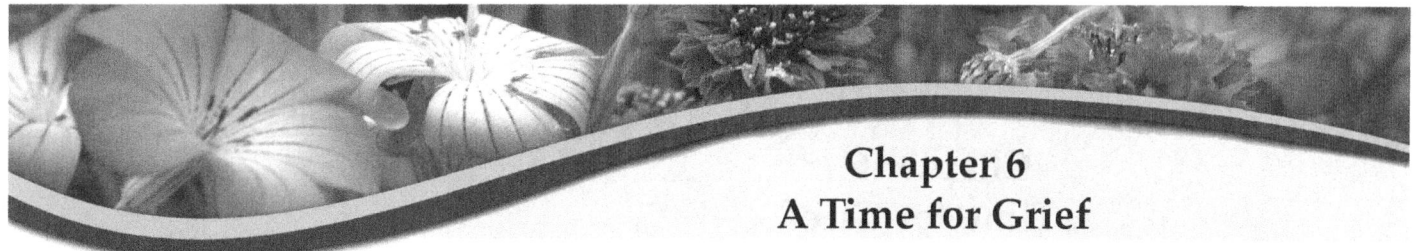

Chapter 6
A Time for Grief

Third to Fourth Month

As the nightmare drags on, there is a decreased tolerance for frustration. A cycle of "good days and bad days" develops. It is during this time that the immune system takes the hardest hit and colds and flu have a heyday with the bereaved, adding their discomfort to the pain of just making it from day to day.

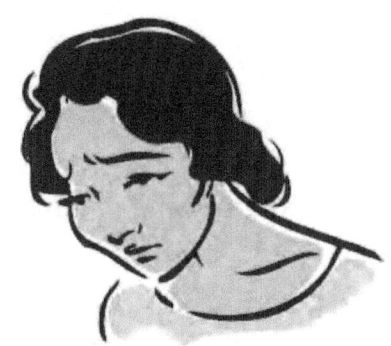

Six Months

This milestone can be excruciatingly painful, resurrecting all the events of the loss and starting the cycle of emotional upheaval all over again. This reaction is also common during holidays, birthdays, and other special occasions.

Twelve Months

The first anniversary of the death can be the hardest day of all for the bereaved. It usually lasts three or four days. If the quality of the grief work done during the year has been high, this may also be the beginning of resolution.

Eighteen to Twenty-four months

This is the time that resolution often occurs. The raw pain has healed and the bereaved is able to bear the pain of separation enough to proceed with life. There is an emotional "letting go" that occurs and the person no longer uses the death as the focal point around which all the rest of life revolves.

"Just the facts, please..."

Chapter 6
A Time for Grief

Aren't there some pretty significant differences in how people respond to the grief process?

Yes, there are. Many factors influence how an individual responds to grief. The following are some of the major ones:

- **Family rules of expression**

As we learned in chapter three, family systems influence the emotional expression of individual family members to a great extent. Some families encourage emotional support between members and others suppress it. In a closed family system, any admission of fear or "negative" emotion is unacceptable.

- **Relationship with the deceased**

The closer the relationship to the one who died, the more intensely the bereaved will sense the loss. This is especially true in the face of closely intertwined experiences, dreams, goals, and future plans. A stressful relationship, in which communication was unhealthy and a high level of dependency was present, will also create a setting for intense grief. Unresolved family issues can exacerbate guilt and prolong the grief process.

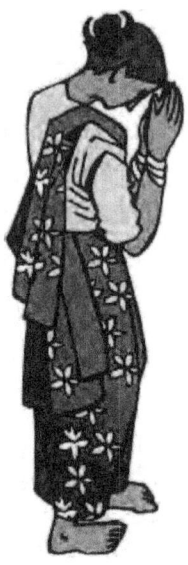

- **Circumstances of the death**

An expected death, with hospice involved to help family members work through the anticipatory grief process, is less likely to precipitate an unhealthy grief reaction than a sudden death by suicide or homicide. The death of an older person who has voiced a readiness to die is sometimes easier to accept than the death of a child who hasn't had a chance to "live" yet.

- **Cultural framework**

One of the most significant factors influencing the grief response is the culture in which the person was raised. "Socially acceptable" grief responses can vary significantly from culture to culture. Some cultures are very emotionally expressive while others tend to repress any show of feelings.

"Just the facts, please..."

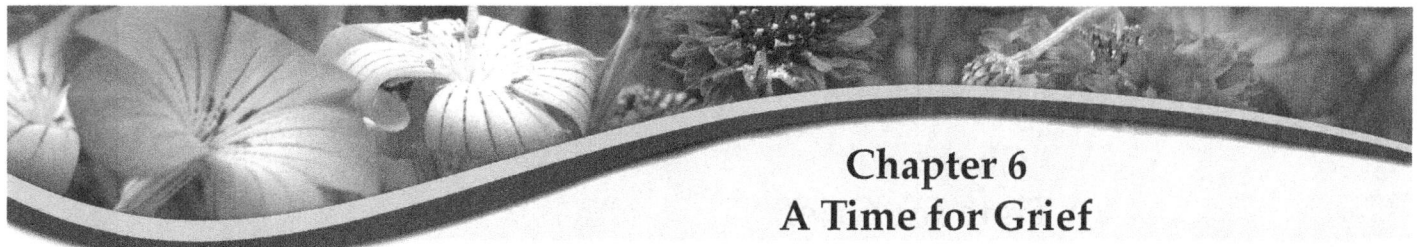

Chapter 6
A Time for Grief

- **Religious beliefs**

The bereaved's spiritual support system has a tremendous impact on her ability to cope with the wrenching pain of separation from a loved one in death. Studies have shown that religious rituals aid in the emotional healing process.

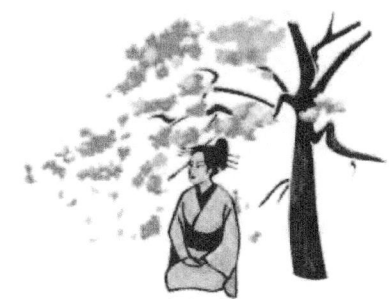

- **Personal coping skills**

Whenever a crisis occurs in an individual's life, they fall back on the coping skills they have developed from early childhood on to adulthood. If their coping skills are based in shame and unhealthy beliefs about themselves, the grieving process will be much more painful and much more likely to develop into abnormal grief.

- **Personality of the individual**

Some personalities are naturally more introspective and serious, investing every event in life with personal meaning. Others are more outgoing and surface in their relationships and tend to heal more quickly from wounds and move on with life. No certain personality type is "good" and "right" any more than any of them are "bad" and "wrong". They are just different.

- **Current life stress**

Stress is cumulative. Some major stressors are death, divorce, moving, having a baby, changing jobs, experiencing a natural disaster, and others. If there are several major stressors already depleting the bereaved's energy, the death could well push her over the brink in her coping ability. There are positive stressors, too. Birth, marriage, job promotions, and other welcomed changes also bring increased levels of stress.

- **Physical health**

A person's health can have a huge impact on their ability to cope with added stressors in their life. A handicap or physical ailment can short-circuit one of the most important stress relievers available to the bereaved: regular outdoor exercise.

- **Support system**

Loving support is crucial to a person coping with the pain of losing a loved one. Those who, before the crisis occurred, established a healthy support network of friends and family cope far more healthfully with the grief process in all its painful phases.

"Just the facts, please..."

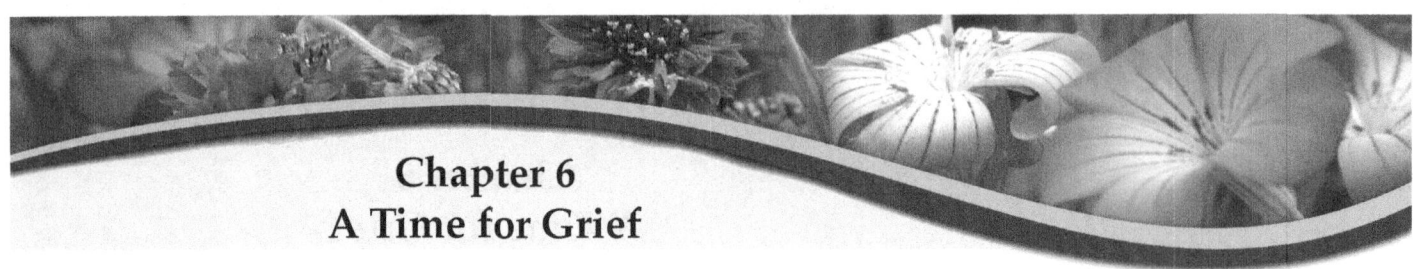

Chapter 6
A Time for Grief

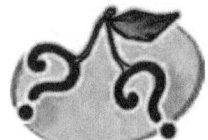 **What are some of the signs that a person is healing and moving on with his/her life?**

There are many signs of healing. It is important to remember, however, when you see these signs of healing, that it is normal and common for someone going through the grief process to experience regression at any point. Some sight, sound, or memory can trigger the pain and sadness without a moment's notice. It is during these painful setbacks that the bereaved needs acceptance and support, not judgment.

Signs of Healing

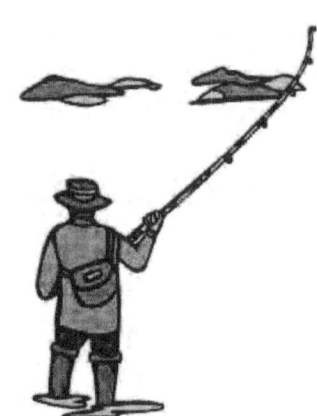

- Able to enjoy time alone

- Actually looking forward to holidays

- Enjoyment of a joke

- Eating, sleeping, and exercise patterns return to "normal"

- A renewed sense of energy and purpose

- A routine develops in daily life

- Able to concentrate on a book or favorite TV program

- Can review both "good" and "bad" memories

- Able to drive somewhere alone without crying the whole time

- Can sit through a religious service without crying

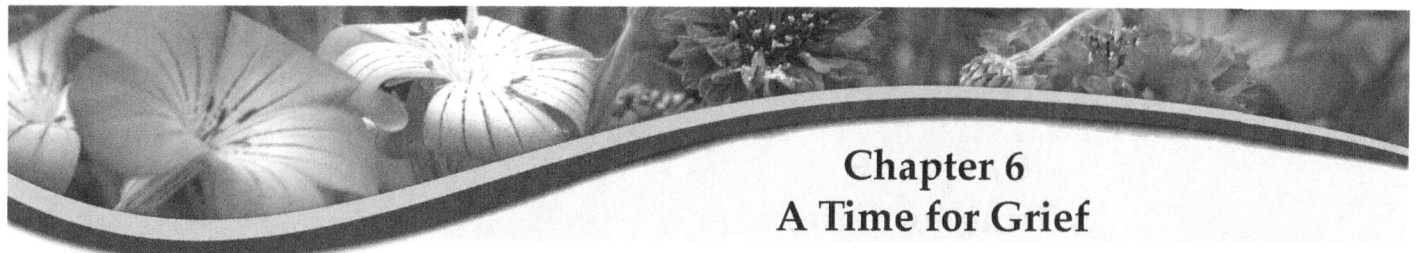

Chapter 6
A Time for Grief

- Establishing new and healthy relationships

- Organizing and planning for the future

- Looking forward to getting up in the morning

- Reinvesting the energy once spent on the deceased in other projects

- Enjoying life's pleasant experiences

- No longer needing daily or weekly trips to the cemetery

- Acceptance of things as they are instead of trying to return to how they were

- Treating own grief "attacks" with patience

- Able to discover personal growth from the grief process

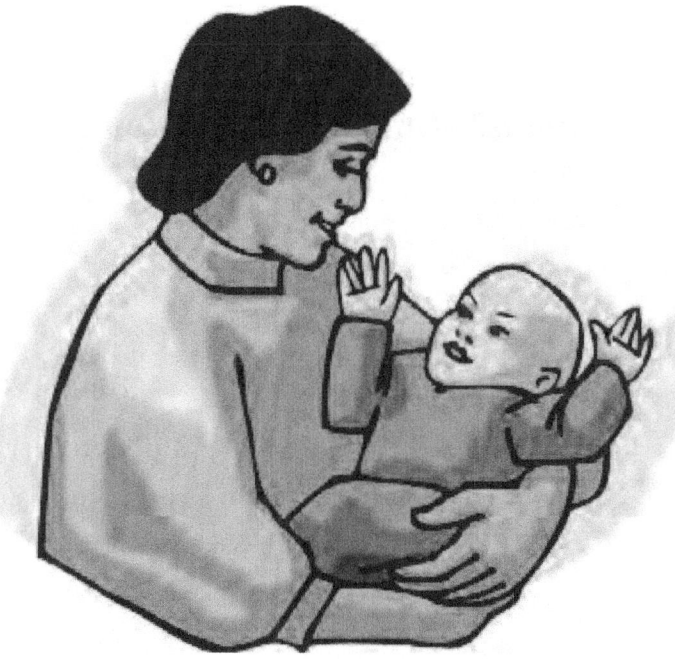

"Just the facts, please..."

**Chapter 6
A Time for Grief**

 *At the Heart of the Matter*

Divide into small groups and discuss the following questions about the "Surviving Grief" story on the video (or write your answers in the spaces provided if you are working through this series on your own):

1. *Have you had an experience of your own with grief? How was it the same and how was it different from the young man's experience in the story?*

2. *How do you feel about the statement, "Don't be afraid of my silences"? What does silence mean to you? How do you respond to silence?*

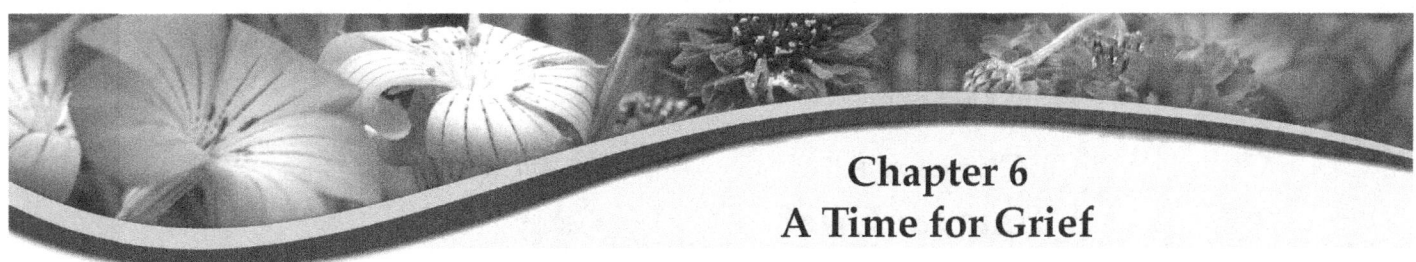

**Chapter 6
A Time for Grief**

3. What actions by your family and others close to you do you feel would be the most comforting and supportive to you if you were in the position of having lost a loved one? What actions or attitudes would feel unsupportive to you?

4. What are your greatest fears about working with someone who is experiencing deep grief?

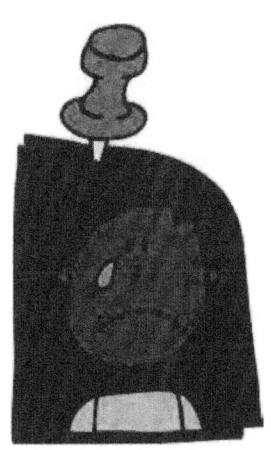

Chapter 6
A Time for Grief

Think of a loss that you have experienced in your life. If you could pick a color that describes that loss, what would it be? Why?

If you feel comfortable doing so, share your "color" and its meaning with the group.

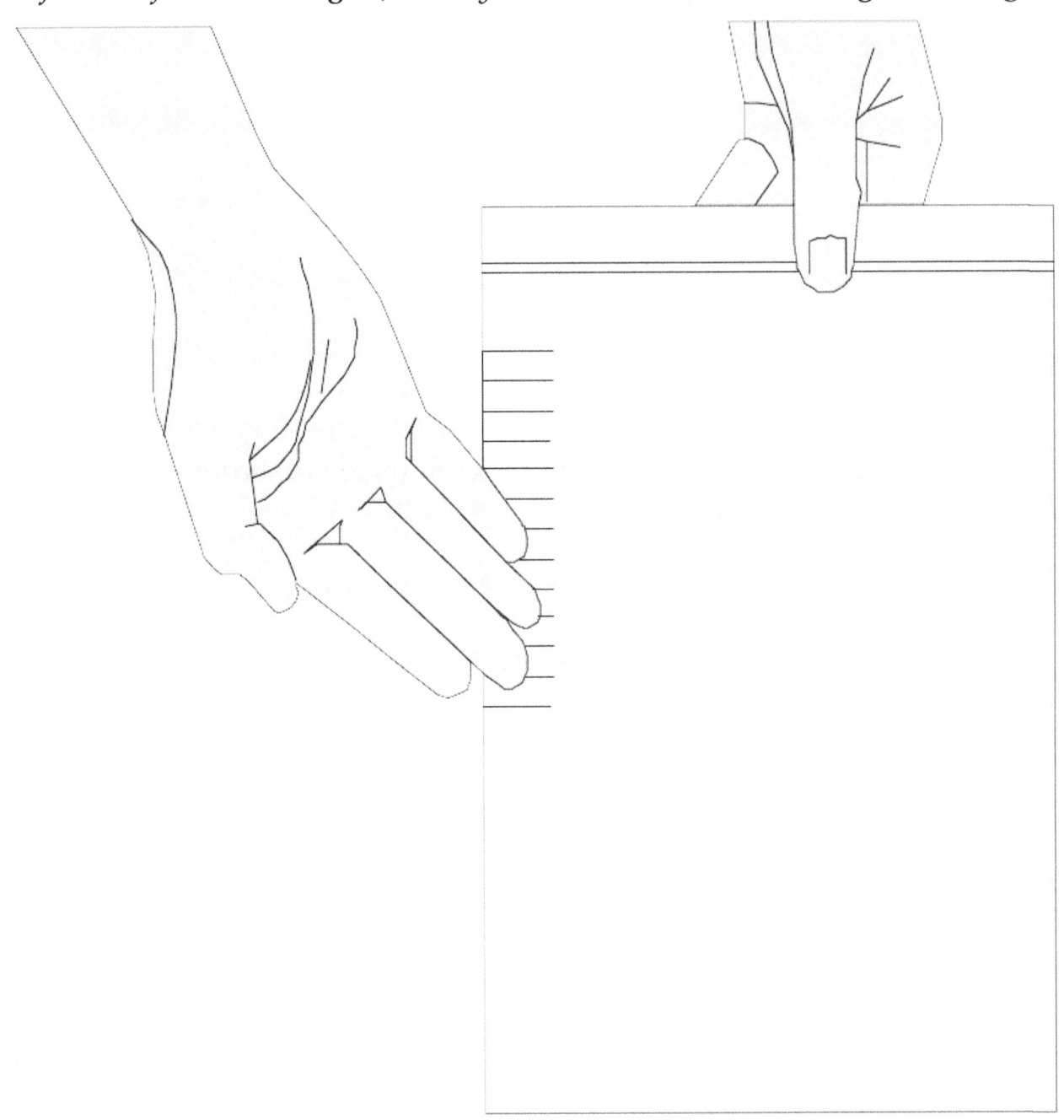

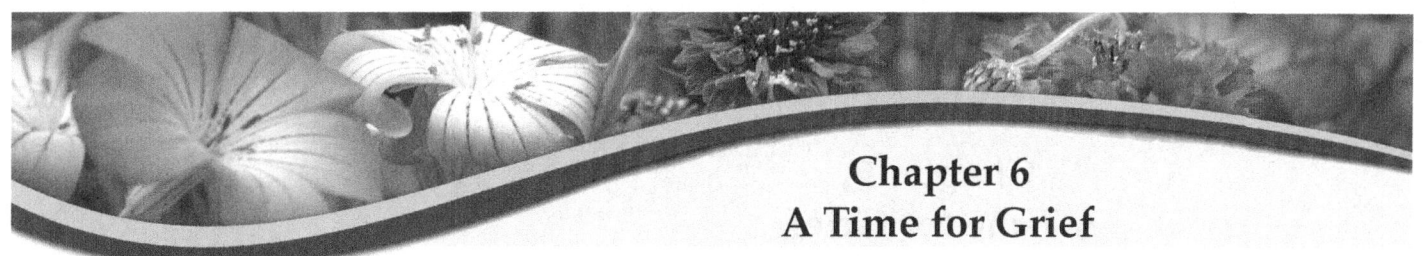

Chapter 6
A Time for Grief

 # Putting it Into Practice

The newly bereaved family has a hard job ahead and you, as a caregiver, can help. Here are some of the things you can do:

- **Help family members understand that their feelings are normal**

- **Practice therapeutic listening**

- **Help family members make difficult decisions**

- **Make sure the family knows that a grief support group is available to them**

- **Encourage family members to reduce stress through:**

Diet

Exercise

Time out / pampering

Breathing techniques

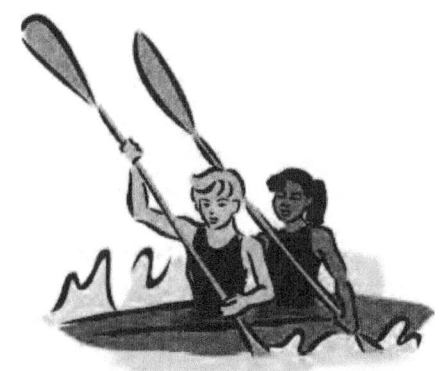

Chapter 6
A Time for Grief

A person who has experienced a major loss often has a hard time sleeping at night. She may find that as soon as she ends a busy day and goes to bed, hoping for a good night's sleep, her mind starts churning, thinking about the loved one she lost. Or she may manage to fall asleep, just to pop wide awake in just a few hours and be unable to go back to sleep. Here are some ideas you can share with her:

- **Try warm milk or herb (decaffeinated) tea with honey before going to bed.**

- **Establish a routine of going to bed at the same time each night and getting up at the same time every morning. Maintain this pattern even on weekends so your body can adjust without confusion.**

- **A hot bath before retiring can be very relaxing.**

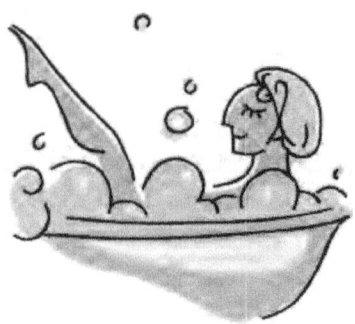

- **Lying down while you watch a boring television program or read a book with lots of relaxing descriptions of scenery (i.e. Michener) may help you nod off.**

- **Avoid naps in the daytime, even if you feel very sleepy then. Take a walk until the urge to catnap passes.**

- **If sleeping in your bed is a painful reminder that your spouse is no longer with you, try sleeping on his side of the bed and using his pillow. It is easier to cope with seeing your side of the bed empty.**

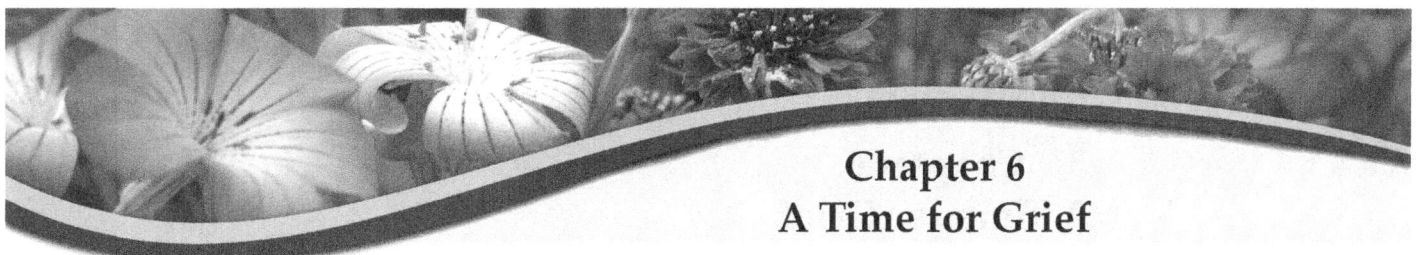

Chapter 6
A Time for Grief

- Avoid stimulants such as coffee, tea, chocolate, and soft drinks that contain caffeine.

- Eat a light meal at supper time instead of a heavy one.

- If it is fear that is keeping you awake at night, do whatever it takes to relieve your fears. Install an alarm system, get a dog, lock your bedroom door, leave a light on, ask a friend to stay over...

- Adjust the temperature in your sleeping room to help you sleep most comfortably. Many times cooler air in the bedroom is more relaxing if you have plenty of covers, but if you have problems with dry mucous membranes, a warmer, more humid environment might help you rest more comfortably.

- Try listening to relaxing music. There are many environmental CDs available now that are very soothing and may help lull you to sleep.

- Don't try to make yourself go to sleep. If none of the usual relaxation enhancers work, get up and do something else for awhile then start the bedtime routine again.

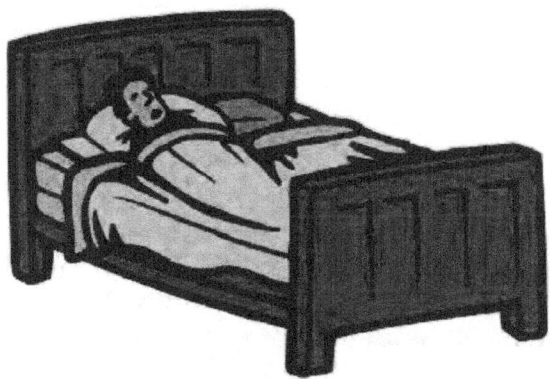

Putting it Into Practice

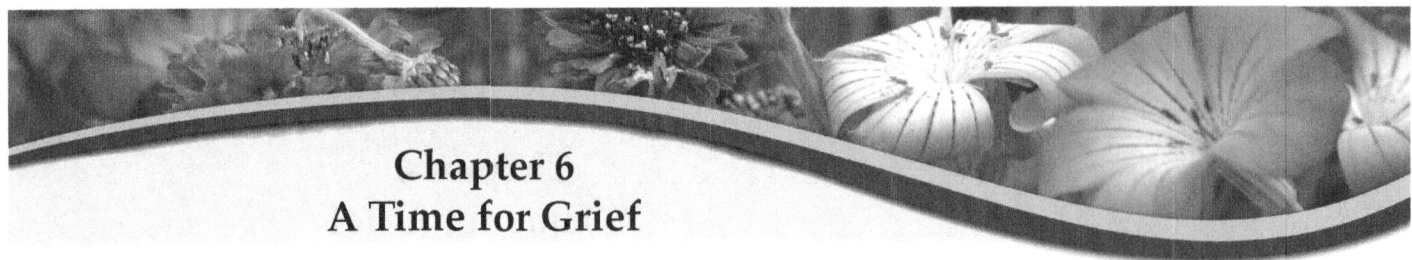

Chapter 6
A Time for Grief

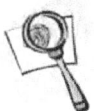 A Closer Look

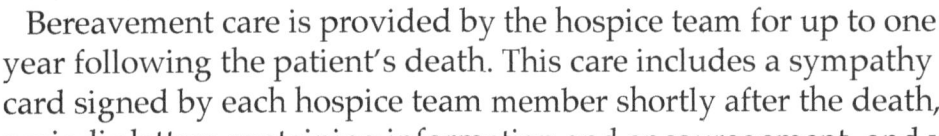

The bereavement coordinator on the hospice team is usually a social worker. This is necessary because of the need to be on the alert for signs of abnormal grieving and to guide the team in how to provide bereavement care in special cases such as those involving children.

Bereavement care is provided by the hospice team for up to one year following the patient's death. This care includes a sympathy card signed by each hospice team member shortly after the death, periodic letters containing information and encouragement, and visits at intervals throughout the year by members of the hospice team who knew the patient and family.

Volunteers often play a significant role in bereavement care as they are among the team members that most often achieve a sense of real closeness to the family. Bereaved family members tend to want to talk about the patient's death to someone who knew him and is familiar with the circumstances surrounding his care.

It is important for the volunteer, or any other member of the care team in touch with the family, to be able to recognize signs of potential difficulties in grieving. These signs of possible abnormal grief should be reported at once to the bereavement coordinator or to the social worker following the family. (They are called "possible" signs of abnormal grief because the line between healthy and unhealthy grief can often be very thin and sometimes indistinguishable. It is the degree of intensity or the length of time a certain symptom persists, rather than the symptom's presence, that is important.)

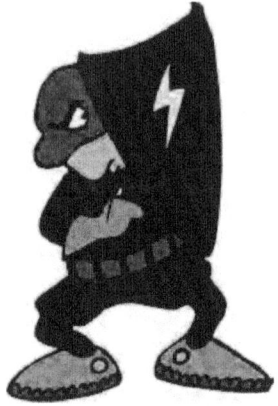

Another important aspect of providing care for the bereaved is keeping current with our own grief. If we, as caregivers, have unresolved grief from our own past and present losses, the likelihood of projecting our issues onto our patients and families is high. The more we look at our own history of personal loss and pain and work through our guilt and grief, the more supportive we can be as caregivers.

Often, when a caregiver has unresolved grief issues of their own, it is easy to become over-involved and over-protective of a patient or family. The flip side of this coin is the tendency to become withdrawn and uninvolved because of a deep fear of exposing our own pain to the light.

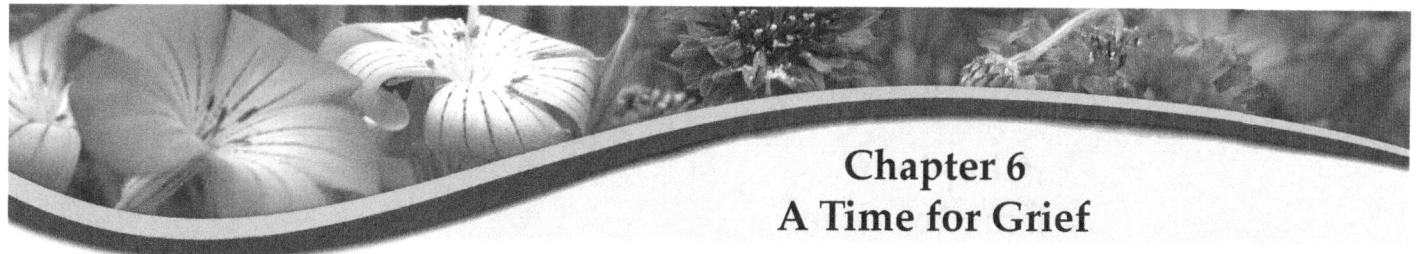

Chapter 6
A Time for Grief

Signs That May Indicate an Unhealthy Grief Response

- Avoiding any thoughts or feelings about the loved one's death

- Significant preoccupation with the death many months after it occurred

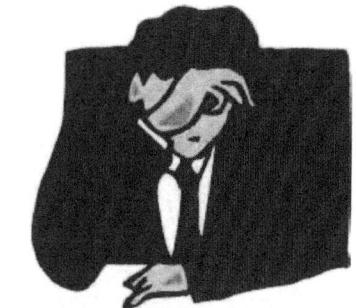

- Large memory gaps

- Flashbacks, hallucinations, and nightmares about the death

- A continuing, significant disinterest in the activities of daily life

- "Worshiping" and over idealizing the person who died, so much that it interferes with daily life even months after the death

- Severe irritability and outbursts of anger toward others in the family and toward coworkers

- Feeling out of control and unable to cope for an extended period of time

- Using alcohol and/or drugs to keep from experiencing the pain of the grief process

- Avoiding all relationships for fear another loss will occur

A Closer Look

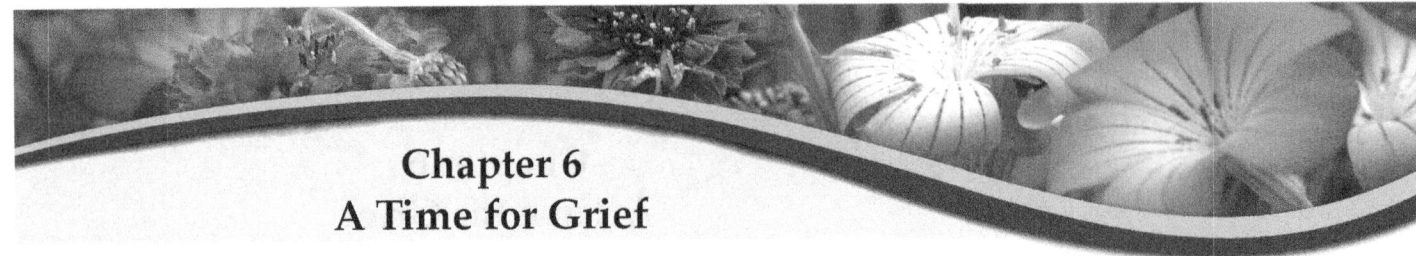

Chapter 6
A Time for Grief

- **Flat affect - no emotion at all, even after the first few weeks following the death**

- **Continuing tension and insomnia that isn't relieved with relaxation techniques**

- **Ongoing physical symptoms such as heart palpitations, severe startle reflexes, cold sweats, and breathing difficulties**

- **The development of new problems sleeping, eating, or relaxing that weren't occurring previously**

- **Feeling guilty about surviving when the loved one died**

- **Talking about suicide, especially if a plan is mentioned**

- **Calmly and methodically giving away possessions**

- **Pronounced detachment and withdrawal from significant others**

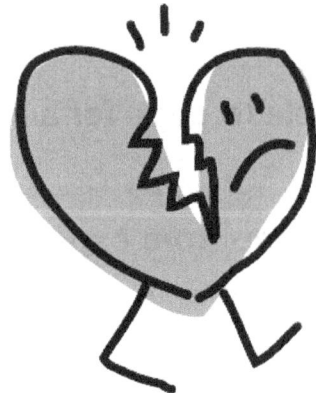

Chapter 6
A Time for Grief

Dealing with Guilt

"It's my fault. I should have been paying closer attention. This would never have happened had I been a better parent." These are the words of a mother in the throes of guilt following a fatal accident involving one of her children. The emotional roller coaster that accompanies such a tragedy is devastating enough without the wrenching pain of guilt. When the self-condemnation begins, the load is crushing.

When a tragedy occurs involving one of our loved ones, whether it is an expected death from cancer or some other disease, or a sudden and unexpected death by accident or attack, it is common for guilt to arise. If we can just blame someone, it feels as if we have some kind of control over the situation. As the feelings of helplessness and hopelessness well up inside, assigning guilt gives us the illusion that we are taking action.

This illusion, however, is not helpful in our healing process. Blame, whether directed toward others or ourselves, is a particularly harmful form of self-deception and takes us all the way **back** to the denial stage of grief.

What does guilt look like in the grief process? How can I tell if it is unhealthy guilt or a conviction of something that I really have done wrong?

First of all, let's look at unhealthy guilt. The following are some of the ways that guilt can paralyze us and prevent healing from taking place:

- **Survivor guilt**

This kind of guilt says that it isn't fair that you are still alive when your loved one isn't. It also kicks in as you grow and change past where your loved one had grown before his or her death. It tells you that to move on and do something new or different with your life is disloyal to the one no longer with you.

- **Depression**

This is not the clinical depression that is caused by a chemical imbalance in the brain nor is it the deep, reality-based sadness that is one of the stages of the grief process. The depression that is instigated by guilt is a downward spiral that feeds on itself. It is fueled by the belief that if only you were a "better person" or had done the "right thing", this terrible loss would not have happened.

A Closer Look

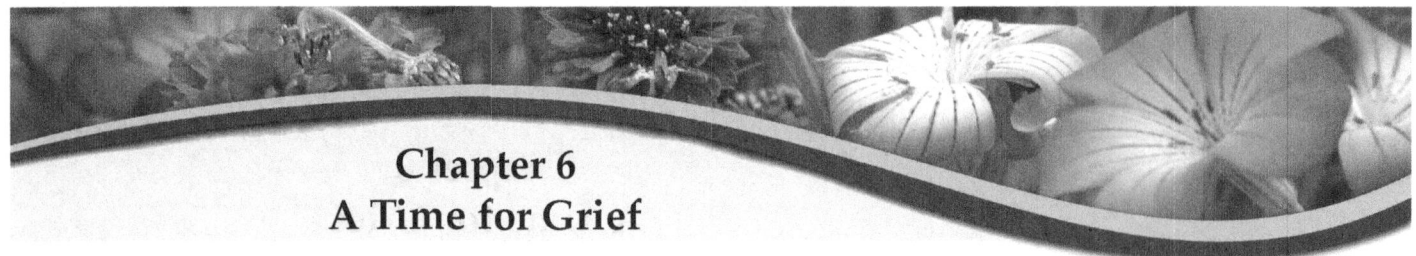

Chapter 6
A Time for Grief

- **Magical thinking**

Magical thinking is a carry-over from childhood when we believed that just by imagining something in our minds we could make it happen. Often, when a parent dies, a child will believe that the death was a result of bad feelings the child carried toward the parent.

- **Blaming**

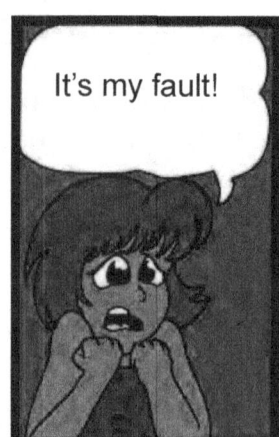

Blaming is a defense mechanism that keeps us stuck by focusing our attention on a "symbol" of our anger. Guilt feelings are incredibly painful and blaming prevents us from seeing reality, thus numbing our pain somewhat. The price tag for this anesthetic, however, is enormous.

Healing can only come as we move through the grief process, facing our feelings and accepting the truth about the loss. Blaming blocks the truth from our conscious minds and keeps us stuck in frozen grief that can last a lifetime if the blaming patterns continue. The toll on our physical, emotional, and spiritual health is tremendous.

- **Victim Mentality**

Victim mentality is learned helplessness. We each ideally possess a healthy balance between weakness and strength. Our weakness tells us that we need each other's help and support. Our strength tells us that with faith in ourselves and others, we could move mountains of despair or difficulty and meet challenges that help us grow.

Physical, sexual, or verbal abuse (criticism) in childhood can throw us out of balance, teaching us to access only our weakness. Because "strength" feels so unfamiliar, we avoid it and choose to stay stuck in helplessness. Guilt and shame are the hallmarks of victim mentality, reinforcing the illusion of weakness and preventing forward momentum.

Healthy conviction lifts up and illuminates, inviting us to a healthier, more complete place. If we have erred, it corrects us in a very specific way that lets us know exactly where the error was and what to do to make it right. It invites us to let go of shame and embrace wholeness. It does not mean that we won't feel the weight of grief or experience the anger or sadness of the grief process. It does mean that we are not carrying the world on our shoulders, responsible for what happens to our loved ones. It also means that we can trust that things will work out in the "right" timing.

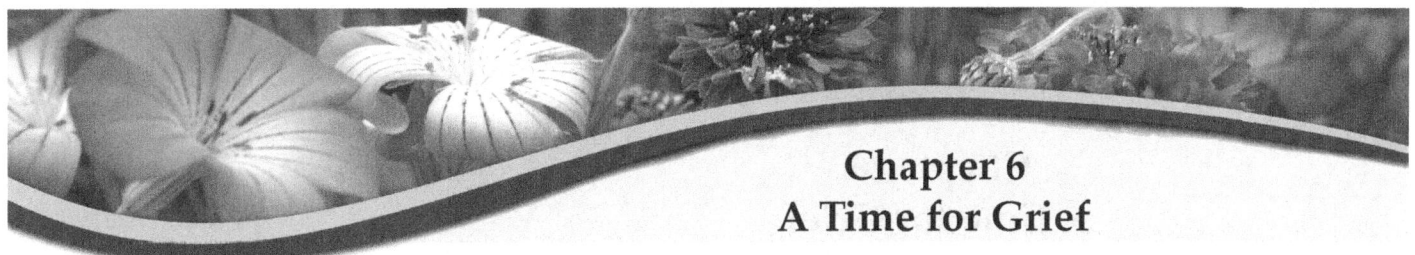

Chapter 6
A Time for Grief

Dealing with the guilt feelings that arise during grief can be a difficult process, one of those "easier said than done" situations. Here are some practical strategies for dealing with guilt:

1. Choose to be open to the truth about your circumstances

The first step in differentiating between unhealthy, destructive guilt and conviction is to ask for the truth. Talk to loved ones who are safe people that you can trust to give you honest feedback. Be willing to look at (and journal about) all the negative and hurtful emotions that guilt provokes and read this aloud to your safe group. Let the pain and confusion come flowing out.

Receive the insights that come as you share and write those down too. You realize that you have something you need to make right or you may realize that whatever happened was not in your "yard" and you are not to take it on.

2. Make amends where necessary and possible

In your meditation, journaling, and sharing time, you may discover something specific that you have actually done to hurt another person. If that person is still alive and it is possible to go to them and ask forgiveness, do so as soon as possible.

3. Forgive others

If someone has hurt you, begin the process of moving through the stages of grief in relationship to the wound. The moment you make a decision to forgive the other person, you step out of denial and into the next stage in the grief process.

Sometimes resolution comes quickly, and sometimes it takes longer. The key is that throughout the forgiveness process, from the anger stage to the acceptance stage, you are committed to loving the person who has hurt you. Your heart is open to healing. You are doing the grief work that makes true reconciliation possible.

If the wound is deep, you may not be able to be in active relationship with the person until healthy boundaries have been established, but that does not mean you aren't in the process of doing the hard work that it takes to create a safe and healthy relationship.

A Closer Look

Chapter 6
A Time for Grief

If the person you need to forgive is your loved one who died, it is still possible to move through the forgiveness process to complete healing. Write letters to your loved one and read them to a trusted friend, a counselor, or to a group you feel safe "processing" in. Allow the emotions to surface and face them honestly. Don't shame yourself for any part of the process. Tears, anger, sadness, frustration, and confusion are all part of the process.

4. Forgive yourself

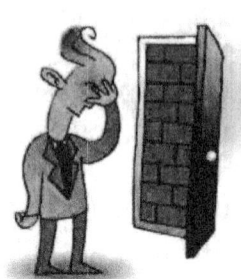

Forgiving ourselves is sometimes the hardest part of letting go of unhealthy guilt. Forgiving ourselves means surrendering control and not hanging on to the illusion that there is something we can do to somehow make things OK again. As crazy as it sounds, refusing to forgive ourselves keeps the "ball in our court" and gives us a sense of control.

5. Create a symbol of finality

We as human beings have a deep innate need for rituals and symbols. Rituals and symbols give our hearts something concrete to hang on to as a reminder of an important transition in our lives. Our ancestors were good at memorializing important events. Men exchanged shoes as a symbol of a vow to each other. In other situations they might shave their heads or build an altar. Rites of passage were honored in many different ways depending on the cultural norms.

In modern society, we don't use symbols as much as our ancestors did. That doesn't mean we can't learn to. Symbols and rituals are a valuable tool in healing.

What symbol or ritual may you need to help you to let go of unhealthy guilt? Perhaps you might need to write out a list of your unhealthy expectations of yourself ("I should be able to go on with my life without crying all the time over my loss…", "I should have been a better wife…") and burn the list in the presence of your trusted friends. Maybe you need to create a memorial fund for your loved one and use it to further a cause he loved and supported. Possibly, it would be meaningful to plant a tree in her memory. Sometimes the lingering sense of guilt you feel is simply the loose ends of unfinished business that need completion through a ritual.

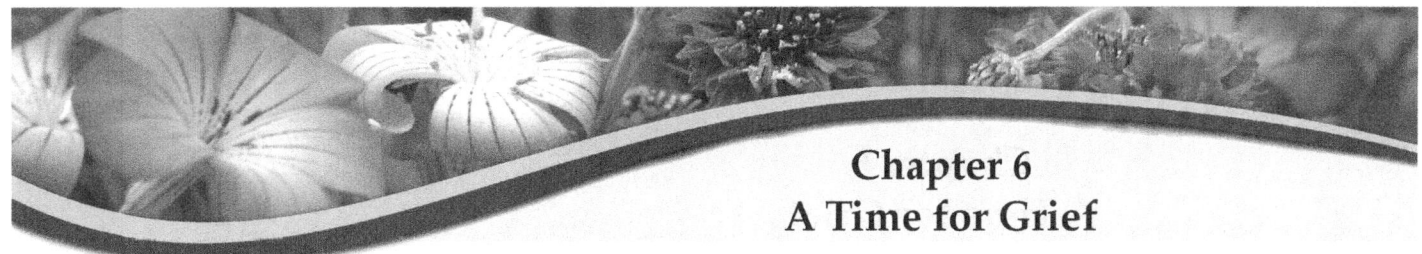

Chapter 6
A Time for Grief

6. Replace the guilt with positive action

In addition to rituals, there are many "positive action" activities you can engage in to move your heart along the path to healing. Journaling is a valuable tool, whether it is done in the form of writing or drawing.

When a young child is upset, mom does "containment" for the child by describing the child's emotions for him. "Johnny, I can see that you are angry that Billie took your truck and won't give it back." The child feels heard and understood and is able to face his own emotion with less fear when it is contained. Journaling is a way to do "containment" for ourselves.

Implementing a balanced program of diet and exercise is another helpful "positive action" tool for dealing with the ravages of unhealthy guilt, especially if the exercise is outdoors in a beautiful place. There's something about being out in the woods or hiking along the seashore that opens the heart to deeper joy and peace.

7. Develop a long-term support system

Nothing is more of a deathblow to unhealthy guilt than being a part of a good solid support system made up of people who have learned to interact with each other in safe, healthy ways. If you are questioning whether or not your feelings of guilt are caused by a thinking error on your part or are truly a conviction that you have wounded someone, take it to your safe group. Talk to them about your feelings. Ask them for feedback. Listen as they share their own struggles. Much of what they say will ring true for you, too, and you will feel uplifted and encouraged knowing you are not alone in your pain.

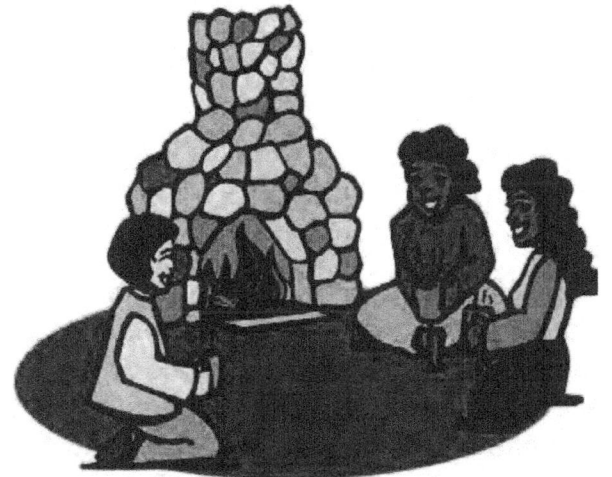

A Closer Look

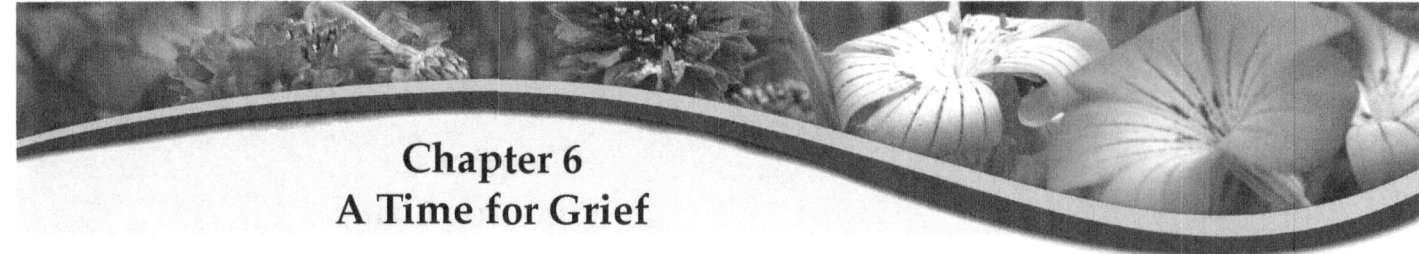

Chapter 6
A Time for Grief

A Child's Grief

When the person who died is one of the child's parents, the child will most likely react in four basic ways:

☹ **Fear**

Fear that he will lose the other parent or that he, too, will die can cause the child to react in an insecure, clingy manner. Other fears include a fear of going to sleep, of being separated from close family members, or of being unprotected. On top of all these fears, he will likely be afraid to share his feelings with others.

☹ **Guilt**

There are many things that children tend to feel guilty about when a parent dies. Guilt can arise from anything at all, so it is sometimes hard to identify the source. There are, however, some basic beliefs that are common to children who have lost parents.

One common belief that causes tremendous guilt in the child is that the death is a punishment for misbehaving. Children at certain developmental stages are very concrete in their thinking and reason from cause to effect in a direct and deliberate way. If something goes wrong, they easily assume they are to blame.

Believing that the parent died because they wished it so, or that they didn't love the parent enough to prevent the death, or that it isn't right for them to be alive when the parent is dead can all cause a heavy load of guilt in the child.

☹ **Anger**

A child whose parent has died is likely to start misbehaving and acting in very aggressive ways at school and at home. The anger that spawns such behavior is often rooted in the child's underlying belief that he has been abandoned. He also may feel that he is unimportant and that his future has been taken away from him. He may feel that he is fighting forces so much bigger than himself that he has no chance of "winning" and be furious at how unfair it all seems.

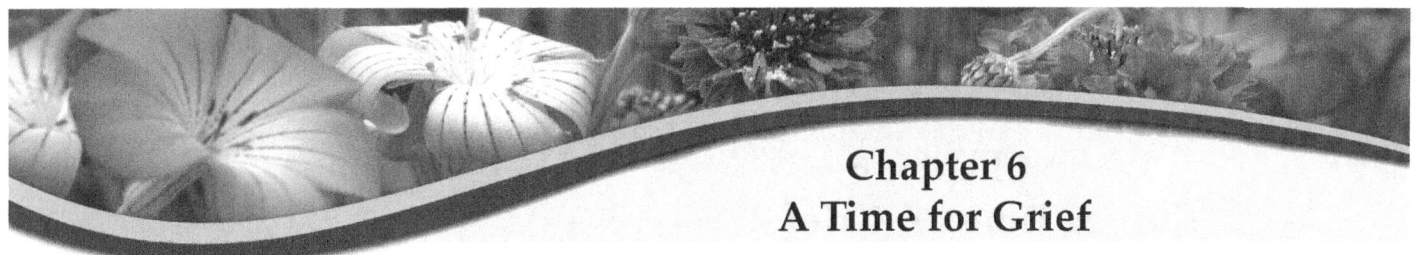

Chapter 6
A Time for Grief

☹ Confusion

In a situation that would bewilder even the most self-possessed adult, imagine the confusion that a child must feel when she has just had her world turned upside-down by the death of a parent. Trying to sort out the overwhelming feelings triggered by such a traumatic event is a daunting task for the child and she probably hasn't had the chance to develop her communication skills to the point of even being able to describe how she feels.

The grieving child will likely be confused about other's expectations of her, about God and religion, about her own emotional reactions, and about her perceptions and memories of the deceased parent's life and death.

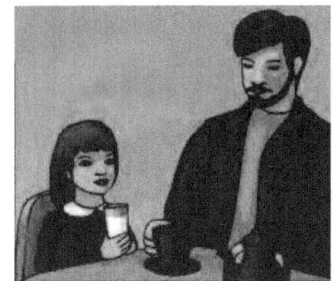

Telling a Child about a Death

It is crucial when telling a child about a death that has occurred, whether it be a parent, sibling, grandparent, or other family member or friend, that the person breaking the news be sensitive and aware of the child's needs.

- Tell the truth about the death

- Use simple and easy to understand language

- Be direct (no euphemisms)

- Lay the groundwork for future explanations when the child is older

- Let the child know they will be involved in rituals surrounding the death (funeral, memorial service)

- Assure the child that their feelings are accepted

A Closer Look

Chapter 6
A Time for Grief

As a hospice volunteer, you may have many opportunities to help a grieving child process the loss of their loved one. Children process grief differently than adults and it is valuable to know how to support them. Here is some additional information about dealing with a child's grief:

- **Respect their natural curiosity but don't give more information than they are ready to handle**

Because children are naturally curious and ask lots of questions (if they feel safe enough to do so) it would be easy to give them too much information that they are not at the maturity level to understand. Give short, age appropriate answers to questions they may ask. Be honest. The child will usually go away and play and think about what you said, then come back and ask another question (or the same question again.) Be patient with repeat questions. These are the ones that the child is having a hard time with.

- **Don't use euphemisms**

Telling a child that their loved one is "asleep" is a bad idea. Kids are concrete in their thinking and processing. If you tell her that Grandpa went to sleep and won't wake up again, she may think that if she goes to sleep, she might not wake up either. Or if you tell her that Daddy went on a long trip and won't be back, she may likely assume that Daddy left because she was bad and Daddy didn't want to be around her any more. Children often think that something they have done has caused the loved one to die.

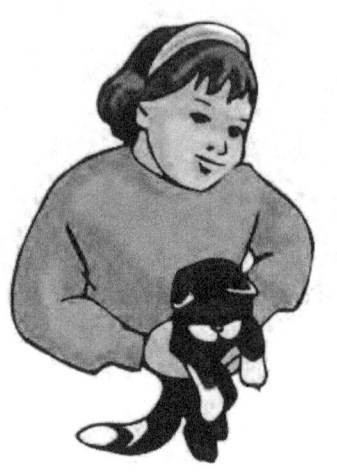

Don't feed into that fear by using unclear descriptions of what is happening with their loved one. You can say, "Daddy was very sick and his body couldn't keep going any more. It's not your fault. He loved you very much and was very sad to think that he wouldn't be with you and Mommy any more."

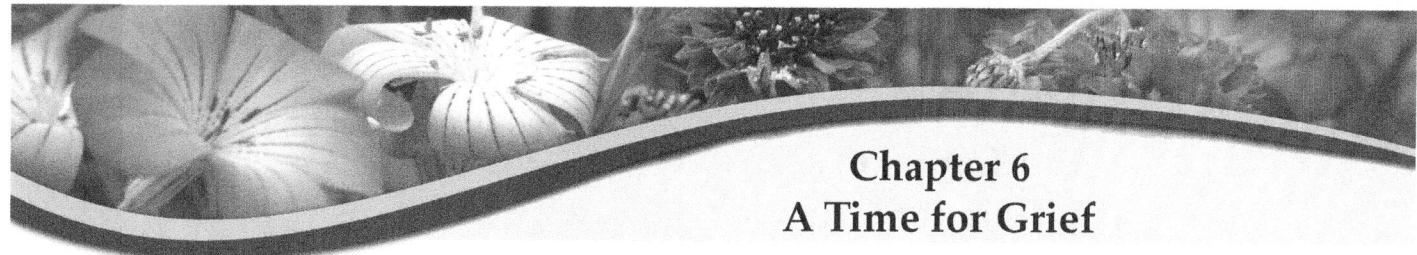

Chapter 6
A Time for Grief

- **Recognize the signs of anxiety**

   Children seldom know how to communicate their anxiety directly. Talking about emotions is a skill that even many adults haven't mastered yet! The way children act out their fear and anxiety will vary depending on their personality or their age and stage of development. They may act in uncharacteristically mean or rude ways. They may cry, throw temper tantrums, yell, bite other children, start wetting the bed, or withdraw.

   They may fear that if one person in the family dies, the other adults will, too. This is a terrifying prospect to a young child who depends on those adults for his survival. If he can't articulate his fears, play "sandbox" games with him using small plastic figures and a small, portable sandbox. Or give him paper and crayons and ask him to draw pictures. If the fears are lurking, they will come out if he feels safe with you.

- **Allow them space for their anger**

   A child could be angry at the patient for being sick, for leaving them, for not paying attention to them, and for lots of other reasons. They may feel guilty for being mad at someone they love and be ashamed to talk about it. They may be afraid of their own anger. Let them know, through your acceptance, through stories you tell, or through games you play with them, that their anger is normal and okay.

- **Spend one-on-one time with them**

   A little concentrated attention can go a long way with a grieving child. Sit with them and talk, take them for a walk, color with them, play computer games, draw, or play with puppets. Children often get shuttled to the background when the family is in crisis, and they will greatly appreciate the focused attention you give them in the middle of it all.

- **Include them in what is going on**

   Even a very young child can be given something to do to "help", even if it is just sitting here in this chair and "babysitting my stuffed animal". A child can wet a washcloth and wipe the patients forehead, bring snacks to visiting family members, or any number of simple tasks that will make them feel included.

A Closer Look

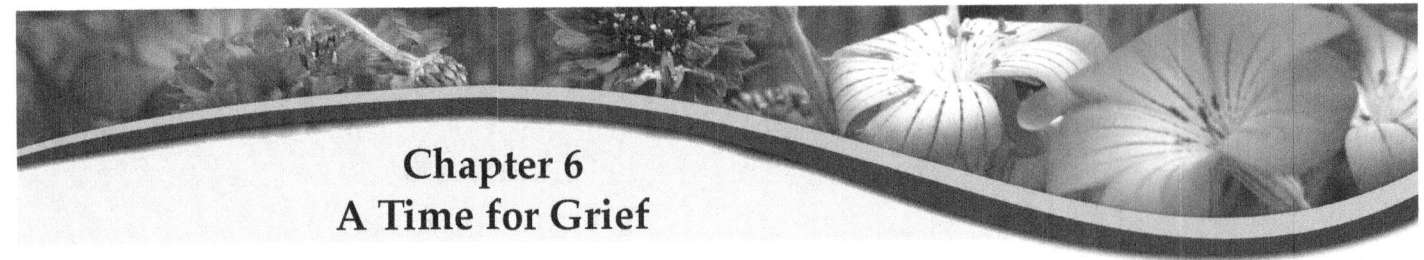

Chapter 6
A Time for Grief

- **Lead by example**

Children pick up our attitudes like small, very absorbent sponges. Children from birth to about ten years old are in their formative years and soaking up their environment and learning cultural "norms" to take with them for the rest of their lives. Death is a normal part of life and if we treat it that way, the children will do the same. This is not to say we like it or are not sad about it, but we accept it. This is far less scary to a child than adults who are secretive, controlling, and communicating fear about the process.

- **Give them something tangible**

A well chosen gift for a young child can give them a positive association to attach to the hospice team (which you represent). A coloring book and crayons, a small stuffed animal, or a special lapel button would let the child know they are noticed and important. (A wonderful coloring book to give is Jennifer Collier's activity book on grief called This Hurts: A Children's Guide-Journal to Death and Grief. It's for children ages 5-9 and is available at www.bordermountain.com.)

- **Set up a "memories table" for the patient and let the child help.**

Set up an area close to the patient's bed and ask friends, family, staff, and anyone else visiting the patient to bring something special that represents the patient and a treasured memory with them. Have the adults give their memory object to the child to place on the table. Tell the child the story, so that he can tell repeat it to the patient and to others who come to visit and see the display.

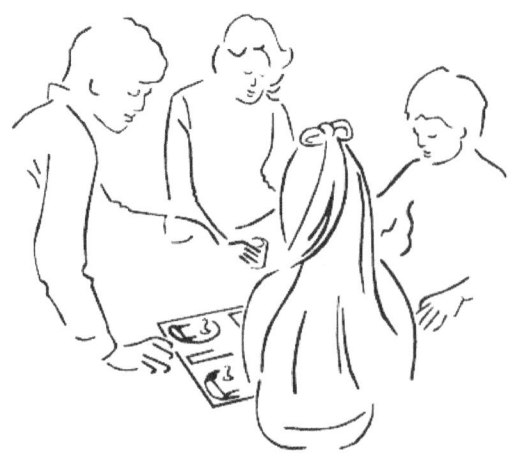

A Closer Look

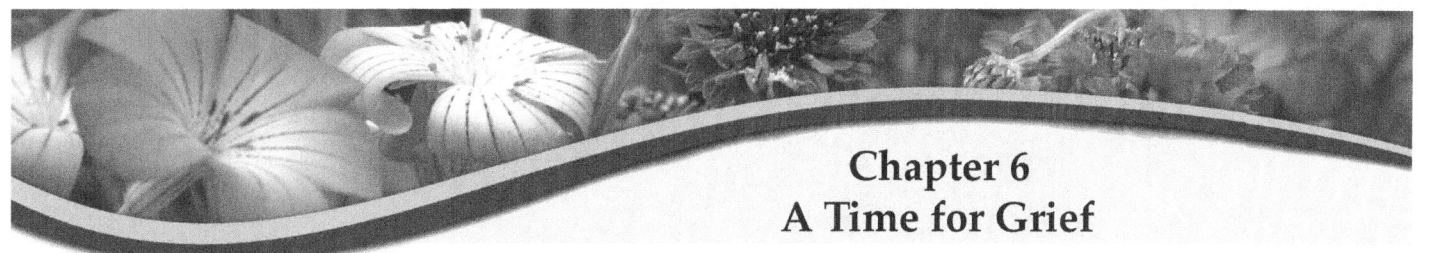

Chapter 6
A Time for Grief

How to Help a Grieving Child Heal

- Don't act as if the parent or loved one did not die

- Encourage the child to express feelings

- Share your memories and feelings about the one who died with the child

- Be affectionate with the child, emotionally and physically

- Reassure the child that his basic needs will be met

- Help the child plan for the future

- Encourage open and honest communication within the family

- Help the child deal with feelings of anger, depression, and bewilderment

- Explore and address the child's feelings of guilt

- Encourage the family to participate in family therapy

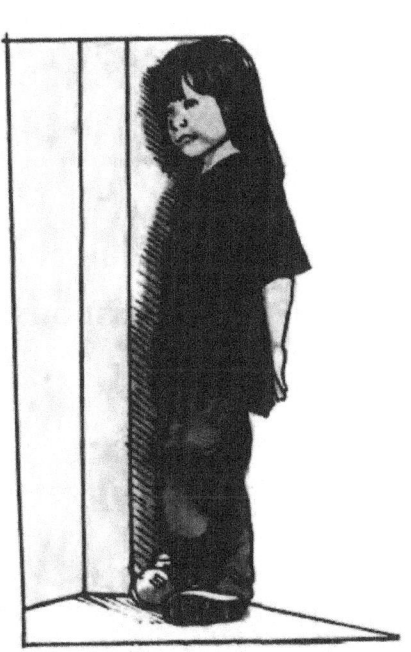

A Closer Look

Chapter 6
A Time for Grief

When an Adult Child Loses a Parent

- **They may be losing a friend, advisor, and consultant as well as a parent**

- **There is often a sense of losing part of one's family history and roots**

- **There can be a significant sense of loss of support and unconditional love**

- **Conflicts and ambivalent feelings about the past may be stirred up**

- **Family roles and responsibilities may change**

- **The grieving adult child may be expected to "get over" the loss more quickly than if it were a spouse who died**

- **It can be a strong reminder of one's own mortality**

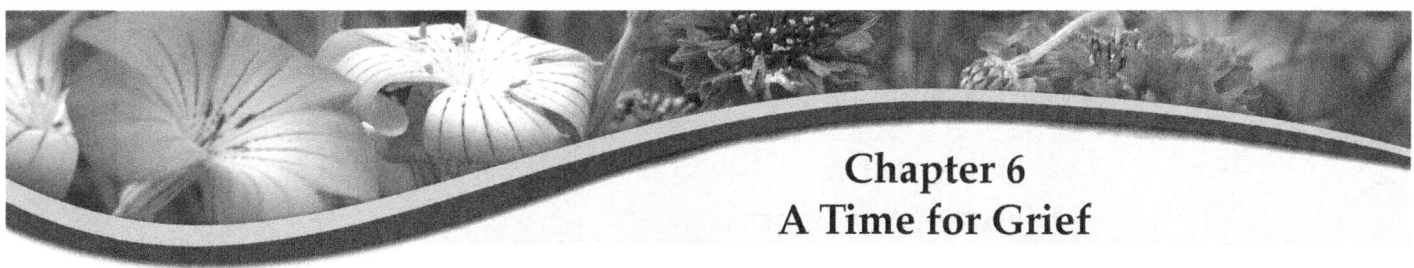

Chapter 6
A Time for Grief

In the box below, draw a picture that represents grief to you.

"To die is not a sin; to not live fully is.

If you do not grieve fully,

you cannot live fully."

G. Wendt

A Closer Look

Chapter 6
A Time for Grief

Losing a loved one is a heavy burden to bear whatever the circumstances, but there are some situations that can make grief even more difficult to deal with. Let's take a look at some of the factors that can complicate grief and hamper healing:

- **When there are deep unresolved issues with the person who died.**

The depth and intensity of grief with any loss is directly proportionate to the impact the person has had on our lives. When there is a strong emotional connection with someone, losing them pulls at the very roots of our soul. When the relationship was positive and there are many happy memories, it feels more natural to engage in rituals that honor the person's memory and, even in the sadness, celebrate the connection we had (and always will have in our heart) with them.

When unresolved emotional issues are present, there is confusion and difficulty engaging in the necessary rituals of grieving. The person may have had a negative impact on our life but it creates an intense connection nonetheless. It will probably require the assistance of a good counselor to work through the complex issues of this kind of grief.

- **When the death was a suicide.**

Anger, guilt, intense searching and pining, and ripping pain are common bedfellows when the death was a suicide. Anger can be directed at the medical profession (for not doing something to prevent the suicide), at the one who died (for abandoning and rejecting you by choosing death rather than staying with you), at God (for not intervening), at yourself (for not being able to stop the suicide), or just at the very fact that it happened at all.

Guilt is present in some form or another with all losses but in the case of suicide, it can be overwhelming. "If only I had listened more…." "If only I had known how much pain she was in…." "If only I had said _____…" "If only I'd gotten home a little earlier…."

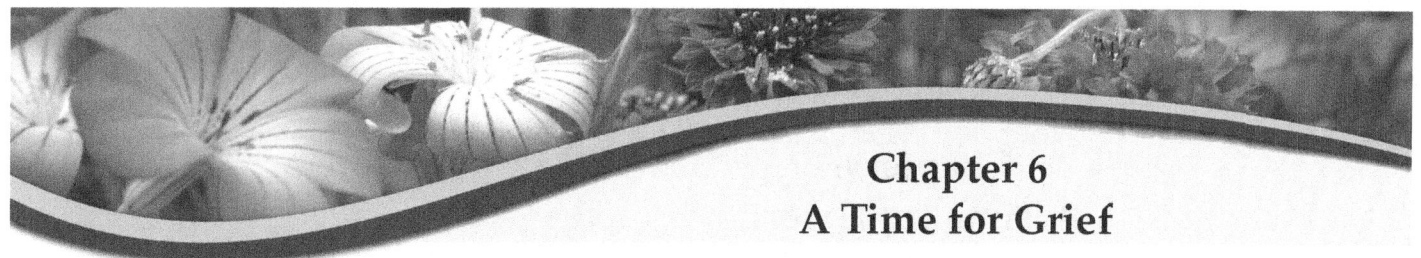

Chapter 6
A Time for Grief

Those who have lost loved ones to suicide often search for the loved one for months, even years after the death. Lois Bloom, in her little booklet "Mourning After Suicide", talks of searching the streets on her way home from work looking for her son who had committed suicide months earlier. She knew "in her head" it was irrational, but her heart kept searching and hoping to see him again.

A good support system is especially important to someone grieving the loss of a loved one through suicide. Many cities have support groups just for processing this kind of grief. The presence of friends and family is also crucial to the healing process. It's important for the person to connect with those who are able to provide loving support.

- **When the person who died was a child.**

There is something about the death of a child that rips at our hearts in a way nothing else can. It doesn't seem right. It feels unfair. It feels as if the future has been snatched away so very prematurely from an innocent victim. We are somewhat prepared to lose our parents as they age and have lived a full and meaningful life. But a child? How can it be time to let them go?

Losing a child can create an intense amount of guilt in the surviving parents. Where did I go wrong? How could I have prevented this from happening? Often, the intense anger and guilt that accompanies the death of a child can cause severe communication problems in the parent's relationship. Private family therapy, in addition to group support, is crucial during this time when life seems to be unraveling at the seams.

- **When the person's body cannot be recovered.**

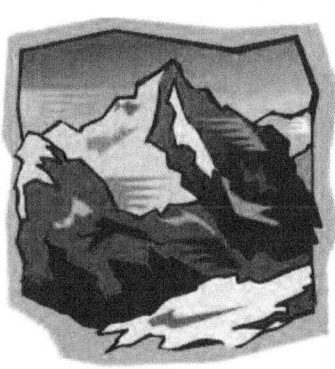

Closure is an important part of healing process. For millennia, humans have been laying out their dead to be viewed and touched to help the living accept the finality of the loved one's death. When the body has been lost at sea or on Mt. Everest or in a fire and cannot be recovered, closure becomes very difficult. There is the lingering feeling that the person isn't really dead and they will show up someday. This lack of closure produces an enormous amount of stress in the griever's body. Emotional energy needed for the healing process is siphoned away into searching and pining.

A Closer Look

Chapter 6
A Time for Grief

If the grieving person has a loved one whose body has not been recovered, he may find it helpful to create a closure ritual just for himself in which he tells his heart that the person is really gone and give his emotions a chance to say a final goodbye. The memorial service is helpful, but he will probably need something more personal just for him, such as burying a symbolic item. Encourage him to take someone with him who understands his need for closure and can support him emotionally as he says his own personal goodbye.

- **When no rituals are performed.**

More and more, families are opting not to have a funeral or a memorial service when a loved one dies. "We have to get on with our lives. The service won't bring them back," they say. Experts in the area of grief and bereavement are alarmed by this trend, which reflects the disconnection and isolation of our society today. The rituals performed are not for the person who died, they are for us. We need a chance to say goodbye to move on with our healing process. We can't reinvest in life if we don't acknowledge and grieve our losses.

Rituals, such as funerals, wakes, candle-lighting vigils, memorial services, flowers at the graveside, and shrines to the lost loved one, are necessary exercises of the heart that connect us to our own emotions about the loss as well as honor the person who died. They give us inner "hooks" to hang our grief on.

If the family opted for no rituals when their loved one died, it is not too late for the grieving person to create her own rituals. If her family won't join her, encourage her to find a trusted friend or two to help her take the necessary steps to creating a ritual that will be meaningful and healing for her heart.

- **When the person was murdered or died as a result of an act of terrorism.**

Intense anger is often the most predominate emotion when someone takes the life of our loved one through murder or terrorism. The anger can be all consuming because the loss is based on the choices of another human being to dehumanize our loved one to the point of taking their life away. Everything in us screams for justice. We want to see the person punished so that some kind of balance can be restored.

A Closer Look

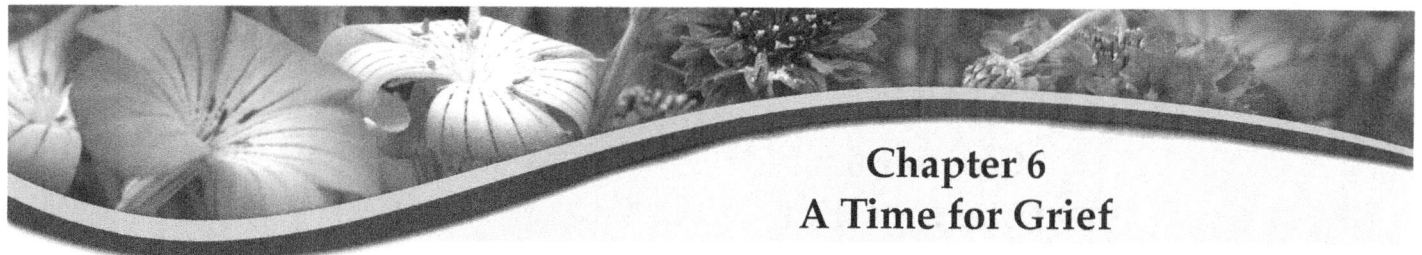

Chapter 6
A Time for Grief

Any act of intimidation from one person to another is dehumanizing. The bully, in his own fear and insecurity, finds a victim upon which to vent his rage toward his own weakness. He destroys an innocent life because of his own issues and everything in us shouts, "Foul play! You didn't even know him! How could you take the life of my loved one so callously and snuff it out as if he were an ant on the ground?"

When a loved one is murdered, the intense grief rises, not only in response to the immediate loss, but also in response to every act of dehumanization that has happened to us or around us since our earliest childhood experiences. Grief is cumulative and unless the grieving person has had a chance to work through childhood abuse issues (parents, teachers, bullies on the playground), his responses to this deep loss will be compounded many times over. This is an opportunity to uncover many hidden wounds with a good counselor that can do a timeline of childhood experiences.

Things to Avoid

In the First year Following a Major Loss

- **Beginning a new romantic relationship**
- **Buying or selling a house**
- **Changing jobs or careers**
- **Adopting a new baby**
- **Moving to another area of the country**
- **Getting a new pet**
- **Making any major financial decisions**
- **Extensive travel**
- **Any kind of gambling, drugs, or alcohol**

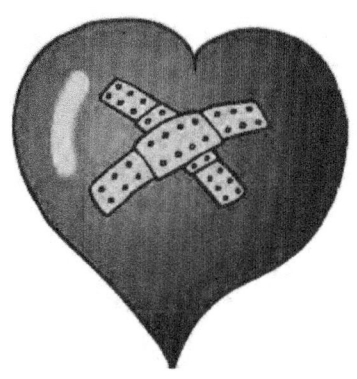

A Closer Look

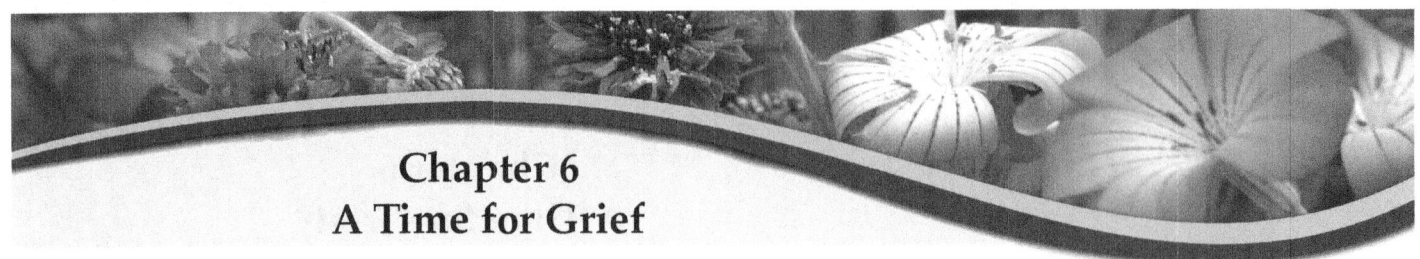

Chapter 6
A Time for Grief

 ## Skill Check

1. Define grief.

2. List the five stages of grief and describe the characteristics of each.

3. What are the physical and emotional symptoms that a bereaved person may experience as the anesthetic of denial wears off?

4. List five factors that affect how a person responds to the grief process.

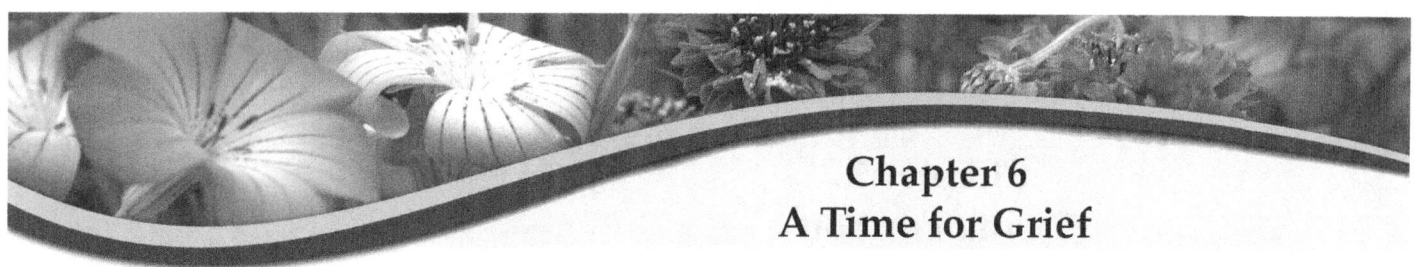

Chapter 6
A Time for Grief

5. How can you tell when a person is healing and moving on with their life?

6. What are some of the signs of a potentially unhealthy grief response?

7. List four basic ways a child may react to a loved one's death and explain how to deal with each.

"Accept the seasons of your heart,
even as you have always accepted the seasons
that pass over your fields."

Kahlil Gibran

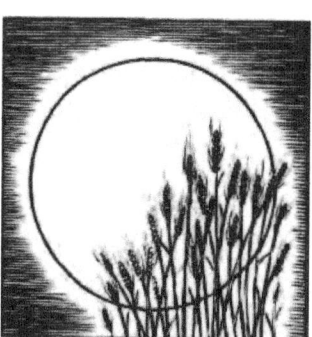

Skill Check

Chapter 7
Caring For You

7. Caring For You

Learning to Give Without Hurting Yourself

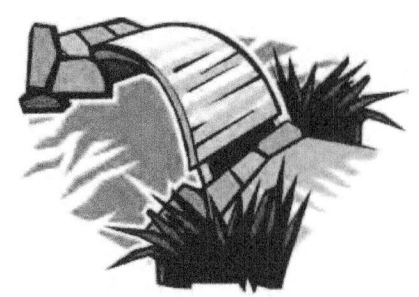

"Just the facts, please..."

Hospice workers are at high risk for burnout within the first year of providing care for the dying. Burnout, a malady characterized by many physical and emotional symptoms, is caused by a burning up of the emotional energy reserves.

Burnout occurs when stress levels stay at an unhealthy intensity for prolonged periods of time without being balanced out by self care techniques. It is a serious condition, because it can prevent its victim from being able to interact healthfully with others.

Physical and emotional signs of burnout may include:

- increased susceptibility to infection
- various illnesses, especially migraine headaches, digestive disorders, and cardiac episodes
- increased risk of injury
- shallow breathing
- muscle pain and tension
- lack of energy
- connective tissue pain
- "blank outs" and poor memory
- shedding tears at the slightest provocation
- weight gain or loss
- insomnia
- excessive sleep
- feeling overwhelmed by ordinary daily tasks
- avoiding friends and activities
- low self-esteem
- anxiety
- irritability with family and friends
- feeling of numbness
- dreading getting up in the a.m.

Once burnout has reached the level of crippling its victim's interactions with others, the only recourse is to retreat and rest. Continuing on in the same care giving role will only make symptoms worse. The best way to deal with burnout is to prevent it in the first place.

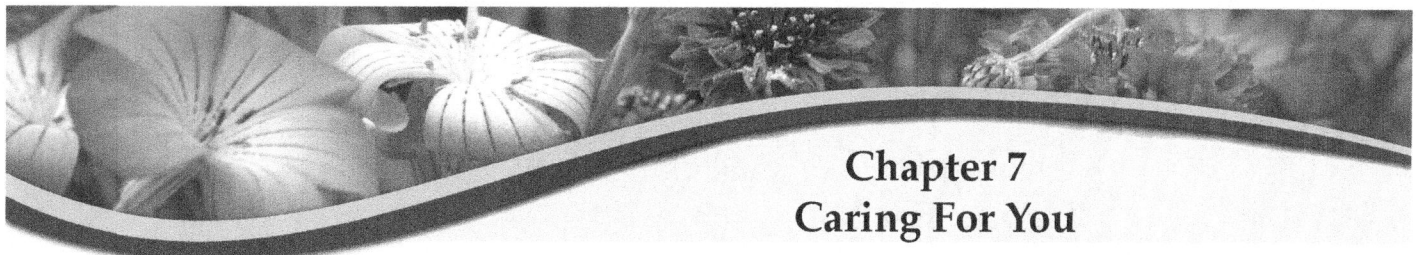

Chapter 7
Caring For You

A Personal Bill of Rights

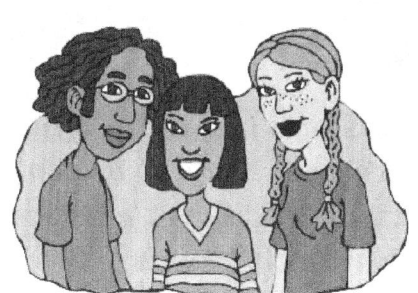

I have the right to ask for what I need.

I have the right to say no to requests or demands I know I can't meet.

I have the right to change my mind.

I have the right to my own feelings, whether they are positive or negative.

I have the right to set my own priorities and make decisions in accordance with them.

I have the right to make mistakes.

I have the right to expect others to deal honestly with me.

I have the right not to be responsible for the behavior, problems, and feelings of others.

I have the right to be afraid and to say so.

I have the right to my own personal space and my own personal time.

I have the right to be angry at someone I love.

I have the right to be in a safe, non-abusive environment.

I have the right to change and grow.

I have the right to be treated with dignity and respect.

I have the right to be playful and to enjoy my life.

I have the right to have my wants and needs respected by others.

I have the right to be happy.

"Just the facts, please..."

Chapter 7
Caring For You

 ## *At the Heart of the Matter*

Personal loss is the underlying cause of burnout, whether the losses are big or small. Since grief tends to be cumulative if there hasn't been sufficient time for healing in between each loss, a series of significant losses can send the griever reeling into a state of serious burnout.

How many losses have you experienced over the course of your life? People don't often recognize that any change we experience in our lives is a loss. Have you had the opportunity to grieve each loss and heal? Because the losses experienced in hospice work are often ongoing and weighty, it's important to do a personal loss inventory and ascertain your level of unresolved grief before you begin working with hospice patients.

My Personal Inventory of Losses

*List the losses/changes you have experienced related to each of the following.
Note the impact each had on you, negative or positive.*

Births (your own, your own children, and others close to you)

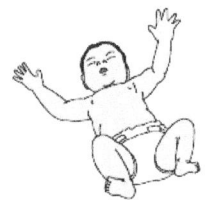

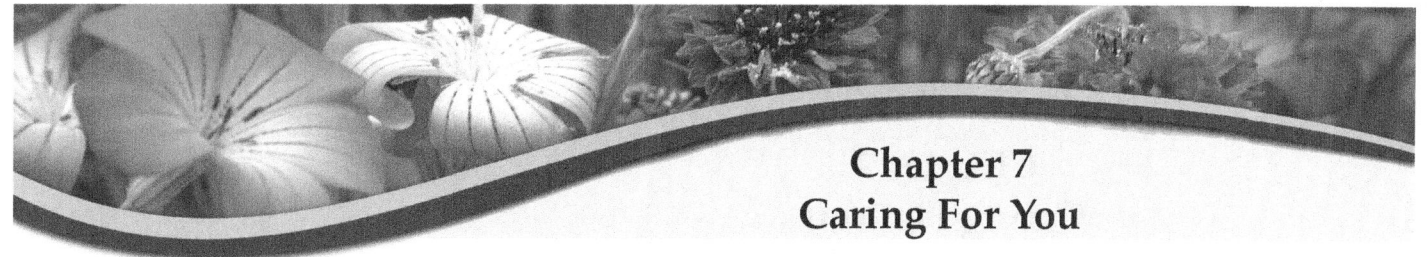

Chapter 7
Caring For You

Relationship changes involving children and parents

Changes in place of residence

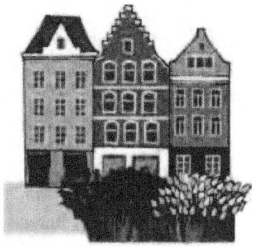

Changes in schools or teachers

Illnesses- short or long term

At the Heart of the Matter

Chapter 7
Caring For You

Holidays, family reunions, birthdays

Marriages and divorces

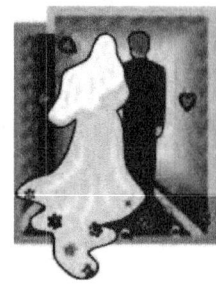

Employment (jobs lost or gained)

Any incidences of assault or abuse

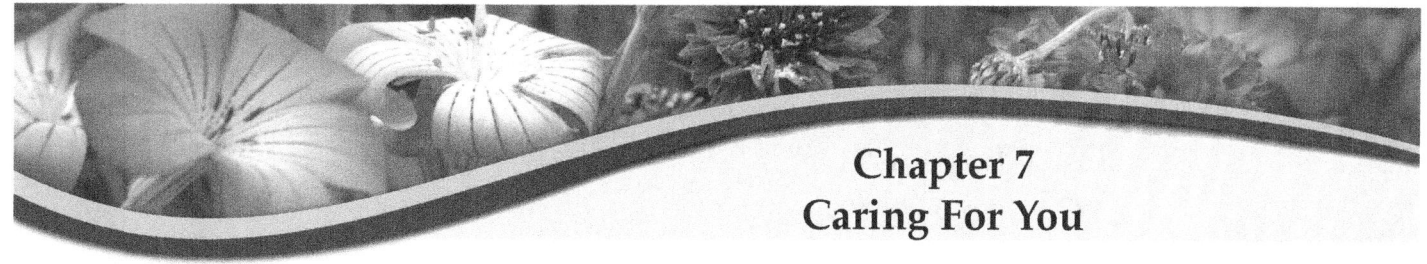

Chapter 7
Caring For You

Aging process

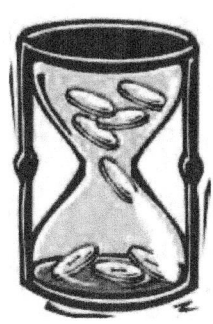

Significant relationships (beginning, ongoing, ending)

Periods of success (often more stressful than failure!)

Financial losses or gains

Chapter 7
Caring For You

Natural disasters experienced (fire, earthquakes, tornadoes, floods)

Retirement

Deaths (family, friends)

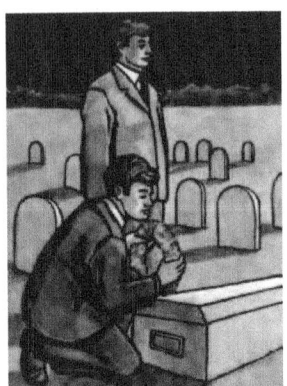

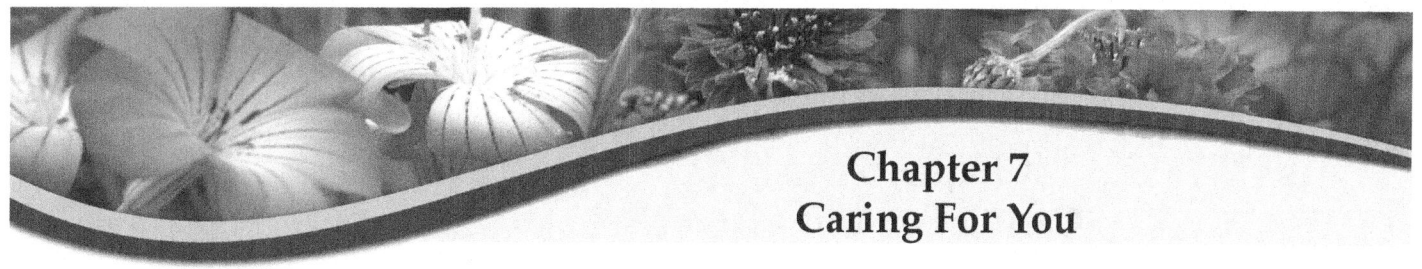

Chapter 7
Caring For You

When you have completed your loss inventory, divide into groups and discuss which losses stand out in your mind as being unresolved (possibly because of being unrecognized as a loss) and un-grieved. In the space below, create a step-by-step plan for yourself, outlining the steps you feel comfortable taking to begin processing through your unresolved grief issues:

At the Heart of the Matter

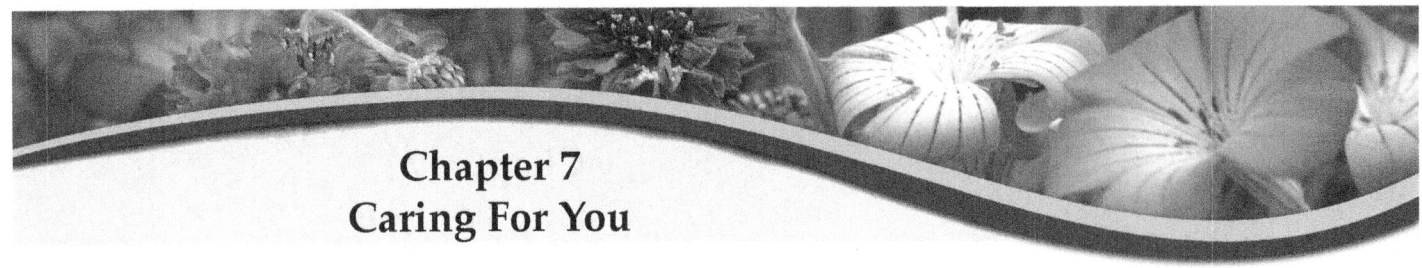

**Chapter 7
Caring For You**

 # Putting it Into Practice

Besides identifying and grieving old losses, there are many other things we, as care providers, can do to take care of ourselves and prevent the painful effects of burnout. Here are some tips:

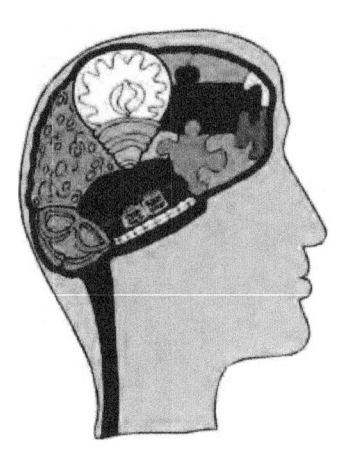

- Use your brain to cut stress. If you understand which side of your brain is experiencing stress, you can actually encourage the other side of your brain to "take over" and help calm the stressed-out side.

- *Clue: If you feel depressed or emotionally "worked up", the stress you're experiencing is in the right side of your brain - the creative, emotional side. Try switching to your left brain by doing something factual like math. The emotional side of your brain will calm down! If your left brain is feeling the stress, it may exhibit itself in feeling time-pressure or a heavy sense of feeling burdened down with the cares of life. Try switching to your right brain by singing or taking a relaxing walk.*

- Find a place all your own where you can go, undisturbed, every day. Use the solitude to relax, meditate, and regroup.

- Learn to accept the praise and gratitude of others. Practice affirming yourself using positive self-talk. Praise others freely, telling them sincerely and openly what you appreciate about them. The endless cycle of giving and receiving love and acceptance energizes and heals.

- Change your routine whenever you can. Getting into a rut can feel "safe" but it can also dull the senses and stifle creativity, which is essential for spiritual health.

Chapter 7
Caring For You

- Say "I choose to" instead of "I should" and "I won't" rather than "I can't." Guilt is a poor motivator, sapping inner strength and creative a feeling of helplessness and hopelessness. Continually remind yourself through your choice of words that you are free to choose the course of your life, that you are not a victim of circumstances.

- Establish a "buddy system". Use it regularly as a source of encouragement, support, and re-direction. Nothing is more valuable than a trusted friend who will not only accept us and cheer us on to greater accomplishments, but will also gently tell the truth about our behavior patterns.

- Remember that when you can't do any more for your patient and their family than you are doing, an attitude of aloofness and indifference is far more harmful to them than just admitting your limitations. A lack of openness and honesty can set up a dynamic in which you expend a tremendous amount of energy avoiding the real issue with them and feeling guilty about your emotional withdrawal.

- Find things to laugh about. Experience joy. Exult in the beauty all around you, from the smile of a child to the brilliance of a sunset over the ocean. These feed the spirit and give life to the body and soul.

- *Ponder this one: If you never say no, what is your "yes" worth?*

Putting it Into Practice

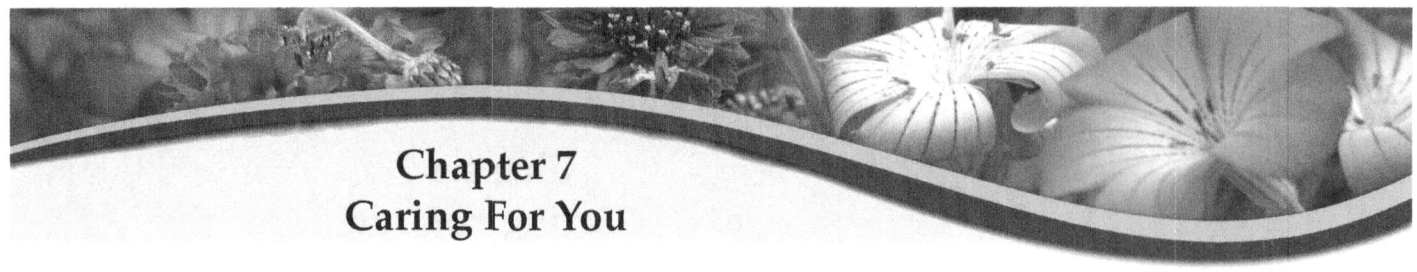

Chapter 7
Caring For You

Self-Nurturing Activities

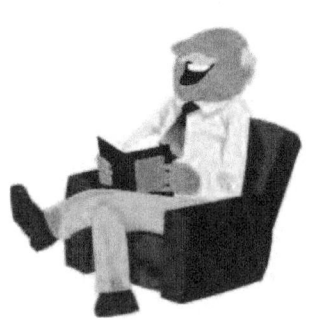

1. Walk in the park
2. Pray
3. Relax with a great book
4. Go to bed early
5. Rent a funny video
6. Sleep out under the stars
7. Play your favorite song
8. Have your nails done
9. Get a massage
10. Buy yourself fresh flowers
11. Go to the zoo
12. Watch a sunset
13. Take a bubble bath
14. Go to the pet store and play with the puppies
15. Get a make over
16. Buy ice cream with sprinkles
17. Wear purple

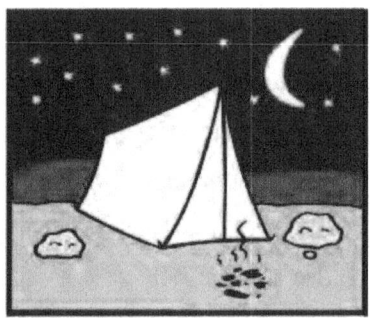

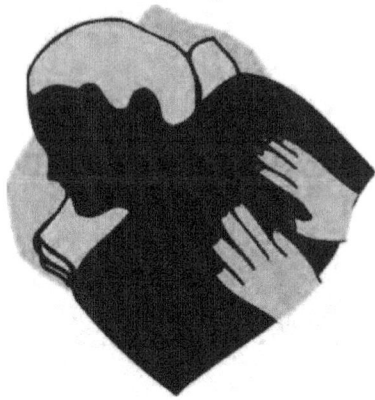

18. Spend the day at the beach
19. Sit in the Jacuzzi
20. Call a friend
21. Hug a teddy bear
22. Go on a picnic in the country
23. Write yourself a love letter and mail it
24. Fix a special meal for yourself and eat it by candlelight

Putting it Into Practice

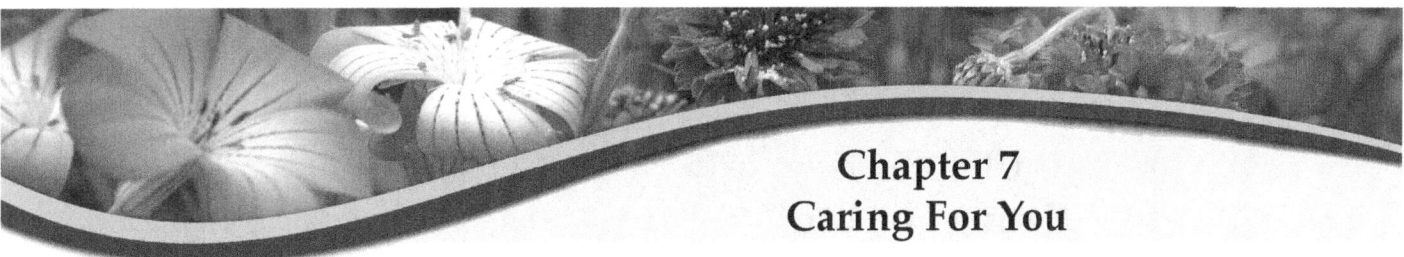

Chapter 7
Caring For You

25. Buy a new outfit
26. Ask a special person to nurture you
27. Play golf with a friend
28. Work out at the gym
29. Join an aerobics class
30. Meditate
31. Sit in a sauna
32. Serve yourself your favorite breakfast in bed

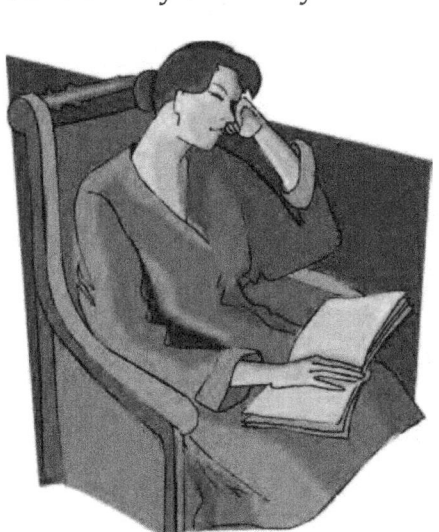

33. Lay on the grass and watch the clouds
34. Go to the library
35. Ride a bicycle down a country road
36. Go to bed early with a cup of hot peppermint tea and toast
37. Look at your photo albums
38. Talk to your cat
39. Take a class in creative writing
40. Sit in the sunshine
41. Warm your robe in the dryer before you put it on
42. Keep a journal
43. Learn to paint with water colors
44. Sit in a quiet, dark room with cucumber slices over you
45. Carry on a conversation with your favorite plant
46. Massage your feet on wooden rollers
47. Read poetry out loud
48. Walk in mud barefoot
49. Sing
50. Run through a sprinkler

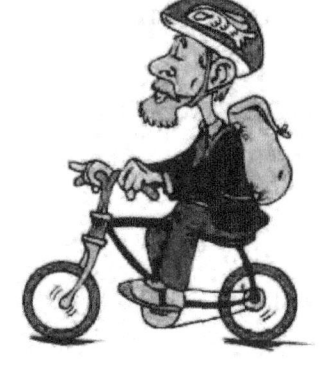

Putting it Into Practice

Chapter 7
Caring For You

When you are feeling stressed:

- **Remind yourself that you can only change those things that you have control over (namely, yourself).**

It's easy to get bent out of shape by circumstances, events, and people that are out of your sphere of influence. Learning to let go of the "if only"s frees up your energy for dealing with those areas in which you really can make a difference.

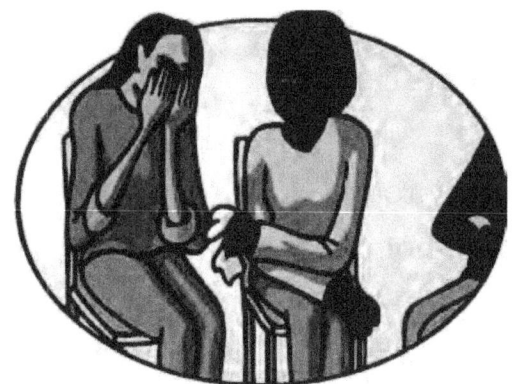

- **Find someone you trust to confide your feelings to.**

Talking your circumstances over with someone who won't try to solve your problem for you, but will listen without judgment, allows you to put things into perspective. Often, this is all it takes for you to find a solution that is right for you.

- **Interpret procrastination as a signal from your subconscious that it's time to lower your stress level.**

Instead of shaming yourself when you can't seem to get anything done because of procrastination, look deeper for the root cause. Perhaps it's time to say "no" for while to allow yourself time to regroup and rest.

- **Develop a reward system for yourself.**

One effective way to cope with current stress is to look back at some point of achievement in the past. Remind yourself of how well you did then and do something to reward yourself. Then establish goals for the future and decide what you will do to reward yourself when you reach them.

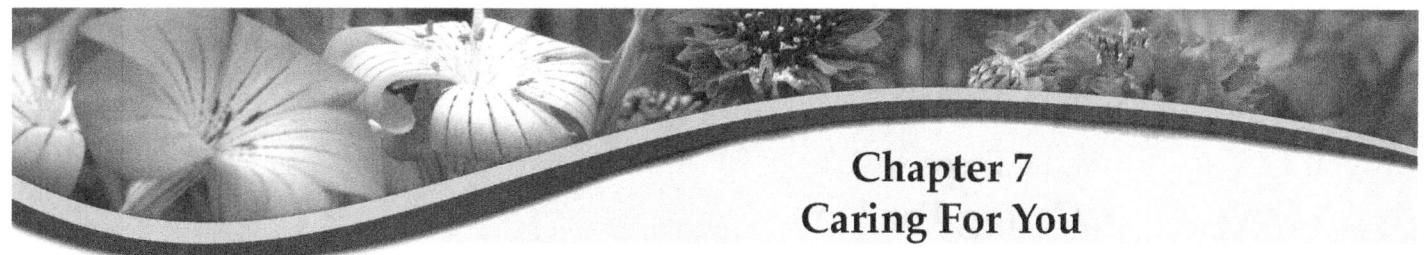

Chapter 7
Caring For You

- **Learn to pace yourself and take one thing at a time.**

Concentrate just on the task at hand and don't allow yourself to be overwhelmed by everything at once. Take time to rest when you need to. And don't forget to exercise!

Are You A Highly Sensitive Person?

In every herd of horses, cattle or deer, there are individuals that serve a special purpose to the group. They are the sensitive ones, those who first smell smoke or the scent of an enemy, and alert the rest of the group to the danger. Research has shown that all of the higher mammal species have this subgroup of sentinels, including humans. They comprise about 15% of any given population.

In centuries and millennia past, the highly sensitive humans became the spiritual leaders and the leading thinkers of the times. Highly sensitive people not only have finely attuned physical senses, such as hearing and sight and smell, they see patterns in society very readily and can make sense of these patterns in ways that others cannot. They are also often highly spiritually attuned and possess a deep level of spiritual insight.

Because of their innate perceptivity and the worldview they have developed as a result, these individuals often lend their energies and insight to causes they believe in. It is likely that most, if not all, of your care team are highly sensitive people. Most end of life caregivers are. You are probably one yourself.

What are the implications for you if you are indeed a highly sensitive? There are many, actually, and you will function much more effectively if you recognize and honor this trait as the valuable gift that it is, and shape your work and home life around it to increase your productivity and happiness on the job and everywhere else.

Putting it Into Practice

Chapter 7
Caring For You

Characteristics of Highly Sensitive People

- Can walk into a room and sense what people are feeling in seconds

- Notice subtleties in tone, inflection and body language in others that most people would miss

- Very sensitive sense of smell and taste

- Often sensitive to perfumes, smoke and chemical odors, even if they're present in very small amounts

- Have a difficult time screening out stimuli and can feel bombarded by visual and auditory stimulation (such as a shopping trip to a department store) and feel exhausted in a short time

- Can struggle with insomnia and anxiety issues when feeling stressed

- Work better on their own time table rather than on a forced schedule since they often need time to decompress after social interactions, especially intense ones

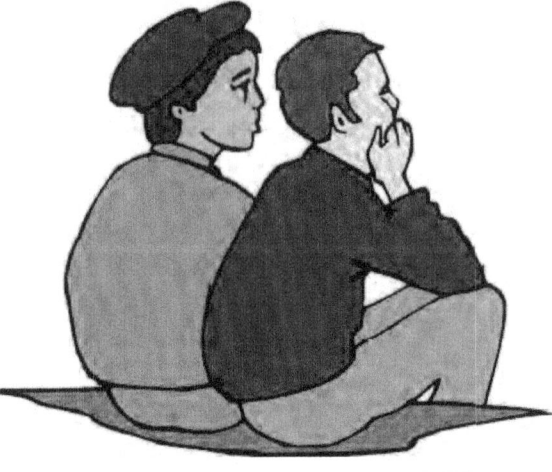

- Need to have a high level of meaning in their work to feel that they are fulfilling their purpose in life

- Are deeply intuitive and tend to see patterns in society that others don't

- Very sensitive to others' presence in their "space", although they won't necessarily see it as an invasion depending on the situation

Putting it Into Practice

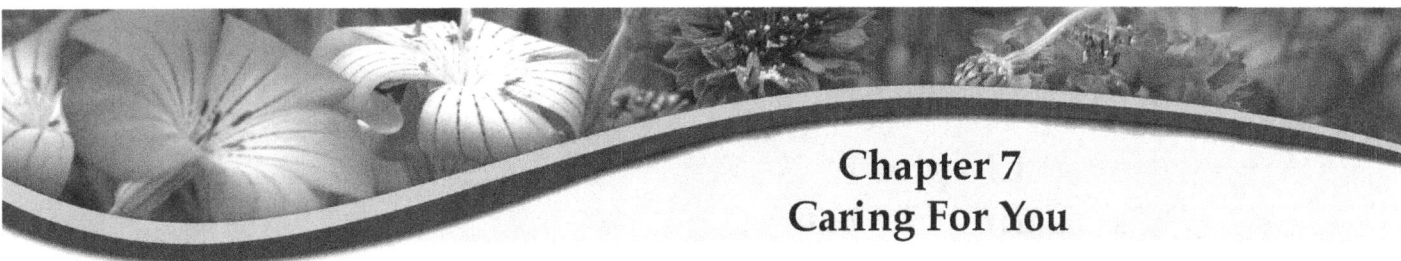

Chapter 7
Caring For You

- Deeply wounded by careless comments or thoughtless gestures

- Tend to cry easily

- Often highly skilled at gift giving or notes of appreciation as they pick up easily on cues about what the other person would find meaningful

- Usually highly spiritually attuned, though they may not talk about it

- Move easily in different cultural settings since it comes naturally to them to notice and adapt to cultural variances

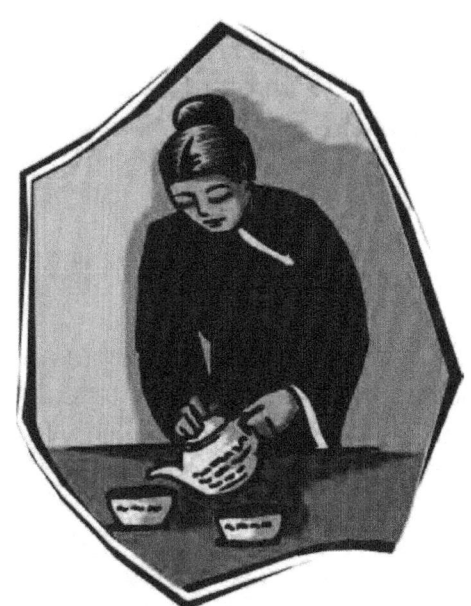

> **If you are a highly sensitive person, be sure you have a place to go that refreshes your heart and mind and feeds your spirit. For you, this isn't a luxury. It is necessity.**
>
> **Spend time outdoors whenever you can. Limit exposure to environments where positive ions predominate. You may want to invest in a negative ion generator.**
>
> **Rest and relaxation isn't optional. You will deplete your stores of energy faster than your non-highly sensitive friends. Guard your rest as the precious treasure that it is.**

Putting it Into Practice

Chapter 7
Caring For You

Review the self nurturing activities in the Putting It Into Practice section of this chapter. Which of these could you incorporate into your life to provide a way to reduce stress and increase well-being and balance in your life? Write about it.

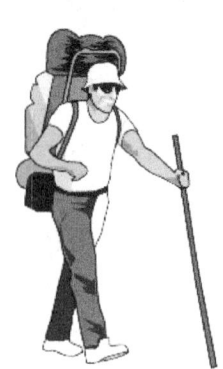

Don't try to change your life all in one grand effort. Habits we have today were formed over a life time. It takes time to create new behavior patterns. Just changing our attitude to reflect the high value we are now placing on nurturing and rewarding ourselves is a great start.

If you are a highly sensitive person (and even if you aren't), small changes in how you talk to yourself every day can make a huge difference in your energy level and attitude for the day. Write love notes to yourself and stick them up around the house. Keep up a streaming conversation with yourself, in the shower, as you are taking a walk, during your commute to your patient's home or facility, about how grateful you are for the good things in your life.

Congratulate yourself on every small thing you do that is successful. And everything is a success in some way. Even if you make a mistake, it is a great successful learning experience. A dropped egg on the kitchen floor in the morning is a great chance to clean the floor well and tell yourself how proud you are of yourself for handling the job so effectively. And, my, doesn't it look nice!

Here are some affirmations to use. Sprinkle them liberally, on a minute by minute basis, throughout your day. They are one of the greatest antidotes to burnout on the planet.

I am my own person	Good things are coming my way
I feel free and safe	I am grateful for my life
I trust myself	I have a relaxed and peaceful body
All is well in my world	My mind is full of possibilities
I am at peace	I am adaptable and calm in the face of change
I can do this	I trust the process
Miracles happen every day	

Putting it Into Practice

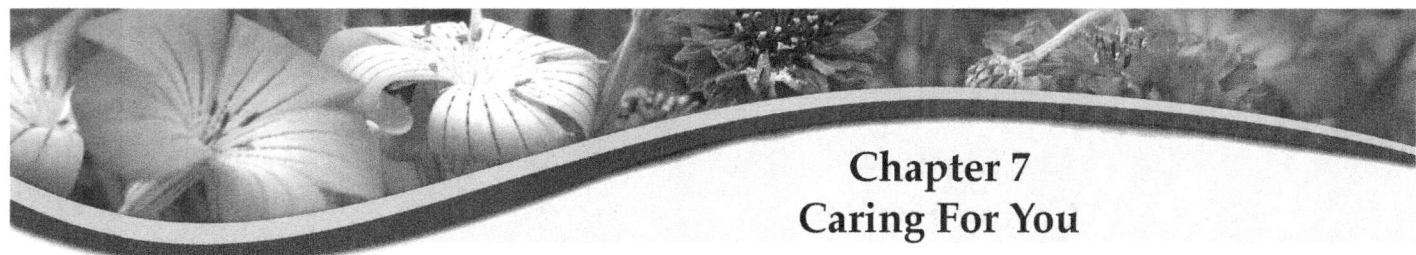

**Chapter 7
Caring For You**

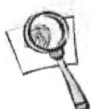 # A Closer Look

Healthy boundaries in our personal lives are the most important factor in interacting with others in a positive way and preventing burnout. A boundary marks the place where you end and someone else begins. When we maintain healthy boundaries, we ask to be treated with respect and we treat others with the same honor.

Giving up our own reality, our own inner world, in order to please, satisfy, or impress others is betrayal of our true self. This lack of genuineness creates feelings of worthlessness and despair because we are actually betraying ourselves. Healthy boundaries help us maintain a healthy self-concept and a strong sense of personal integrity even in the face of someone treating us badly. Our self-worth doesn't come from "out there", it comes from knowing who we are and what we stand for as individuals.

Boundaries don't separate and distance us from others. Quite the contrary. They make it safe for us to be close to those we care about. When we know our own boundaries we can have healthy intimacy without becoming confused by intermingling others' needs, wants, and desires with our own. We can see clearly what belongs to us, in the emotional realm, and what belongs to them.

Individuals who have been abused as children by having their boundaries repeatedly ignored, often grow up to have either absent boundaries (where they allow others to use and abuse them emotionally or physically) or rigid boundaries (in which case they become controlling and fixed in their determination not to let anyone "too close" for fear of being annihilated emotionally again).

Flexible boundaries are the most effective. It's very possible to express what we want and need clearly and directly, while also being sensitive to how our words will affect others. We can be assertive with others without being aggressive. We can be both tender and strong, firm and respectful.

Past wounds are most often the culprits when we find ourselves unable to stand up in the face of present mistreatment. It's helpful to ask ourselves (when feelings of anger and helplessness signal a boundary invasion), *"When did I first feel like this?" What happened in my early childhood that was an assault to my boundaries?"*.

Once we identify the early assault, we can remind ourselves that we are no longer in the position of helpless child and we don't have to be abused. We can gently, but firmly, set clear guidelines as to how we expect to be treated. If the abuser refuses to treat us with respect, we can remove ourselves from the negative environment.

Chapter 7
Caring For You

Healing from early childhood wounds doesn't happen in a vacuum or without deliberate effort. Every caregiver would benefit from a safe group and a good personal counselor with which to process early boundary invasions.

Signs of Unhealthy Boundaries

- Telling everything about yourself
- Talking intimately with someone the first time you meet them
- Falling in love with someone you just met
- Falling in love with anyone who reaches out to you
- Being totally preoccupied with a person - thinking only of their needs and ignoring your own
- Acting on first sexual impulse
- Being sexual for your partner, but not for yourself
- Going against your personal values to please someone else
- Not noticing when someone has inappropriate boundaries
- Not noticing when someone invades your boundaries
- Touching someone without being sure its OK with them
- Accepting things you don't want (food, sex, gifts, touch)
- Taking as much as you can get, just because you can
- Giving as much as you can give, just for the sake of giving
- Allowing someone to take as much as they can from you
- Letting others direct your life
- Letting others define who you are
- Letting others describe your reality for you
- Believing others can anticipate your needs
- Expecting others to fill your needs automatically
- Falling apart so others will take care of you
- Self-abuse: sexual and physical abuse, drug abuse, food abuse

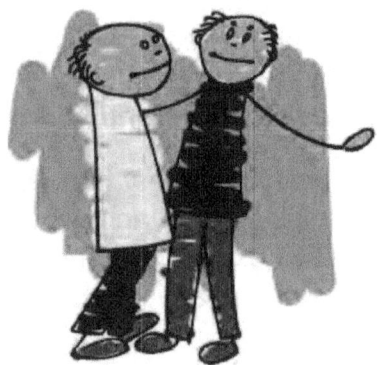

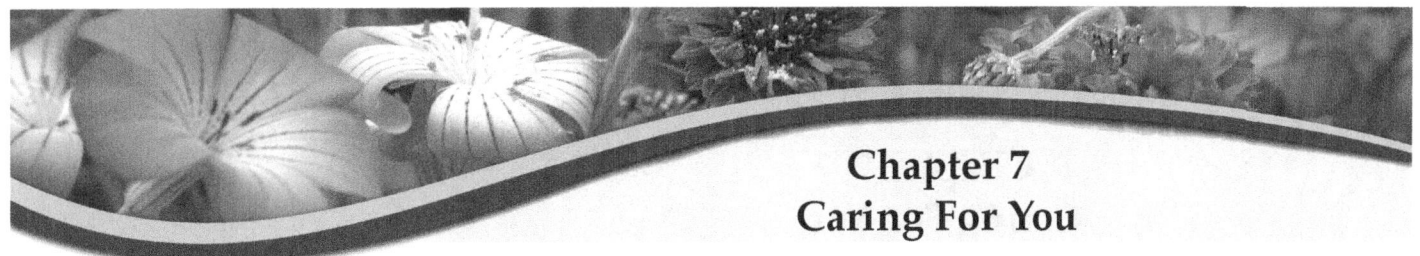

Chapter 7
Caring For You

Characteristics of a Safe Group*

Finding a safe group to process emotions and learn healthy interpersonal skills is an important part of good self care. So how can you tell if a group is safe? Here are a few characteristics that may help you in identifying the group for you:

- Individual members each honor confidentiality.
- They don't "preach", shame, or give unsolicited advice.
- Each member is on a healing journey of their own.

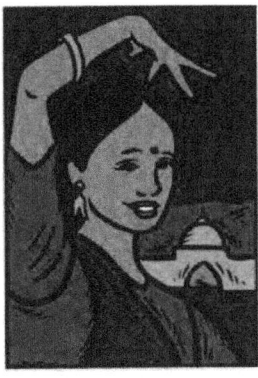

Personal Traits of Safe People*

- Safe people are willing to admit their weaknesses.
- Safe people are truly spiritual, not just religious.
- Safe people are confrontable.

- Safe people are humble.

- Safe people don't just apologize, they take action to change their hurtful behavior.

- Safe people face their problems and deal with them instead of avoiding them.

- Safe people are always "open to audit" and are willing to earn trust, not demand it.

- Safe people take responsibility for themselves and their problems instead of blaming others.

A Closer Look

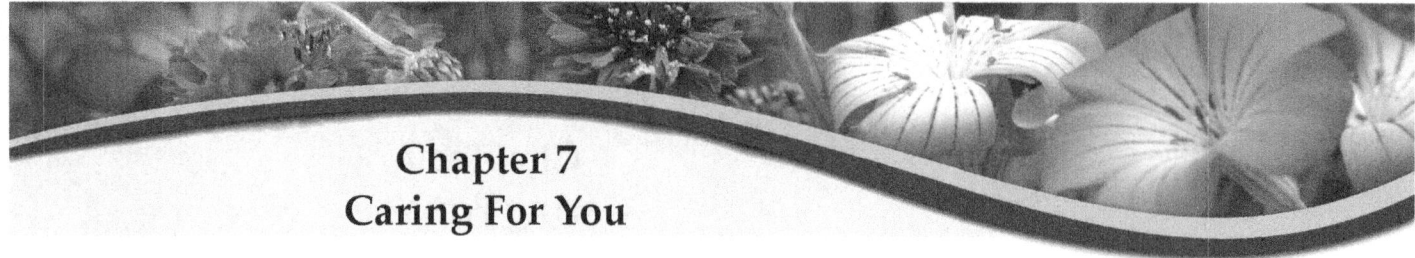

Chapter 7
Caring For You

- Safe people are committed to honesty and truth about themselves.

- Safe people are willing to grow and change.

Interpersonal Traits of Safe People*

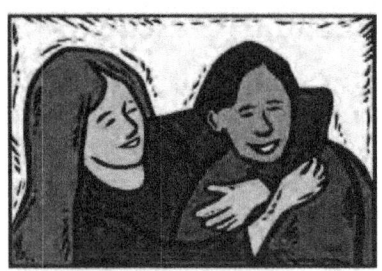

- Safe people nurture connection with others instead of avoiding it.

- Safe people think in terms of relationship ("we" instead of always "I").

- Safe people encourage, respect, and honor the other's freedom.

- Safe people are willing to lovingly confront instead of avoiding telling the truth by engaging in flattery.

- Safe people are forgiving instead of condemning.

- Safe people relate to others as equals, avoiding the parent/child role.

- Safe people are consistent over time.

- Safe people are a positive influence on us, helping us grow.

- Safe people honor confidences.

- Safe people are NOT perfect, but they value their relationships enough to do the painful work of growth so that intimacy becomes possible.

* Adapted from Safe People by Henry Cloud and John Townsend, Zondervan Publishing House, Grand Rapids, Michigan, 1995.

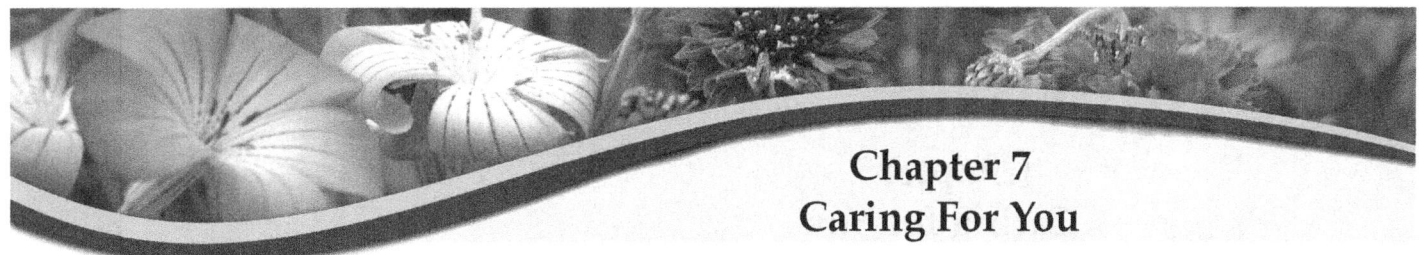

Chapter 7
Caring For You

One important way to relate safely to others when someone might be running over your boundaries is to use "I" messages. This is a helpful skill to develop when setting healthy boundaries both personally and professionally.

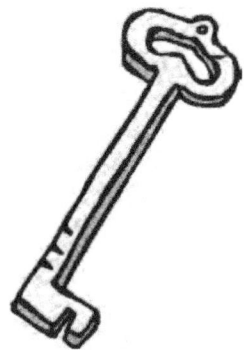

"I" Messages

The Key to Setting Healthy Boundaries

(when yours have been violated)

1. What you are feeling

2. A description of the offensive behavior

3. The reason you feel as you do

4. The expected outcome

- Voice tone is emotionally neutral (adult to adult)

- There is no blame

- The focus is not shifted to the other person

- There is clear ownership of your own feelings

A Closer Look

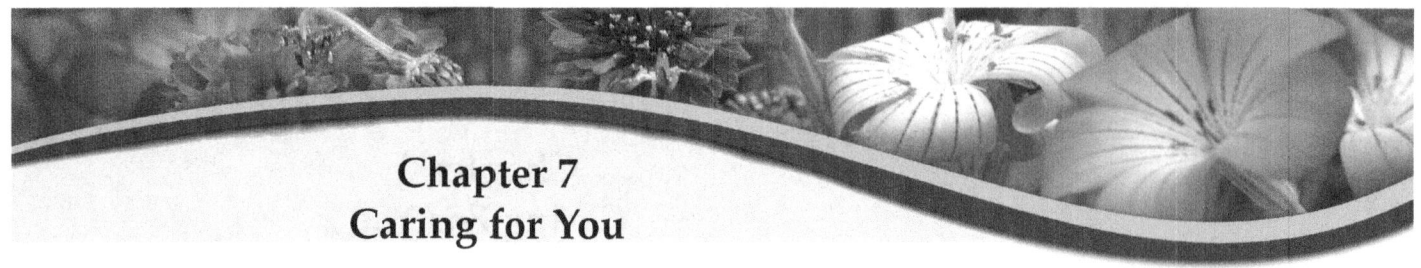

Chapter 7
Caring for You

Healthy boundaries are a foundational component in healthy self care. Unless you, as a hospice volunteer, know how to set boundaries for yourself, burnout is inevitable. There are too many opportunities, when dealing with death and dying, to burn the candle on both ends and give more than is healthy. The need is great, the work is compelling, and it feels good to be highly thought of and appreciated.

Divide into teams of two people each and role play the following scenarios. Take turns with your teammate being the one asking and the one responding. Try to remember to use "I" messages to form your responses.

1. Ruby Smith, your patient's wife, has asked you to sit with Marvin, the patient, while she gets her hair done. She agrees to be back by 4 pm. Your high school age son has a soccer game at 5 pm that you promised him to attend. At 4:30 pm, Mrs. Smith calls you to say she ran into an old friend and lost track of time talking to her. She would like to go to get coffee with the friend. How do you respond?

2. You were up until 3 am with the family of an actively dying patient. You receive a phone call at 7 am from the hospice chaplain, Dan, asking if you can come this morning and teach a segment of a class on the spiritual benefits of touch. You have been studying this topic and feel passionate about it. How do you respond to him?

3. One of your patients, Mary Landers, is actively dying. Her daughter lives out of town and is notified by the hospice nurse that her mother could die at any time. She delays her arrival for several days and arrives just after her mother dies. You are there with the family, offering support. She turns to you and starts shouting that you were with her mother and didn't do anything to save her and that it is your fault that she died. What do you say?

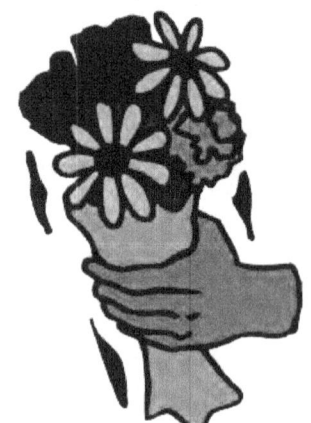

A Closer Look

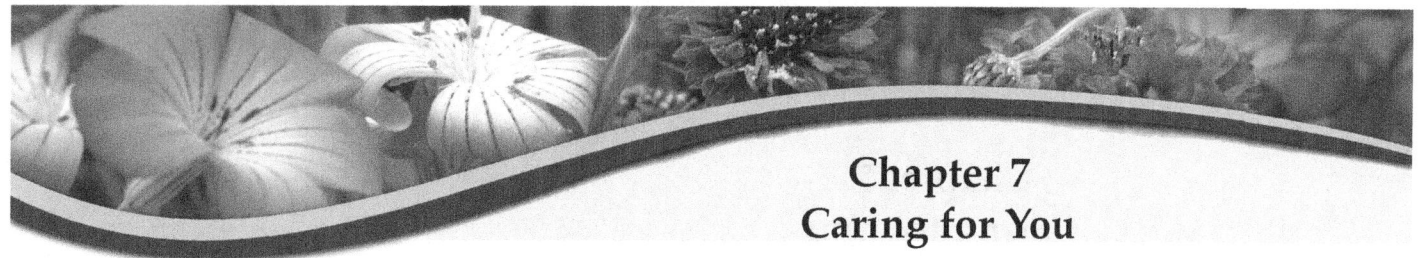

Chapter 7
Caring for You

Preventing Caregiver Burnout

As a hospice volunteer, you have a responsibility to yourself, as well as to the hospice team, to your patients, and to their families to take care of yourself. Burnout is not just a word in the dictionary, it is real and it hurts. Burnout can cost you your job, your relationships and your health. It is much better to prevent it than to try to heal it once it happens.

What measures do I need to take today to refocus my attention to my own health in the following areas?

Mentally

Physically

Emotionally

Spiritually

A Closer Look

Chapter 7
Caring for You

Signs "on the job" that indicate that you may be at risk for caregiver burnout:

- Feeling that you are the only one that can help your patient
- Finding yourself unable to distance from the patient/family
- Dreading visits with your patient/family
- Insensitivity (others may point this out to you after the fact)
- Inappropriate humor (have to laugh to keep from crying)
- Feeling angry, irritable, and touchy a majority of the time (everyone has bad days - if you're having a bad month, you may want to take a look at yourself and see what other signs of burnout you may be exhibiting)

What helps:

- Maintain your professional distance while keeping your caring attitude
- Know your boundaries and maintain them
- Don't compromise them even if others on the team try to pressure you to
- Know when to say "no"
- Don't be afraid to pamper, nurture, spoil, and reward yourself frequently

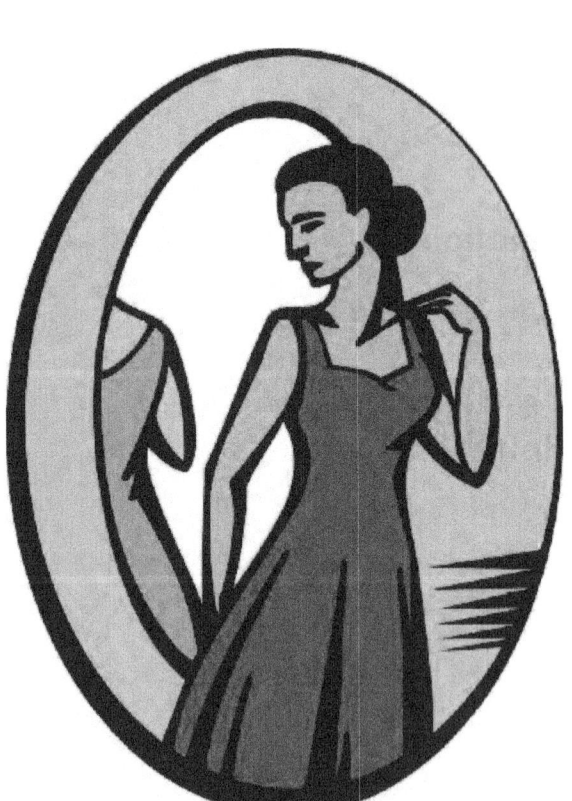

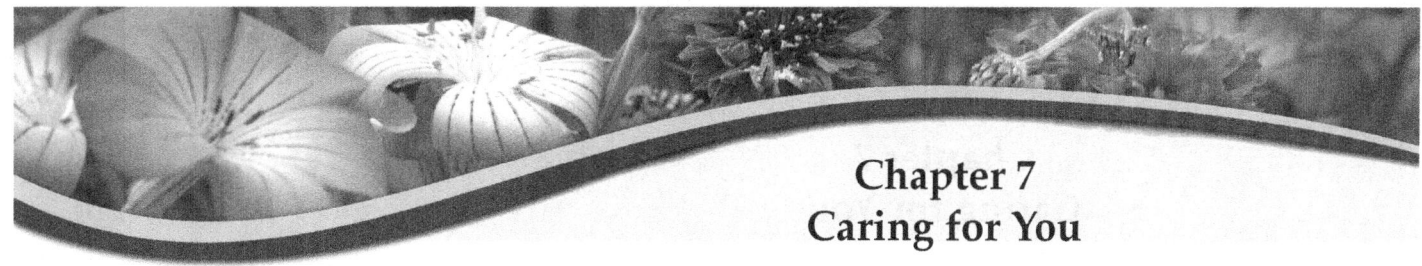

Chapter 7
Caring for You

Ask yourself the following questions:

How do I view death?

What fears do I have in facing my own death in light of the losses I've experienced?

Who in my life can I rely on regularly to be able to process my feelings about my own mortality as they are triggered by experiences with my patients as they are dying?

A Closer Look

Chapter 7
Caring for You

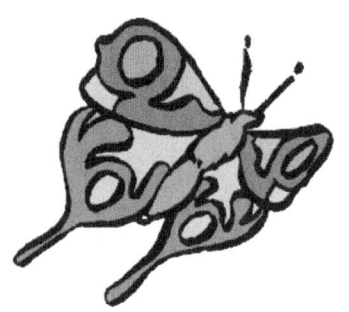

To Let Go...

Does not mean to stop caring,
It means you can't do it for someone else.
Is not to cut myself off,
It's the realization I can't control another.
Is not to enable,
But to allow learning from natural consequences.
Is to admit I am powerless,
Which simply means the outcome is not in my hands.
Is not to try to change another,
It's to make the most of myself.
Is not to care for,
but to care about.
Is not to fix,
But to be supportive.
Is not to judge,
But to allow another to be a human being.
Is not to be in the middle arranging all the outcomes,
But to allow others to affect their own destinies.
Is not to be protective,
It's to permit another to face reality.
Is not to criticize or regulate anyone,
But to try to become what God has planned for *Me*.

To LET GO is to FEAR LESS

Author Unknown

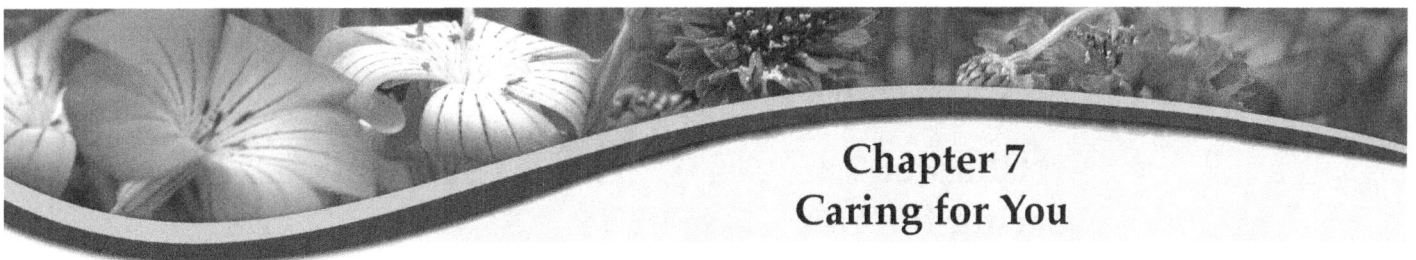

Chapter 7
Caring for You

Autobiography in Five Short Chapters

Chapter One
I walk down the street.
There is a deep hole in the sidewalk.
I fall in.
I am lost...I am helpless.
It isn't my fault.
It takes forever to find a way out.

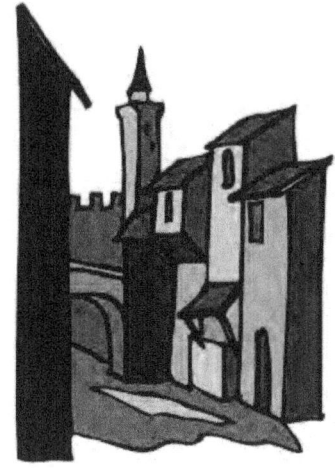

Chapter Two
I walk down the same street.
There is a deep hole in the sidewalk.
I pretend I don't see it.
I fall in again.
I can't believe I am in this same place.
But it isn't my fault.
It still takes a long time to get out.

Chapter Three
I walk down the same street.
There is a deep hole in the sidewalk.
I see it is there.
I still fall in...it's a habit...but,
my eyes are open, I know where I am.
It is my fault.
I get out immediately.

Chapter Four
I walk down the same street.
There is a deep hole in the sidewalk.
I walk around it.

Chapter Five
I walk down another street.

Portia Nelson

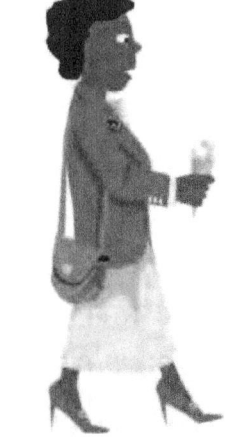

A Closer Look

**Chapter 7
Caring for You**

Skill Check

1. Define burnout.

2. List ten symptoms of burnout.

3. How does personal loss contribute to burnout?

4. Circle the answer you believe to be correct:

T or F   Getting into a rut feels safe and helps promote spiritual health.
T or F   One way to cut stress is to switch to a side of the brain that isn't so tired.
T or F   Using a "buddy system" creates tension and should be avoided.
T or F   An attitude of aloofness and distance protects you from burnout.
T or F   Laughter and beauty feed the spirit and restore the body and soul.
T or F   Procrastination may be a signal of un-grieved loss in your life.
T or F   You should only talk your problems over with someone who will give answers.
T or F   Past wounds often prevent us from being able to stand up to mistreatment.
T or F   Flexible boundaries cause more stress because they make life unpredictable.
T or F   Giving up our own reality to please someone else is a form of betrayal.

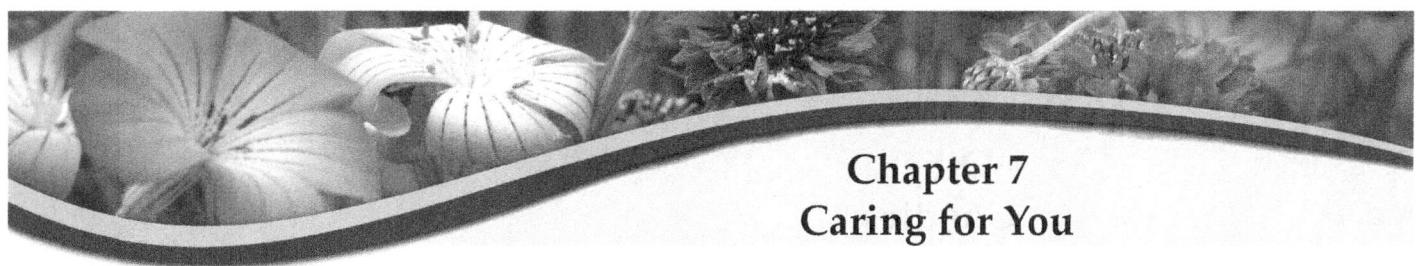

Chapter 7
Caring for You

5. What are the four components of a healthy "I" message?

6. Describe fifteen signs of unhealthy boundaries.

7. List 20 self-nurturing activities that you would like to do to relieve your stress.

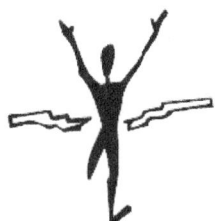

*There will never be another now,
I'll make the most of today.
There will never be another me,
I'll make the most of myself.*

Anonymous

Skill Check

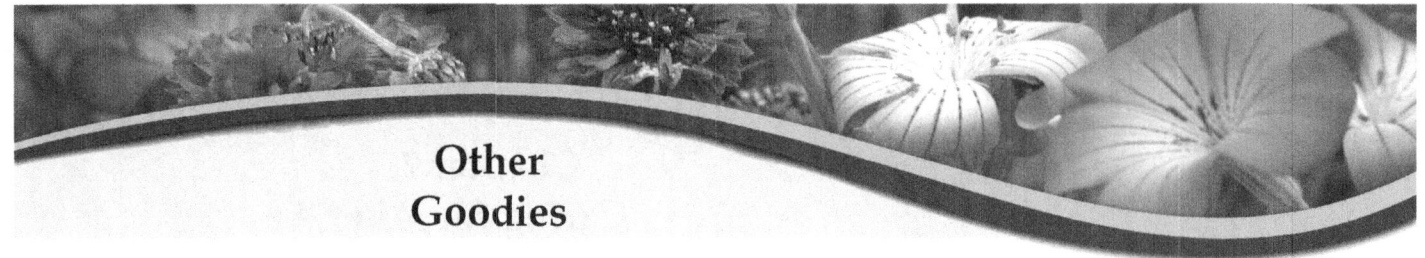

Other Goodies:

Safety and Other Information You Need to Know

About Hazardous Materials

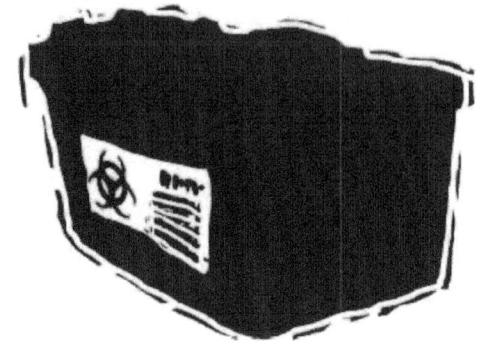

A hazardous material is any material that poses a threat to your life or your health.

1. Sharps: Hypodermic needles, suture needles, lancets must be disposed of in a puncture proof sharps container. Do not recap or cut needles! Do not try to jam a needle into an already full container.

2. Chemicals: Cleaning supplies can cause damage to respiratory tissue or to skin. Make sure the area in which you are working is well-ventilated. Use gloves when handling toxic chemicals. Make sure all containers that contain these chemicals are clearly labeled and stored out of reach of children or adults with vision problems who may not be able to read the label.

3. Infectious Waste: Hazardous body wastes must be disposed of in a double red bag and taken to a disposal site according to your agency's policy.

4. Chemotherapeutic Agents: Most hospice patients will not be continuing on chemotherapy, If you are in contact with these agents however, remember that they are very toxic. Avoid inhalation or direct contact with skin. Wear gloves. Place sharps or unused chemotherapeutic drugs in a leak proof sharps container.

5. Radioactive Waste: Usually not encountered in the home. Follow facility protocol for handling and disposing of these materials if the situation arises.

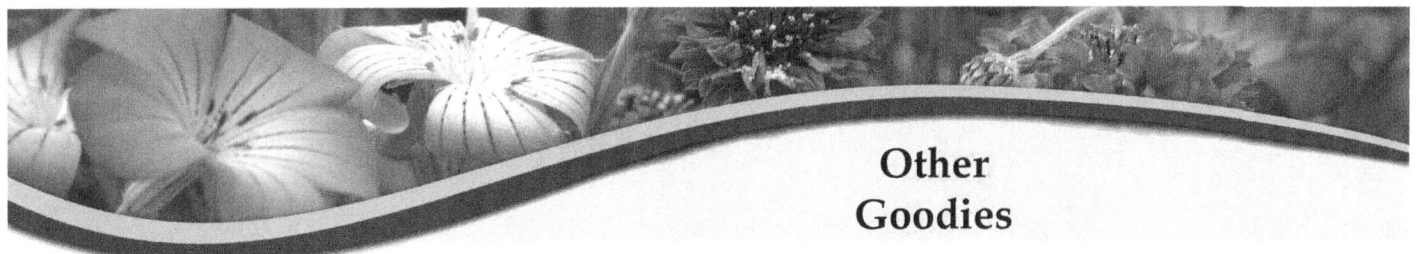

Other Goodies

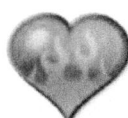 ## Fire Safety

Fires do not happen randomly. In almost every case, they are a result of well known causes and are preventable. Early detection of these potential sources of fire is an important part of preventing them altogether:

- **Smoking near oxygen**
- **Heaters or heat sources that are too close to bedding or other flammable materials**
- **Worn and torn cords on electrical appliances**
- **Wires that cross under rugs or over windows or doorways**
- **Overloaded electrical outlets**
- **Unsafe, malfunctioning appliances**
- **Flammable or spark-producing toys**

Fire Safety Factors

- Make sure all doors, stairways, and hallways are unobstructed.
- Identify all exits as soon as you enter the area - make sure all exits are clearly marked.
- Check to make sure emergency lighting is working properly.
- Check for cords in doorways or down stairs.
- Do not allow smoking in the vicinity of oxygen use or near gas or flammable liquids.
- Ensure that flammable liquids are stored in safety cans and disposed of in designated containers.
- Clean up spills immediately.
- Do not overload electrical outlets.
- Keep combustible materials away from heaters and furnaces.
- Do not allow trash to accumulate.
- Do not use portable heaters in the patient care area.

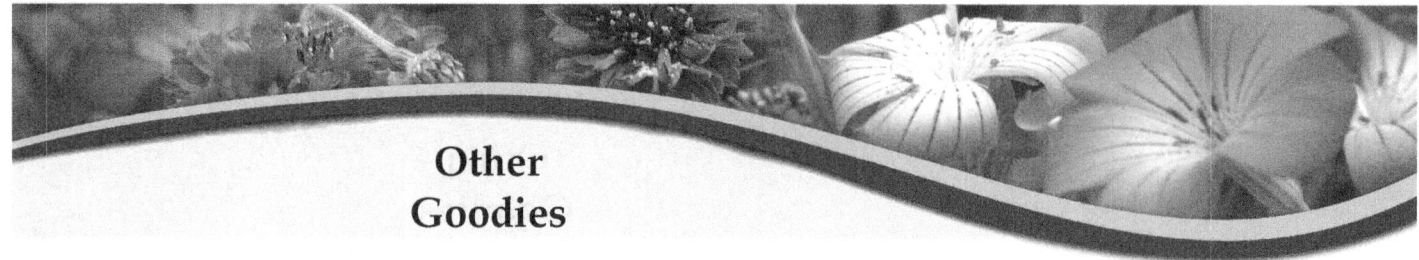

Other Goodies

What to Do in Case of Fire

Remember the mnemonic **RACE**:

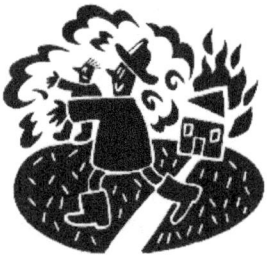

> **R**emove the patient.
>
> **A**lert the fire department by sounding the alarm. Call 911.
>
> **C**ontain the fire by closing doors to stop air movement.
>
> **E**xtinguish the fire if you can do so safely by using a fire extinguisher or smothering it with a blanket.

Patient Removal in Case of Fire:

- **Cradle Drop**

1. Place a blanket on the floor next to the patient's bed, then grip patient under the shoulders and knees.

2. Slide the patient to the edge of the bed.

3. On one knee, lower the patient's legs, then his/her body, to the blanket.

4. Pulling the patient out headfirst, using the blanket as a sled.

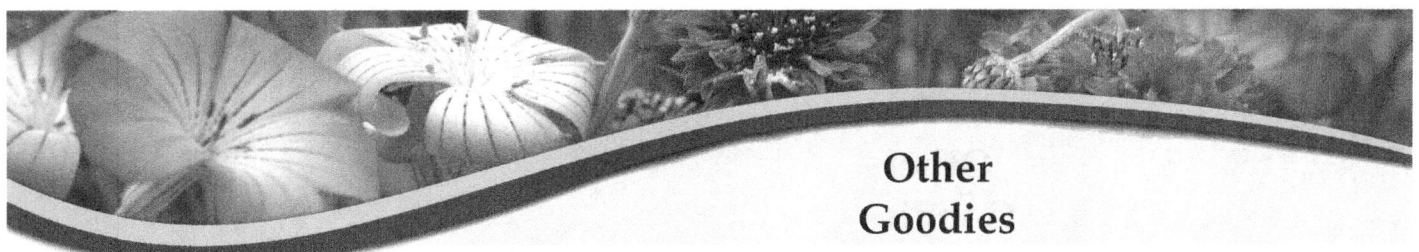

Other Goodies

- **Back Carry**

1. Cross the patient's arms and grab both of his/her wrists.

2. Pull up on the patient's arms as you turn to step under them and cross them in front of you.

3. Lean forward and step to the head of the bed. The patient will roll out onto your back.

4. To put the patient down, lean the patient against a wall and slide him/her to the floor as you drop to one knee.

- **Hip Carry**

1. Put the patient's arm over you back and slide your arm under the patient's back.

2. Lean backward, into the patient's abdomen, and grip the patient behind his/her knees.

3. Hold the patient snugly against your back, then lean forward to carry him/her.

4. To put the patient down, lean him/her against the wall and slide him/her down to the floor as you drop to one knee.

- **Swing (Two Rescuers)**

1. Each rescuer grasps the other's shoulder with one hand as the patient places his/her arms around both of their shoulders.

2. Reaching under the patient, each rescuer grasps the other's wrist.

About Fire Extinguishers

There are three kinds of fire extinguishers. It is important to know which kind is available to you and what kinds of fires to use them on:

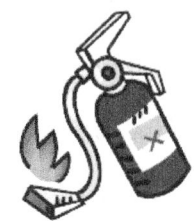

- **Class "A" Fire Extinguishers**

These extinguishers are filled with water. They are used to penetrate and cool ordinary combustible materials such as paper, wood, plastics, mattresses, and clothing.

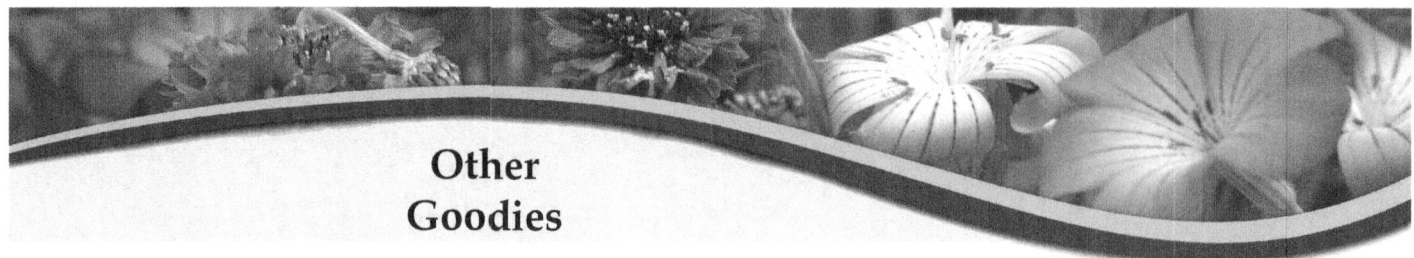

Other Goodies

- **Class "B" Fire Extinguishers**

These extinguishers are filled with a carbon dioxide extinguisher, foam, and dry powder. They smother a fire by separating oxygen in the air from the burning substance. They are used on fires involving flammable liquids, greases, etc.

Caution: Using a Class A extinguisher on a Class B fire could spread it and make it worse.

- **Class "C" Fire Extinguishers**

These extinguishers have carbon dioxide and/or dry powder in them that acts as a non-conducting medium. They are used on electrical fires or fires involving electrical equipment.

Some points to remember when using extinguishers on a fire:

- **Always stay between the fire and your exit**

- **If you use the extinguisher, make sure it gets recharged immediately**

- **Use dry powder extinguishers sparingly– they are very messy**

- **The dry powder extinguisher is considered "universal"- it can be used to put out any kind of fire**

- **To use a fire extinguisher:**

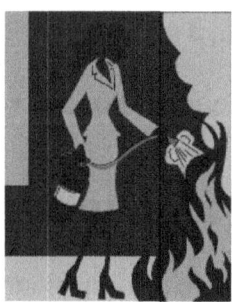

1. Pull the pin

2. Aim the nozzle of the extinguisher at the BASE of the fire

3. Squeeze the handle

4. Sweep the nozzle from side to side at the base of the fire until the fire goes out

5. Shut off the extinguisher

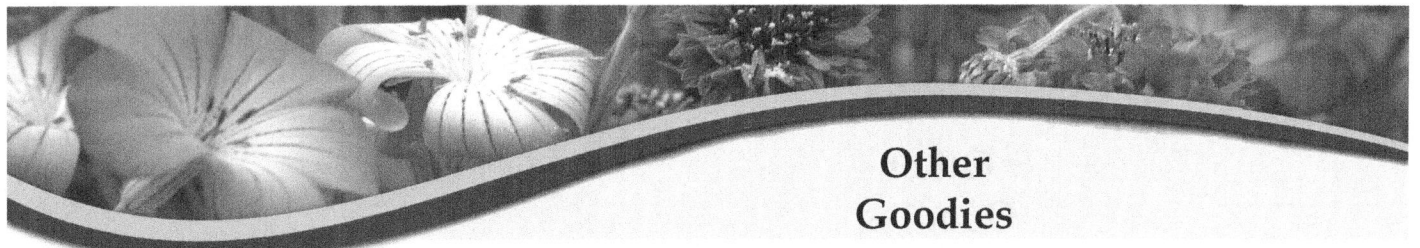

Preventing Violence in the Workplace

It is a chilling fact that violence in the workplace has increased astronomically in the past thirty years. Unheard of until the late 1970s, five states in the U.S. in 1992 reported homicide as the leading cause of workplace death for all workers, both men and women. 1.7 million Americans were victims of workplace attacks each year from 1993-1999, according to National Institute for Occupational Safety and Health (NIOSH) stats.

Here are some of the danger signals that could indicate the potential for violence in the workplace:

1. Use of drugs and alcohol that has noticeably increased. You smell alcohol on the person's breath at work, or he or she exhibits strange behavior that could indicate drug use. Examples include*:

- Cycles of increased energy, restlessness, and inability to sleep (often seen in stimulants)
- Abnormally slow movements, speech or reaction time, confusion and disorientation (often seen in opiates, benzodiazepines and barbiturates)
- Sudden weight loss or weight gain
- Cycles of excessive sleep
- Unexpected changes in clothing, such as constantly wearing long sleeved shirts, to hide scarring at injection sites
- Suspected drug paraphernalia such as unexplained pipes, roach clips or syringes
- For snorted drugs, chronic troubles with sinusitis or nosebleeds
- For smoked drugs, a persistent cough or bronchitis, leading to coughing up excessive mucus or blood
- Progressive severe dental problems (especially with methamphetamine users)
- Cycles of being unusually talkative, "up" and cheerful, with seemingly boundless energy.
- Increased irritability, agitation and anger
- Unusual calmness, unresponsiveness or looking "spaced out"
- Apathy and depression

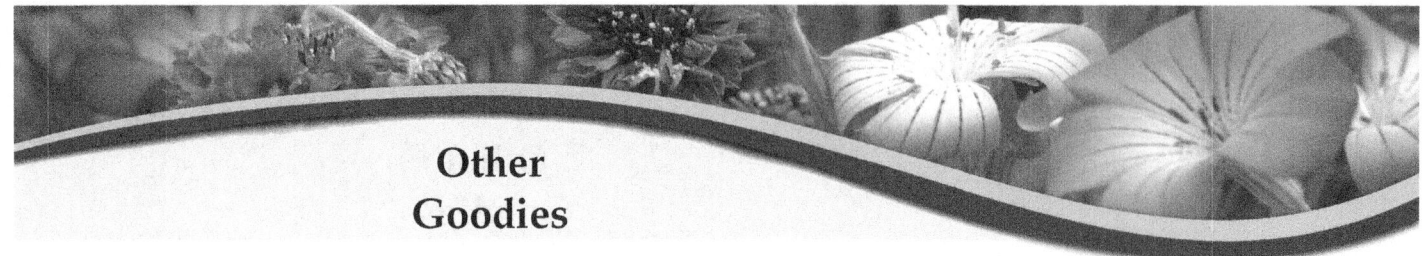

Other Goodies

- Paranoia, delusions
- Temporary psychosis, hallucinations
- Lowered threshold for violence

(*these signs and symptoms of active drug use are from an article by Joanna Saisan, MSW, Jeanne Segal, Ph.D, and Deborah Cutter, Psy.D. on the website www.helpguide.org)

2. An unexplained increase in absenteeism for no apparent reason (such as health problems or a death in the family)

3. A noticeable change in attention to personal appearance and hygiene

4. Withdrawal from co-workers and signs of depression

5. Explosive outbursts of anger or rage without provocation

6. Makes threatening gestures or comments or otherwise verbally abuses co-workers and supervisors

7. Repeated comments about death and suicidal urges

8. Frequent, vague physical complaints

9. Obvious instability in emotional responses

10. Behavior that seems paranoid

11. Makes frequent reference to incidents of violence in the news or in the community

12. Apparent increase in mood swings

13. Speaks of having a plan that will "solve all my problems"

14. Very resistant to, and unhappy about, any changes in company policies and repeatedly violates them with angry self-justification

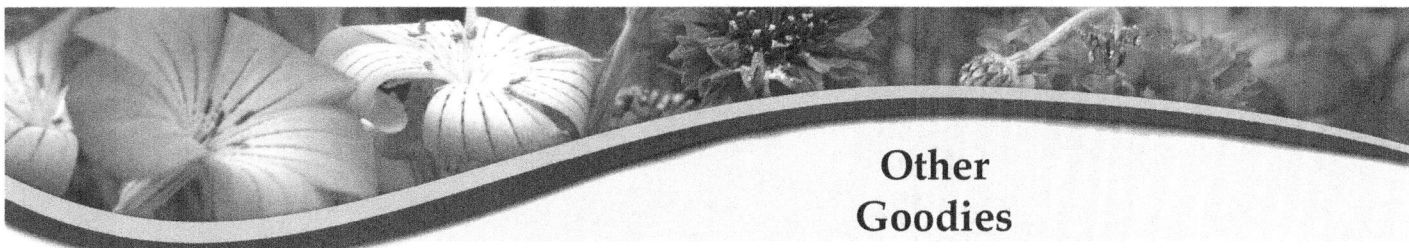

Other Goodies

15. Makes unsolicited comments about firearms and other dangerous weapons

16. Takes a predominantly empathetic position when speaking of individuals committing violence

17. Demonstrates a fascination with watching/reading violent and/or sexually explicit movies or publications

18. Involved in escalating relationship problems– spouse recently left, etc.

19. Recently made a large withdrawal from or closed his/her account in the company's credit union

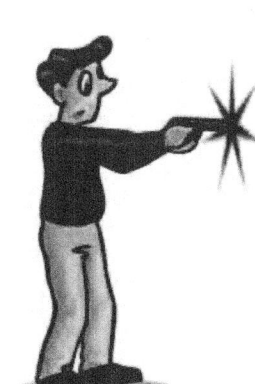

Studies done on acts of violence in the workplace have revealed common characteristics among perpetrators. Although there are always exceptions, the following is a composite profile created from these findings:

- White male, 35—45 years old
- Can't seem to keep a job for long
- Doesn't have much in the way of family support, tends to be a loner
- Chronically disgruntled with everything in his life
- Does not take responsibility
- Tends to blame everyone else for problems
- Unable to receive constructive criticism, reacts defensively
- Tends to identify with violence, in the news/films/books/television
- History of serious drug/alcohol use
- Fascination with weapons

The bottom line is that all of us deserve a safe work environment. This issue must be addressed to ensure that all workers understand the signs of potentially dangerous behavior and have a way to report it confidentially. If your organization does not already have a program for confidentially handling reports of harassment, abuse, and suspicious behavior, today is a good day to start one. It is important that the person handling the reports be a neutral party so the person reporting can do so without fear of being labeled a "troublemaker" and having their employment status affected.

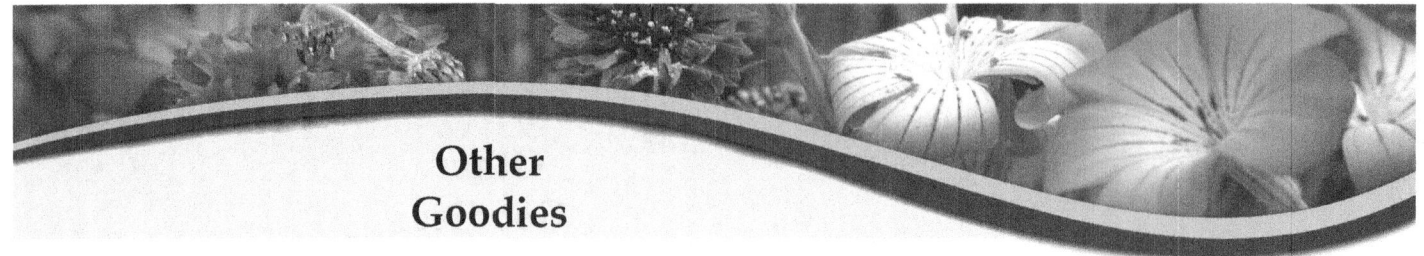

Other Goodies

Sexual Harassment and the Law

Sexual harassment in the workplace is not only distasteful, it's illegal. It is a violation of a person's civil rights according to the Title VII of the Civil Rights Act of 1964. When an employee repeatedly makes unwelcome sexual advances, including requests for sexual favors and other verbal or physical conduct of a sexual nature, to another employee, against his or her wishes, this is considered sexual harassment.

A recent report from the U.S. Equal Employment Opportunity Commission (EEOC) states that sexual harassment has occurred "when submission to or rejection of this conduct explicitly or implicitly affects an individual's employment, unreasonably interferes with an individual's work performance or creates an intimidating, hostile or offensive work environment."

Some behavior patterns that could be considered sexual harassment include:

- Unwelcomed comments or jokes of a sexual nature
- Inappropriate gestures
- Offensive, sexually oriented words on clothing
- Unwelcomed bodily contact with a coworker including touching, scratching or patting their back, grabbing them around the waist, putting hands inside their clothing in any way (including pockets), or interfering in any way with their ability to move ("cornering" them in their cubicle or office space, etc.)
- Unwanted flirting or asking repeatedly for dates
- Sending sexually oriented emails or text messages
- Displaying sexually suggestive objects, pictures, or posters
- Playing or singing sexually suggestive music

Again, be sure there is a mechanism in place in your organization for individuals to be able to confidentially report anything that feels to them to be a violation of their rights to a comfortable and safe work environment. Employees and volunteers not only deserve it, it's the law!

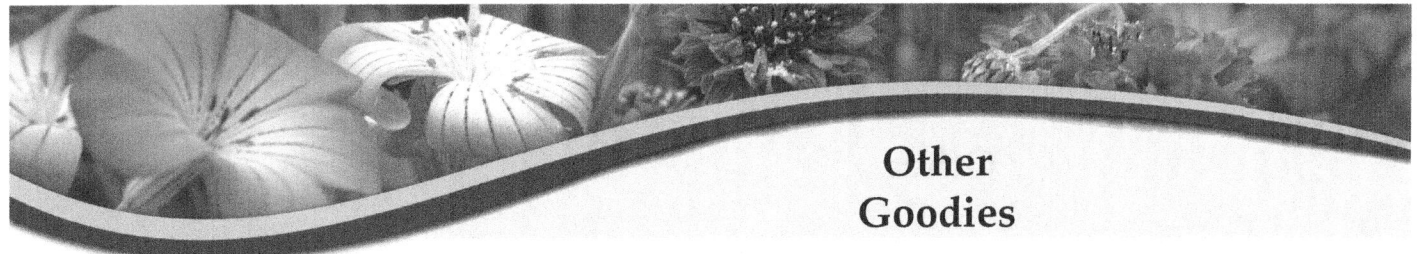

Other Goodies

Tax Deductions for the Volunteer

The following are expenses that can be deducted for volunteer work if your agency is non-profit. The volunteer cannot deduct the value of volunteer time or services, but my deduct out-of-pocket expenses directly related to their volunteer service (if they itemize deductions).

- Mileage and car expenses (not general repair)

- Bus/cab fares

- Parking tolls

- Long distance phone charges

- Supplies needed to perform duties

- Dues or fees for professional organizations

- Special uniform, if required

- Value of non-cash contribution of property

- Travel expenses (including meals and lodging) only if the trip has no significant element of personal pleasure, recreation, or vacation and it is not reimbursed by the hospice

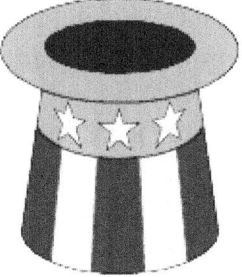

Keep detailed records of dates, places, amounts, etc. For more information contact the **IRS** or **Points of Light Foundation, 736 Jackson Place, Washington D.C 20503**.

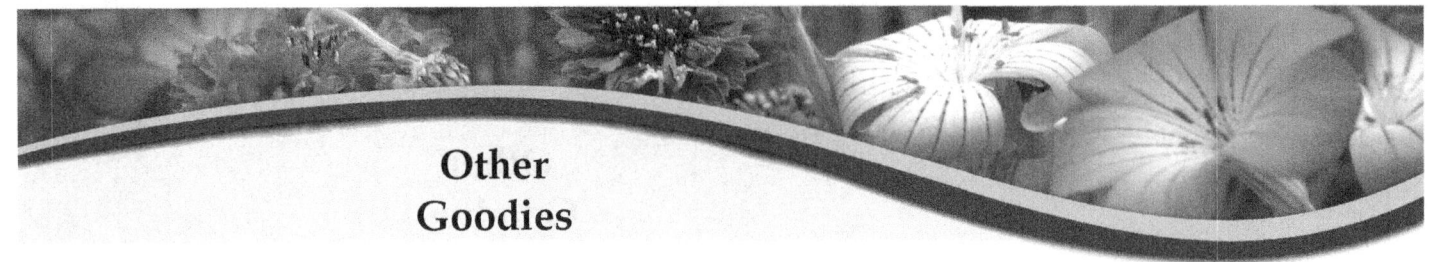

Other Goodies

Bibliography

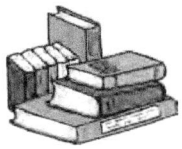

Aron, Elaine N. *The Highly Sensitive Person: How to Thrive When the World Overwhelms You.* New York: Broadway, 1996. Print

Bloomfield, Harold H., Melba Colgrove, and Peter McWilliams. *How to Survive the Loss of a Love.* Allen Park, MI: Mary /Prelude, 2004. Print.

Brand, Paul W., and Philip Yancey. *The Gift Nobody Wants.* New York: Harper Perennial, 1995. Print.

Branden, Nathaniel. (1990). *How to Raise Your Self-Esteem.* New York: Bantam.

Brinkman, Rick, and Rick Kirschner. *Dealing with People You Can't Stand: How to Bring out the Best in People at Their Worst.* New York: McGraw-Hill, 2002. Print.

Buscaglia, Leo F. *Love.* New York: Fawcett Crest, 1983. Print.

Cassel, Eric J. *The Nature of Suffering and the Goals of Medicine.* New York: Oxford UP, 1994. Print.

Chapman, Gary D. *The Five Love Languages: How to Express Heartfelt Commitment to Your Mate.* Chicago: Northfield Pub2004. Print.

Charlesworth, E.S., & Nathan, R.C. (1984). *Stress Management: A Comprehensive Guide to Wellness.* New York: Ballantine Books.

Cloud, Henry, and John Townsend. *Safe People: How to Find Relationships That Are Good for You and Avoid Those That Aren't.* Grand Rapids, MI: Zondervan Pub. House, 1995. Print.

Davidson, Glen W. (1984). *Understanding Mourning: A Guide for Those Who Grieve.* Minneapolis, MN: Augsburg Publishing House.

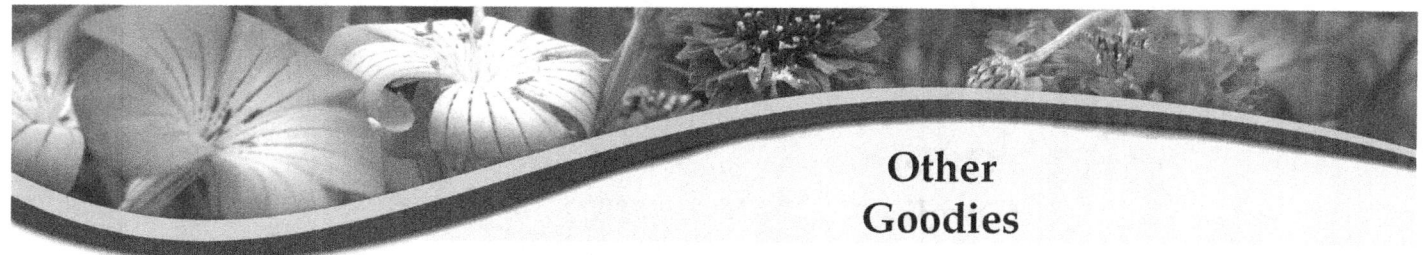

Other Goodies

Deits, Bob. *Life after Loss: a Personal Guide Dealing with Death, Divorce, Job Change, and Relocation.* Tucson, AZ: Fisher 1988. Print.

Doka, Kenneth J., and Joyce Davidson. *Living with Grief When Illness Is Prolonged.* Washington, D.C.: Hospice Foundation of America, 1997. Print.

Doka, Kenneth J. *Living with Grief after Sudden Loss: Suicide, Homicide, Accident, Heart Attack, Stroke.* Washington, DC: Hospice Foundation of America, 1996. Print.

Engel, Beverly. *The Emotionally Abusive Relationship.* Hoboken, NJ: John Wiley & Sons, 2002. Print.

Evans, Patricia. *The Verbally Abusive Relationship.* Holbrook, MA: Adams Media, 2003. Print.

Florence, Susan Squellati. *When You Lose Someone You Love: a Journey through the Heart of Grief.* Spencer, MA: Exley Publications, 2003. Print.

Gaffney, Donna A. (1989). *The Seasons of Grief.* New American Library.

Hay, Louise L. *You Can Heal Your Life.* London: Hay House, 2007. Print.

Hsieh, Tony. *Delivering Happiness: a Path to Profits, Passion, and Purpose.* New York, NY: Business Plus, 2010. Print.

Jaeger, Barrie. *Making Work Work for the Highly Sensitive Person.* New Yorl: McGraw-Hill, 2004. Print.

Jewett, Claudia L. (1982). *Helping Children Cope with Separation and Loss.* Harvard: Har-vard Common.

Karr, Catherine L. (1992). *Taking Time For Me: How Caregivers Can Effectively Deal With Stress.* Prometheus Books.

Kubler-Ross, Elisabeth. *On Death and Dying.* New York: Scribner Classics, 1997. Print.

Kushner, Harold S. (1981). *When Bad Things Happen to Good People.* New York: Avon Books.

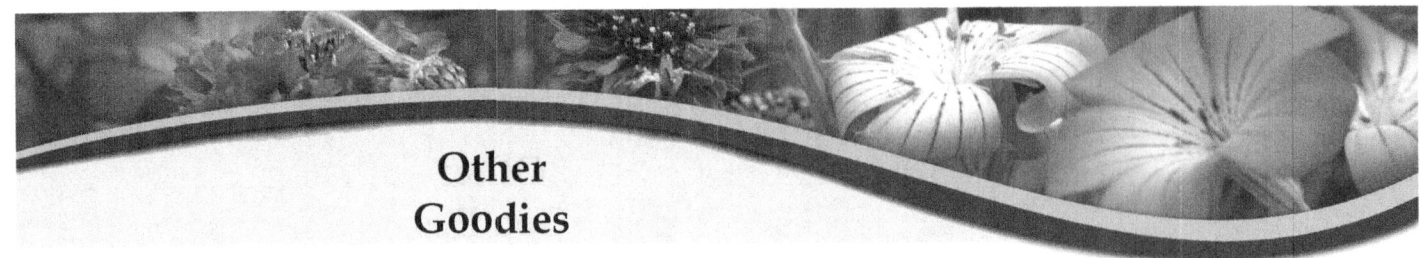

Other Goodies

LaHaye, Tim F. *Transformed Temperaments.* Wheaton, IL: Tyndale House, 1982. Print.

Larson, Dale G. *The Helper's Journey: Working with People Facing Grief, Loss, and Life-threatening Illness.* Champaign, IL: Research, 1993. Print.

Larson, Earnie. (1988). *Old Patterns, New Truths.* Hazeldon.

Lightner, Candy, and Nancy Hathaway. *Giving Sorrow Words: How to Cope with Grief and Get on with Your Life.* New York, NY: Warner, 1990. Print.

Lord, Janice H. (1992). *Beyond Sympathy: What to Say and Do for Someone Suffering an Injury, Illness, or Loss.* Ventura, CA: Pathfinder Publishing.

McClelland, Susan. (1990). *If There's Anything I Can Do.* Gainesville:Triad.

McGraw, Phillip C. *Self Matters--Changing Your Life from the Inside Out.* New York: Simon & Schuster Source, 2001. Print.

Pipher, Mary Bray. *Another Country: Navigating the Emotional Terrain of Our Elders.* New York: Riverhead, 1999. Print.

Rando, Therese A. (1984). *Grief, Dying, and Death: Clinical Interventions for Caregivers.* Champaign, IL: Research Press Company.

Rando, Therese A. (1988). *Grieving: How to Go on Living When Someone You Love Dies.* Lexington Books.

Seamonds, David A. (1981). *Healing for Damaged Emotions.* Wheaton, Illinois: Victor Books.

Secunda, Victoria. *Women and Their Fathers: the Sexual and Romantic Impact of the First Man in Your Life.* New York, NY: Delta, 1993. Print.

Siegel, Bernie S., and Yosaif August. *Help Me to Heal: a Practical Guidebook for Patients, Visitors, and Caregivers.* Carlsbad, CA: Hay House, 2003. Print.

Smith, Kathleen. (1978). *The Stress of Sorrow.* Dallas: Southwest Book Services.

Solomon, Muriel. *Working with Difficult People.* Paramus, NJ: Prentice Hall, 2002. Print.

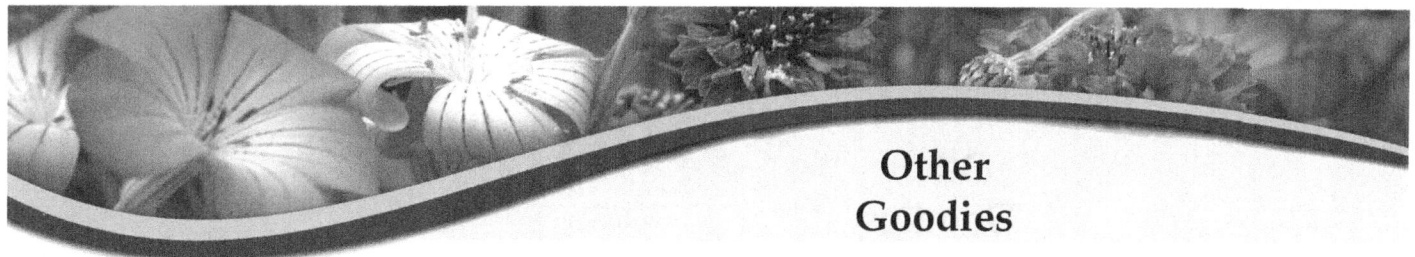

Other Goodies

Tada, Joni Eareckson., and Steve Estes. *When God Weeps: Why Our Sufferings Matter to the Almighty.* Grand Rapids, MI: ZondervanPublishing House, 1997. Print.

Tappan, Frances M. *Healing Massage Techniques: a Study of Eastern and Western Methods.* Reston (Va.): Reston Publ. Comp, 1980. Print.

Tatelbaum, Judy. *The Courage to Grieve: the Classic Guide to Creative Living, Recovery, and Growth through Grief.* New York: Harper, 2008. Print.

Towns, James E., Ph.D. (1984). *Growing Through Grief.* Anderson, IN: Warner Press.

Whitfield, Charles L. *Boundaries and Relationships: Knowing, Protecting, and Enjoying the Self.* Deerfield Beach, FL: Health Communications, 1993. Print.

Worden, J.W. (1982). *Grief Counseling and Grief Therapy.* Springer Publishing.

Yancey, Philip. *Where Is God When It Hurts?* Grand Rapids, MI: Zondervan Pub. House, 2001. Print.

Zonnebelt-Smeenge, Susan J., and Robert C. De Vries. *Getting to the Other Side of Grief: Overcoming the Loss of a Spouse.* Grand Rapids, MI: Baker, 1998. Print.

Some of my favorite titles:

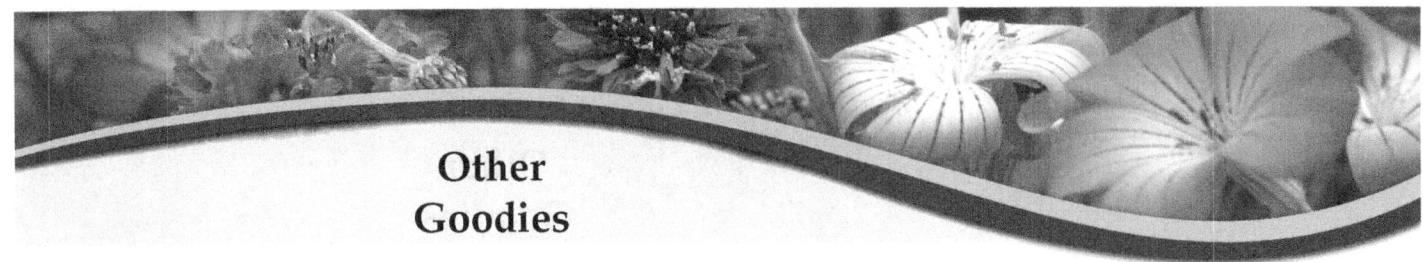

Other Goodies

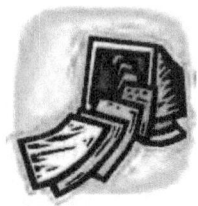 **Some Great Web Resources**

www.aarp.org/relationships/grief-loss/—American Association of Retired People Grief and Loss program includes online articles, publications, support groups, and discussion boards on coping with the loss of a family member.

www.abcd-caring.org—Americans for Better Care of the Dying (ABCD) aims to improve end-of-life care by learning which social and political changes will lead to enduring, efficient, and effective programs. They work with the public, clinicians, policymakers, and other end-oflife organizations to make change happen.

www.accesshelp.org—Aircraft Casualty Emotional Support Service provides peer grief support and resource information to those who have lost loved ones in air disasters.

www.afsp.org—American Foundation for Suicide prevention is dedicated to advancing knowledge of suicide and the ability to prevent it.

www.alivealone.org—Designed to benefit bereaved parents whose children have died by providing a self-help network and newsletter to promote communication and healing.

www.aoa.gov—U.S. Government clearinghouse with many key links and articles to web sites on areas of interest in aging. Contains information about state and local agencies, federal sites, metasites (sites containing many links), and resources for the elderly.

www.babysteps.com—Named after the baby steps that form the long and difficult road to recovery from the loss of a child.

www.bereavedparentsusa.org—Bereaved Parents of the USA offers support, care, and compassion for bereaved parents, siblings, and grandparents.

www.beyondindigo.com—Stories, advice, and info about care giving/terminal illness.

www.climb-support.org—By and for parents who have experienced the death of one or more children during a multiple pregnancy, at birth, and through childhood.

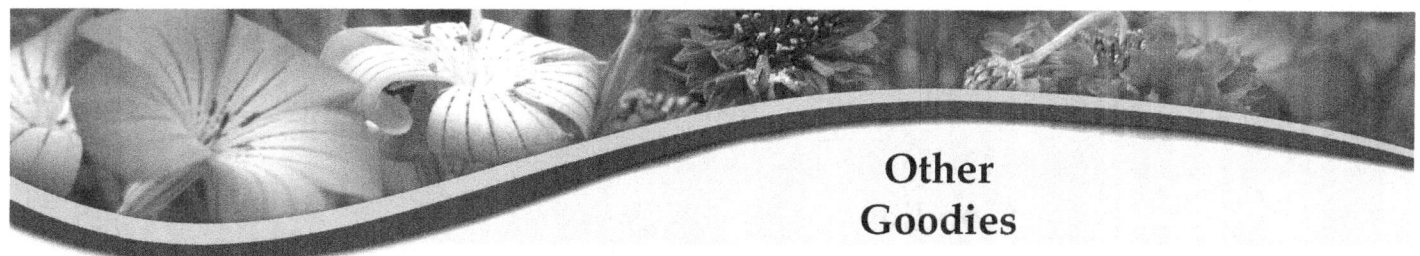

Other Goodies

www.comfortzonecamp.org—No charge nonprofit camp for siblings and children (age 7-17) coping with the loss of a sibling or parent

www.compassionatefriends.org—Grief Support after the death of a child.

www.compassionbooks.com—Grief Resources: Over 400 resources reviewed and selected by knowledgeable professionals to help children and adults through serious illness, death, loss, grief and bereavement.

www.compassionconnection.org—Contains articles and readings for all who have suffered a loss.

www.finalpassages.org—Dedicated to a compassionate and dignified alternative to current funeral practices.

www.griefnet.org—Offers e-mail support groups for the bereaved including parents, siblings, and grandparents. It also offers a wide variety of bereavement related content including a comprehensive resource guide of bereavement organizations and a sister website for bereaved children.

www.growthhouse.org—This award-winning web site is an international gateway to resources for life-threatening illness and end of life care. Its search engines offer access to the net's most comprehensive collection of reviewed resources for end of life care. Over one hundred health care web sites offer remote access to their database to complement their own content.

www.groww.org—Offers wide variety of grief and bereavement resources.

www.hospicefoundation.org—Includes information about hospice care and programs including bereavement support for families using hospice.

www.hospicenet.org—Provides information and support to patients and families facing life-threatening illnesses.

www.madd.org—Mothers Against Drunk Drivers has a mission to stop drunk driving, support victims of violent crime, and prevent underage drinking.

www.misschildren.org—Mothers in Sympathy and Support provides emergency support to families after the death of their baby or young child.

www.nationalshare.org—SHARE's mission is to serve those who are touched by the tragic death of a baby through miscarriage, stillbirth, or newborn death.

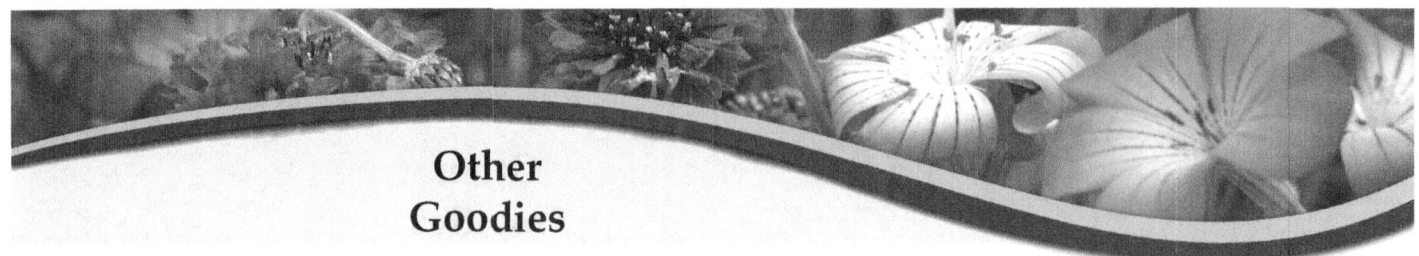

Other Goodies

www.nhpco.org The NHPCO is the largest nonprofit membership organization representing hospice and palliative care programs and professionals in the United States. The site has a searchable engine for hospices around the country by state and county, as well as facts and figures about US palliative care, job openings, and educational opportunities for professionals.

www.nowilaymedowntosleep.org—When a baby or infant has died, Now I Lay Me Down to Sleep, through its nationwide network of professional photographers, will arrange a tasteful private sitting at the hospital with no charge for any services or pictures.

www.pomc.com—Provides support and assistance to all survivors of homicide victims while working to create a world free of murder.

sids-network.org—Sudden Infant Death Syndrome Network offers latest information, as well as support, for those who have been touched by the tragedy of SIDS/OID (other infant death).

www.survivorsofsuicide.com—Survivors of Suicide helps those who have lost a loved one to suicide to resolve their grief and pain in their own personal way.

www.taps.org—Made up of, and provides services to, all those who have lost a loved one while serving the country in the Armed Forces.

www.starrtraining.org/tlc—Dedicated to helping traumatized children and families restore a sense of safety and reduce the effects of trauma; information available about trauma, resources, and training for professionals.

www.twinlesstwins.org—Serves in support of twins (and all multiple births) who suffer from the loss of companionship of their twin through death, estrangement or in-utero loss.

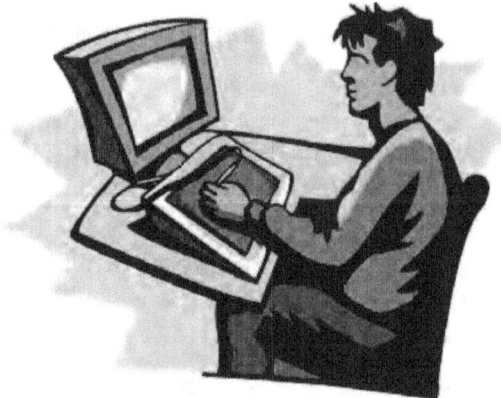

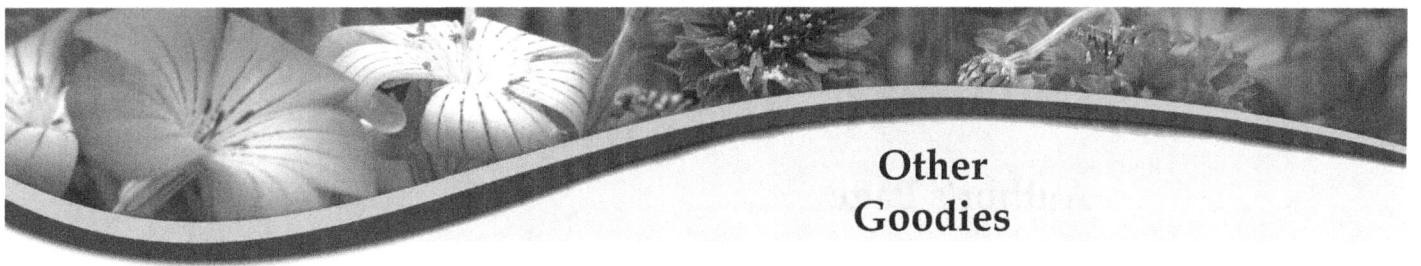

Other Goodies

Timeless Touch

Frail wilted hand clasping a walker,
Holding a quivering cup, reaching for another's hand..
Empty, dangling, dark veins pressing,
Mottled onionskin fabric, signature of senescence.

Are you really alive?
Once pudgy infant hand gleefully reaching skyward,
Vernal little girl hand, Clasping mother's hand,
soft caressing hand, with sensuous touch.
Firm mother's hand, full of child's hand.
Where have you gone?.

Frail ashen hand, who do you reach for now?
Whose secure hand clasp? What lover's hand enthrall?
What child's hand enclose? With whose love connect?
Are you always empty now?

Frail wilted hand, take my hand.
In just a moment, my hand shall wither too.
But as we touch, may some deeper love,
Transcending time, pass through these entwined hands.
For this moment alive.

Larry Bogart M.D.

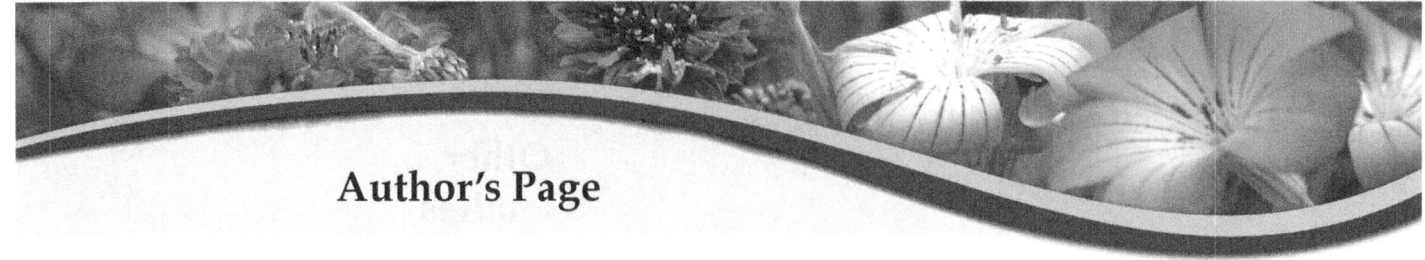

Author's Page

*I'd love to hear your suggestions, comments or questions.
Feel free to email me at* **bordermountain@msn.com**

Visit our sister websites:

www.bordermountain.com *for ordering end of life training materials and grief resources for kids and adults*

www.bordermountain.org *to keep up on progress with our seminars, film projects, and Camp David in the U.S. Virgin Islands, our retreat center in development.*

Blessings on your work with people at end of life.

May all the love you give away come back to you

a hundredfold and more.

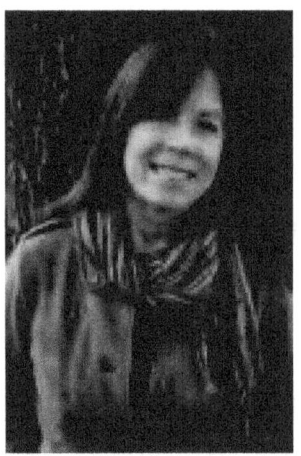

JoAnne Chitwood, R.N., CHPN

Made in the USA
Coppell, TX
12 February 2026